Cases on Healthcare Information Technology for Patient Care Management

Surendra Sarnikar
Dakota State University, USA

Dorine Bennett
Dakota State University, USA

Mark Gaynor
Saint Louis University School of Public Health, USA

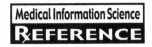

Medical Information Science
RxEFERENCE

Managing Director:	Lindsay Johnston
Editorial Director:	Joel Gamon
Book Production Manager:	Jennifer Yoder
Publishing Systems Analyst:	Adrienne Freeland
Development Editor:	Christine Smith
Assistant Acquisitions Editor:	Kayla Wolfe
Typesetter:	Christy Fic
Cover Design:	Jason Mull

Published in the United States of America by
Medical Information Science Reference (an imprint of IGI Global)
701 E. Chocolate Avenue
Hershey PA 17033
Tel: 717-533-8845
Fax: 717-533-8661
E-mail: cust@igi-global.com
Web site: http://www.igi-global.com

Library of Congress Cataloging-in-Publication Data

Cases on healthcare information technology for patient care management / Surendra Sarnikar, Dorine Bennett, and Mark Gaynor, editors.
     pages cm
  Summary: "This book highlights the importance of understanding the potential challenges and lessons learned from past technology implementations of health information technologies"-- Provided by publisher.
  Includes bibliographical references and index.
  ISBN 978-1-4666-2671-3 (hardcover) -- ISBN (invalid) 978-1-4666-2702-4 (ebook) -- ISBN (invalid) 978-1-4666-2733-8 (print & perpetual access) 1. Medical informatics--Case studies. 2. Nursing services--Administration--Case studies. I. Sarnikar, Surendra, 1977- editor of compilation. II. Bennett, Dorine, 1957- editor of compilation. III. Gaynor, Mark, 1956- editor of compilation.
  R858.C37 2013
  610.285--dc23
                                              2012029416

British Cataloguing in Publication Data
A Cataloguing in Publication record for this book is available from the British Library.

All work contributed to this book is new, previously-unpublished material. The views expressed in this book are those of the authors, but not necessarily of the publisher.

Table of Contents

Detailed Table of Contents

Chapter 1
Doing and Understanding: Use of Case Studies for Health Informatics
Education and Training... 1

Cynthia LeRouge, Saint Louis University, USA
Herman Tolentino, Centers of Disease Control & Prevention, USA
Sherrilynne Fuller, University of Washington, USA
Allison Tuma, Saint Louis University, USA

This chapter provides an introduction to the pedagogy of using the case method particularly for instruction in the health informatics context. The thoughts and insights shared in this chapter are inspired by basic theories, published methods, and lessons learned from the authors' collective experiences. They illustrate the case teaching experience by engaging the reader in an exercise to highlight the basic phases of the case method process and challenges of the process. The case referenced in this exercise (provided in the Appendix to this chapter) has been used on multiple occasions by authors of this chapter, and they draw on their experiences in using this case to illustrate points throughout the exercise. The authors close the chapter by providing the reader with strategies and considerations in using the case method.

Chapter 2
Individual, Organizational, and Technological Barriers to EHR
Implementation 35

Matthew J. Wills, Indiana University East, USA

This case examines the adoption and implementation of an electronic health record in a regional medical center in Midwest, USA. A background of the organization is provided, including a discussion of the organization's inception, financials, and organizational structure. A brief literature review of technology adoption, use, and performance is presented, followed by a discussion of data analysis techniques and results. A detailed overview of specific technology, management, and organizational concerns is presented along with challenges and solutions. The objective of this case is to highlight the challenges and opportunities during electronic health record adoption and implementation. The hope is that educators and students alike will appreciate the complexity of health information technology adoption and implementation through specific examples of challenges and solutions. While the information contained in this case is indeed specific to one organization in the USA, the lessons learned are broadly applicable to healthcare organizations throughout the world.

Regional Health made a commitment as part of quality and patient safety initiatives to have an electronic health record before the federal government developed the concept of "meaningful use." The "One System of Care, One Electronic Chart" concept was a long-term goal of their organization, accomplished through electronically sharing a patient's medical record among Regional Health's five hospitals and other area health care facilities. Implementing a hybrid electronic record using a scanning and archiving application was the first step toward the long-term goal of an electronic health record. The project was successfully achieved despite many challenges, including some limited resources and physician concerns.

Chapter 4

Broadlawns Medical Center (BMC) is a teaching acute care community hospital of 200 beds located in Des Moines, Iowa. As other safety net providers across the nation, the hospital operates in a difficult environment with a growing number of uninsured patients and simultaneously dwindling tax support. By 2005, George Washington University and several Joint Commission reports had publicly highlighted the hospital's challenges of financial sustainability and the provided quality of care. The hospital's senior management team decided to adopt an Electronic Health Record (EHR) system in an attempt to gain access to real-time performance data. The EHR adoption project posed many organizational, managerial, and technological challenges but also provided numerous eventual benefits. BMC had not only successfully resolved the stated problems of healthcare quality, financial stability, and patient satisfaction scores, but also became one of the national leaders in healthcare information technology.

Research Medical Center is a regional medical center that meets the needs of residents of a rural area in the Midwest. It is part of a large healthcare system. The primary care hospital implemented the Electronic Health Record (EHR). The endeavor to implement Health IT applications including Computerized Physician Order Entry (CPOE), EHRs, nursing documentation, and paperless charts, adverse drug reaction alerts, and more were introduced with the corporate initiative. The core applications were clinical and revenue cycle systems, including CPOE. The planning, implementation, and training was developed by the parent operating company and efforts to engage the local physicians were minimal. There were over 300 physicians involved. The physicians were primarily not hospital employees. They had the ability to choose to adopt the EHR and adapt their social, work, and technology practices, or to avoid usage. Follow up research indicated the change management and support efforts were not successful for the physician stakeholder.

Electronic Health Records (EHR) are a system of Health Information Technology (HIT) components including clinical documentation, medication orders, laboratory and diagnostic study results, management, and evidence based clinical decision support. In this case, a patient's care is compromised because of incomplete documentation of medical information and lack of integration among data collection systems. The patient has had over fifty years of medical care in a U.S. government health system followed by care in a private primary care setting. Effective implementation and utilization of EHRs in primary care settings, will positively affect patient safety and quality of care. Appropriate use of EHR provides challenges to clinicians, HIT developers, and healthcare administrators. Provision of quality patient care utilizing HIT is challenging to use and implement, but when patients receive healthcare from multiple sources, the challenge becomes even greater. The need for integrated EHR systems is evident in the geriatric population (Ash, et al., 2009), where the ability to provide data to new clinicians may be affected by cognitive decline in this population. Management of health and chronic conditions in the geriatric population requires an ongoing commitment to HIT implementation for safer and more effective care.

Chapter 7

Electronic Medical Records (EMR) in academic medical centers often have additional complexity to them due to structural and organizational differences. Often the hospital operates independent of the medical school such as the physicians often work for the medical school, while the nurses and other ancillary departments work for the hospital. Such differences require special consideration when making changes to an EMR. The case study concerns an academic medical center where there are two ways to access the EMR. One methodology is to use a clinical computer on clinical floors within the hospital. A second methodology is the use of Citrix servers to access the EMR. Due to organizational differences, the EMR users access the system via two separate sets of Citrix servers. The hospital's support staff controls one set of Citrix servers and the academic support staff controls the other set. Physicians and mid-level providers utilize the academic Citrix servers, but nursing and other ancillary departments use the hospital's Citrix servers. With the servers controlled by separate teams, careful coordination is needed to ensure uniformity across the servers for a consistent user experience.

Chapter 8

Improving the opportunity to access care by infectious disease specialists and improve the overall quality of care received is the core mission demonstrated by this clinic through the on-going and continued development of their telehealth services program. This focus does not remove the need for the clinic to adhere to sound business practices. Instead, this case demonstrates that both focuses can be appropriately accomplished. Current regulatory issues will continue to pose challenges, but these barriers are not significant enough to shut down the enthusiasm for continuing this service or for future expansion plans. This study will discuss the benefits of telehealth not only to patients, but also to the clinic practice as a whole.

Chapter 9

The manner in which health care is delivered to patients has evolved significantly through the years. Technology has played an important role in that evolution. This case study explores one way health care organizations are investing in advanced health care technologies to deliver services to patients when the patients are not in the same room as the providers. This study explores the implementation of an eConsult program, also known as telemedicine, at Avera Medical Group Pierre. This study will discuss the process of implementing an eConsult program, the equipment needed to provide eConsults, privacy, and billing concerns, and the facility's future plans for expanding the telemedicine services they offer. Overall, this case study strives to show that implementing telemedicine can be a relatively easy process of embracing technology, which can greatly benefit patients.

Chapter 10

Alice Noblin, University of Central Florida, USA
Kelly McLendon, Health Information Xperts, USA
Steven Shim, Harris IT Services, USA

Florida began the journey to health information connectivity in 2004 under Governor Jeb Bush. Initially these efforts were funded by grants, but due to the downturn in the economy, the state was unable to support growth in 2008. The American Recovery and Reinvestment Act of 2009 provided funding to further expand health information exchange efforts across the country. As a result, Florida is now able to move forward and make progress in information sharing. Harris Corporation was contracted to provide some basic services to the health care industry in 2011. However, challenges remain as privacy and security regulations are put in place to protect patients' information. With two seemingly opposing mandates, sharing the information versus protecting the information, challenges continue to impede progress.

Chapter 11

Elizabeth J. Forrestal, East Carolina University, USA
Leigh W. Cellucci, East Carolina University, USA
Xiaoming Zeng, East Carolina University, USA
Michael H. Kennedy, East Carolina University, USA
Doug Smith, The Community Partners HealthNet, Inc., USA

Health-Center-Controlled Networks (HCCNs) are collaborative ventures that provide health information technologies to Community Health Centers (CHCs). Community Partners HealthNet (CPH), Inc. is a HCCN. CPH's member organizations are non-profit health care organizations that provide primary health care to individuals in medically underserved areas. As non-profits, they must regularly seek grant funding from foundations and state and federal agencies to provide quality, accessible health care. Consequently, initiatives to adopt and implement Health Information Technologies (HIT) require individual CHCs to carefully consider how best to incorporate HIT for improved patient care. This case study describes CPH, discusses the collaboration of six individual CHCs to create CPH, and then explains CPH's on-going operations.

The Coordination of Rare Diseases at Sanford (CoRDS) registry has been started to provide a central repository of data for participants suffering from a number of rare diseases and to provide those participants with a resource to learn more about their disease and, in a future enhancement, connect with others that are afflicted. The second purpose of the registry is to provide a resource for researchers to identify and recruit potential participants for their research studies. This case study will focus on the technical aspects of setting up a registry and providing access to participants and their medical team, who will enter data about their disease, and researchers, who will access de-identified data to include in their research. Security of the external website and access to Protected Health Information (PHI) are the main areas of concern with this registry.

The use of Information Systems (IS) in healthcare organizations is increasing. A variety of information systems have been implemented to support administrative activities such as scheduling systems, insurance and billing, electronic prescriptions, pharmaceutical dispensaries, and patient health records and portals. To make a fundamental difference in the delivery of patient care, systems that support important clinical healthcare decision processes are needed that leverage the clinical knowledge embedded in patient medical records. The aggregation of clinical data from multiple sources is difficult due to data interoperability issues. The VHA case study of the CISCP system illustrates a program that effectively leveraged clinical data from multiple surgical programs to build a system to support decision-making at many organizational levels. The technical and organizational practices from the VHA case provide important lessons to address interoperability issues when building other healthcare information systems.

Utilization and application of the latest technologies can save lives and improve patient treatments and well-being. For this it is important to have accurate, near real-time data acquisition and evaluation. The delivery of patient's medical data needs to be as fast and as secure as possible. Accurate almost real-time data acquisition and analysis of patient data and the ability to update such a data is a way to reduce cost and improve patient care. One possible solution to achieve this task is to use a wireless framework based on Radio Frequency Identification (RFID). This framework can integrate wireless networks for fast data acquisition and transmission, while maintaining the privacy issue. This chapter discusses the development of an intelligent multi-agent system in a framework in which RFID can be used for patient data collection. This chapter presents a framework for the knowledge acquisition of patient and doctor profiling in a hospital. The acquisition of profile data is assisted by a profiling agent that is responsible for processing the raw data obtained through RFID and database of doctors and patients. A new method for data classification and access authorization is developed, which will assist in preserving privacy and security of data.

Advances in technology have accelerated self-care activities, making them more practical and possible than before using these technologies. The utilization of new Health Information Technologies (HIT) is becoming more and more apparent in self-care. Many patients incorporate the use of PDAs in diabetes self-care (Forjuoh, et al., 2007; Jones & Curry, 2006). Mobile phones are used in diabetes self-management by diabetes patients (Carroll, DiMeglio, Stein, & Marrero, 2011; Faridi, et al., 2008; Mulvaney, et al., 2012). Also, reminders based on SMS cell phone text messaging are used to support diabetes management (Hanauer, Wentzell, Laffel, & Laffel, 2009). Given the current advances in the field of health care, health care technologies, and handheld computing, this case explores the possible primary usages of mobile phones, PDAs, and handheld devices in self-care management. More specifically, the case illustrates how such technologies can be used in diabetes management by patients and health care providers.

Clinical practitioners need to have the right information, at the right time, at the right place, which is possible with mobile healthcare information technology. This chapter will help in understanding the need for mobile device usage across six different roles in healthcare: physicians, nurses, administrative staff, pharmaceutical staff, emergency staff, and patients. Research indicates that even in this advancing digital age, there are more than 98,000 deaths because of preventable medical errors. This can be abated with proper utilization of mobile devices in the healthcare sector. Utilization of technology in the process of sharing information may help in improving the decision making, and thereby reducing the medical errors and costs involved. This chapter illustrates the implementation and the application of mobile devices in healthcare from six different user perspectives, and summarizes the advantages, challenges, and solutions associated with mobile information technology implementation in healthcare.

Chapter 17

Millions of people around the world have diabetes. It is the seventh leading cause of death in US. An advancement of technologies may serve as the backbone for controlling diseases. Computerizing healthcare is expected to be one of the powerful levers essential for significant transformation in the quality and cost of delivering healthcare. Data management and technology is essential for providing the ability to exchange data and information at the right place in the right time to the right people in the healthcare process, to enable informed decision-making, and to achieve better health outcomes. Clinical Decision Support System (CDSS) provides guidance specific to the patient, including importing/entering patient data into the CDSS application and providing relevant information like lists of possible diagnoses, drug interaction alerts, or preventive care reminders to the practitioner that assists in their decision-making. This chapter has focuses on the use of CDSS for diabetes prevention.

Preface

The importance of Health Information Technology (HIT) studies continues to grow as health care organizations make significant investments in health information technology such as Electronic Health Records (EHR), Health Information Exchanges (HIE), Computerized Provider Order Entry (CPOE), ePrescribing, and Clinical Decision Support Systems (CDSS), among others. The need for HIT studies and growing need for HIT workforce has led to the development of health information technology programs at several universities. As health care organizations continue to make large investments in health information technology, it is important to understand the potential challenges and lessons learned from past implementations.

The overall objective of this book is to provide a comprehensive set of cases that describe the challenges faced in various stages of health information technology implementation in different types of health care organizations. It is written for professionals who want to improve their understanding of the process, challenges faced, and lessons learned in the implementation, application, and adoption of Health Information Technologies. The cases span a wide variety of health care organizations from large health care systems to small independent rural health care centers, and describe a wide range of health information technologies. The cases also cover a range of Health IT issues such as security, privacy, adoption, change management, and return on investment.

We believe the cases in this book will be useful for practitioners, researchers, and students working in the field of health care information management and technology. The cases provide insight and support practitioners by providing an understanding of potential challenges to HIT implementation in a variety of health care organizations. For students and educators, it provides a rich set of cases describing HIT implementations that complement the theoretical knowledge gained in HIT course work. This case collection will also serve as a valuable data set for building theory as well as validating IT implementation and adoption theories in the health care context.

The book begins with an overview of the case method for teaching health informatics. In Chapter 1, the authors discuss the case method of teaching and provide examples of successful application of health informatics teaching cases. The chapter includes extensive guidance on various styles of case teaching and a detailed process for using case studies for health informatics education and training. The process presented in the chapter is based on published literature on case-based teaching methods as well as the authors' collective experience in using the case method for teaching.

In recent years, electronic health records have been the major focus of information technology investments in the healthcare industry. While many organizations in the United States have implemented or plan to implement electronic health records, their adoption by clinicians remains a major issue. This issue is the focus of Chapter 2, which describes the implementation of electronic health records at a large medical center in the Mid-Western United States. The case provides an in-depth description, along with survey data, of the individual, organizational, and technological barriers faced by the organization in its electronic health record implementation process. The case includes a discussion of the findings in the context of adoption theories and other research studies on the adoption of information technology in healthcare.

Large electronic health record implementations, such as those in multi-hospital, multi-clinic organizations, spread across multiple states involve additional complexities and challenges when compared to single entity organizations. Such a complex implementation and its associated challenges and solutions are discussed in Chapter 3. The chapter details the implementation of Electronic Health Records at Regional Health, a health organization that includes multiple hospitals, clinics, and specialized healthcare centers such as rehabilitation, cancer care, and behavioral health. As organizations implement electronic health records, integrating current patient data held in paper records into the electronic records is among the most challenging aspects of the implementation. This case particularly focuses on scanning and archiving paper records as a first step towards building an electronic health records infrastructure.

Improving quality of care and reducing healthcare costs are among the key objectives in implementing electronic health records, and Chapter 4 describes a case where they were the driving criteria for the adoption of an EHR. The case describes the cost and quality challenges at a rural safety net hospital and the EHR-based strategy adopted by the organization to overcome those challenges. The case includes a description of the EHR implementation process from a financial, business process, and strategic perspectives, and is set at the Broadlawns Medical Center, which was recognized as the "Most Wired Hospital" in the Small and Rural Hospital category by the Hospital and Health Networks Magazine. A unique aspect of the case is the emphasis on the strategic use of EHR for monitoring real time performance data and improving financial, clinical outcome, and patient satisfaction measures.

One of the main challenges in electronic health record implementations is identifying stakeholders, understanding their needs, and ensuring stakeholder involvement in the implementation process. This is especially critical for physician acceptance of the electronic health record systems. Chapter 5 describes the case of an EHR implementation with specific focus on stakeholder identification and change management. The case is set at a medical center in MidWest US and describes the adoption issues encountered at the organization due to the failure to adopt effective change management practices and stakeholder involvement in the implementation process. A unique aspect of the case is the focus on the effects and changes in the underlying organizational cultural climate due to the EHR implementation. The case includes survey data that helps pinpoint specific problems related to technology, implementation process, and project management that lead to the adoption problems.

Understanding the impact of electronic health records on quality requires an understanding of the clinical process and the use of information systems for achieving the process objectives. Chapter 6 focuses on providing such an understanding. It includes a case scenario that describes the clinical utility of integrated and readily available information that can be provided by different health information technologies including computerized provider order entry and clinical decision support systems. The case details through the use of examples the clinical decision problems that can be supported using various health information technologies. The case also describes the shortcomings of information technology and potential for their improvement by analyzing different health information technologies within the context of a clinician's workflow. It describes how design limitations can hinder the flow of critical clinical information, but when technology is designed with attention to clinical workflow, it can significantly enhance care processes by enabling better information flow.

Clear and effective communication is essential for the successful implementation of information technology projects, and especially critical for large multi-stakeholder projects, such as the implementation of electronic health records. In Chapter 7, the authors describe the implementation complexities and communication issues that can arise during electronic medical record implementation at academic medical centers due to the structural and organizational complexities of such organizations. Academic medical centers have differences in structure and organization as they often include hospitals that operate independent of medical schools, and this issue requires special attention and consideration in health information technology implementation projects. The case includes a description of the communication issues leading to problems with the infrastructure design, and consequent impact on user experience and system maintenance.

One of the leading uses of technology in healthcare has been to provision health-care services to remote and underserved areas through the use of telehealth. Chapters 8 and 9 describe challenges and issues in implementation of telehealth programs. Telehealth is especially useful in making specialist healthcare services available in remote and underserved areas. The case in Chapter 8 describes the implementation of a telehealth program to provide underserved rural areas with access to infectious disease specialists. In this case, the authors provide an overview of benefits of the program not only to the core mission of providing quality care, but also from a business and clinical practice perspective. The case provides a detailed discussion of the impact of expanding services on clinical resource and operation management as well as the regulatory issues related to telehealth implementations.

The case study in Chapter 9 describes an eConsult program, also known as tele-medicine, at a regional clinic that is a part of a large integrated healthcare system. The case includes a detailed description of the equipment required for the program, the implementation process, and the benefits of the program for patient care. The case describes the benefits of establishing standard procedures for implementa-tion process as organizations gain experience in technology implementations. The main differentiating aspect of telemedicine is that the patient encounter with the physician is through a technology medium as opposed to a face-to-face encounter. Therefore, significant attention needs to be given to ensuring a robust technology infrastructure. In this case, the authors present details that bring out the challenges in implementing telemedicine by focusing on the differences between electronic consults and face-to-face consulting in terms of the patient consultation process and medical technology used for patient consultations. This is an area that needs special attention as primary care clinics in underserved areas implement telemedicine for expanding access to specialist services.

As an increasing number of healthcare organizations implement electronic health records, the logical next step is to develop infrastructure to allow for the electronic exchange of records to enable faster and more comprehensive information sharing between patient care providers for providing a better quality of care. The develop-ment of a health information exchange is the focus of the case in Chapter 10, which describes the evolution of the Florida Health Information Exchange and the chal-lenges in implementing the exchange that arises from the opposing mandates of sharing of information versus protecting the information. The case demonstrates the importance of legal policy and trust agreements for the successful implementation of inter-organizational health information technologies.

Shared health information technology infrastructures can help organizations reduce costs associated with their implementation and use. This is especially a ma-jor consideration for Community Health Centers, which serve as safety net health care providers for vulnerable patient populations and rely predominantly on grant funding for their operations. Community Health Centers can potentially achieve economies of scale by forming a Health-Center-Controlled Network, a collaborative venture that provides health information technology services to member community health centers. Chapter 11 describes the formation of a Health-Center-Controlled Network, the Community Partners HealthNet, formed through the collaboration of six individual Community Health Centers. The case includes a detailed description of the environment and background leading to the formation of the Community Partners HealthNet, and also describes challenges in planning for sustainability and ongoing operations, which is a critical issue due to the financially challenging environment in which community health centers operate.

The majority of the information technology investments have focused on information technology for supporting core clinical processes of a healthcare organization, such as electronic health records. However, there is significant potential for the use of various information technologies for supporting specialized healthcare processes. In Chapter 12, the design and operation of a disease registry for rare disease is described. The case describes the technology, implementation, and challenges involved in creating a disease registry that can not only be used for patient care but also for clinical research. The case also illustrates how information technology can be used to solve difficult healthcare problems such as helping patients suffering from rare diseases.

The increasing adoption of electronic health records leads to the generation of large amounts of data that can then be analyzed and leveraged for further improving the quality of care. The case study in Chapter 13 describes the implementation of a decision support system that leverages data from multiple systems to support clinical decision processes. The chapter specifically focuses on interoperability challenges that arise when integrating and aggregating data from multiple systems. The case describes several challenges that are unique to the healthcare industry and arise due to the dynamic nature of the healthcare operating environment.

A key requirement arising out of the dynamic operating environments in healthcare is the need to access and update patient data in real-time. Chapter 14 describes an innovative solution using radio frequency identification for the real-time acquisition and updates to patient data. The chapter includes descriptions of cases where the technology can be applied to acquire patient data, locate the nearest available physician, and enable the physician to access the patient data using a computing device. Given the ubiquitous nature of wireless and RFID networks, the chapter also includes a specific focus on security- and privacy-related aspects of the technology.

While many information technology applications in healthcare have focuses on applications that can be used by clinicians to provide care for patients, information technology can also be leveraged for enabling self-care by patients. Chapter 15 focuses on the application of new advances in handheld and mobile phone technologies to diabetes self-care. The chapter summarizes the evolution of the handheld and mobile technology for diabetes management by reviewing several studies that describe the implementation, use, and outcomes of using mobile technology for diabetes self-management. The chapter includes a discussion on the challenges faced due to technological limitations of the devices as well as operational challenges when a healthcare organization adopts large-scale uses of mobile devices for patient care management.

Given the massive growth and large-scale adoption of mobile devices such as smartphones by the general population, there is potential to use mobile technology in many healthcare applications. Chapter 16 describes the potential uses of mobile devices in six different scenarios that involve various clinical workflows. The chapter includes a detailed analysis of each workflow, mobile technology uses for individual tasks within the workflow, and an implementation process for automating specific tasks within the workflow with mobile technologies. In addition, the chapter includes a detailed list of advantages of mobile technology in healthcare and potential challenges that can arise during implementation.

In order for information technology to help in the improvement of health outcomes, it needs to be designed and implemented based on an in-depth understanding of clinical and care provisioning process. The final chapter in this book begins with an in-depth description of the clinical processes for diabetes care and presents an overview of how clinical decision support systems can be used to support all aspects of diabetes care including screening, prevention, and treatment. The chapter includes a mapping between various types of clinical decision support systems and the different clinical decision processes they can support.

Chapter 1
Doing and Understanding:
Use of Case Studies for Health Informatics Education and Training

Cynthia LeRouge
Saint Louis University, USA

Herman Tolentino
Centers of Disease Control & Prevention, USA

Sherrilynne Fuller
University of Washington, USA

Allison Tuma
Saint Louis University, USA

EXECUTIVE SUMMARY

This chapter provides an introduction to the pedagogy of using the case method particularly for instruction in the health informatics context. The thoughts and insights shared in this chapter are inspired by basic theories, published methods, and lessons learned from the authors' collective experiences. They illustrate the case teaching experience by engaging the reader in an exercise to highlight the basic phases of the case method process and challenges of the process. The case referenced in this exercise (provided in the Appendix to this chapter) has been used on multiple occasions by authors of this chapter, and they draw on their experiences in using this case to illustrate points throughout the exercise. The authors close the chapter by providing the reader with strategies and considerations in using the case method.

DOI: 10.4018/978-1-4666-2671-3.ch001

INTRODUCTION

I hear and I forget, I see and I remember, I do and I understand—Confucius *(Chinese philosopher and reformer, 551–479 BC).*

The effective practice of health informatics requires a systems approach to reach solutions to complex, real-life situations in everyday work. The practice of health informatics is faced with complexities of multijurisdictional, multidisciplinary, multicultural partner-based approaches to problem solving. This practice context can be simulated in the academic setting through the use of case studies.

Case studies provide a learner-centered, interactive and dynamic environment that stimulates class discussion, and they allow participants to think innovatively and collaboratively develop complex solutions within the boundaries of a classroom (Barnes, Christensen, & Hansen, 1994). However, instruction by using case studies also has its challenges related to participant engagement, group dynamics, cultural perspective, case propriety, and ensuring crucial learning messages are effectively articulated. These challenges are not addressed merely by providing cases as a resource. Thus, some guidance is based on past studies of the case method and practical experience is needed.

This chapter will reflect past research involving the case method as well as experiential and reflective health informatics case-study experience. This chapter will hopefully help readers develop a more complete understanding of content related to the health informatics case, but also the case analysis process and mechanics of the case method of instruction.

BACKGROUND: WHAT IS CASE-BASED TEACHING?

Cases are factually based, complex stories written to stimulate classroom discussion, collaborative analysis, and problem solving. Case teaching involves interactive, student-centered exploration of realistic and specific situations with a focus on resolving questions that often have no right answer. Case-based teaching differs from Problem-Based Learning (PBL), which is often used in medical education; PBL has a known answer and the decision pathway to that answer is vital (e.g., specific diagnosis or treatment) (Schneider, 2006).

Case teaching is an effective method for student practice of competencies difficult to teach by using traditional lecture approach. Figure 1 provides a comparison of the case method to the lecture method. Cases complement classroom lectures and allow students to improve mastery of theories and their application, enhance decision-making skills, and improve critical, analytical, and reasoning skills.

Figure 1. Comparison of lecture and case method

Lecture		Case Method
Knowledge acquisition	⟵————⟶	Knowledge application
Abstract	⟵————⟶	Concrete
Concepts	⟵————⟶	Practices
Lecture	⟵————⟶	Discussion

Cases have been used extensively in teaching in a variety of domains including public policy, law, and business education; in fact, some curricula are taught by using cases exclusively. In the health domain, however, limited adoption of case-based teaching has been used. The value of case-based teaching is increasingly being recognized in the multidisciplinary field of health informatics given its complex blend of technical, social, legal, and ethical dimensions.

Using cases in the classroom is a means for teaching principles in the context of the current rapidly changing environment such as health care settings today (e.g., particularly attributable to technology advancements and increasing application). This method of teaching is useful for stimulating new ideas about old problems, encouraging creativity and independent thinking, providing content for exploring leadership (and followership) roles, and bringing the real world into the classroom. Case-based learning provides a nonthreatening context in which students can explore leadership and followership roles.

Examples of Successful Application Health Informatics Teaching Cases

Cases have been successfully incorporated into health informatics courses in a variety of settings in the United States and internationally. They are quite popular with students, especially if the cases are based on real situations that are familiar to them. Case studies, when strategically integrated within a defined curriculum, can contribute to building capability beyond competencies (Elwyn, Greenhalgh, & Macfarlane, 2001). The following are some examples of the successful use of cases in HIT education.

The Public Health Informatics Fellowship Program (PHIFP), a two-year, applied, competency-based program at the U.S. Centers for Disease Control and Prevention (URL: http://www.cdc.gov/phifp) has developed and used case studies to illustrate Public Health Informatics (PHI) concepts and principles involving real-world settings. PHI fellows typically come from diverse training and experience backgrounds (e.g., public health, medicine, nursing, veterinary medicine, engineering, library science, epidemiology, statistics and information, and computer science and technology) and cultures. As these training and experience backgrounds present challenges in the implementation of the didactic and applied components of the PHIFP curriculum, they also present unique opportunities for fellows to effectively participate in contexts where multicultural, multidomain problems arise during collaborative problem solving.

Faculty from the University of Washington have used unpublished cases, developed by Tolentino, with students from the Mekong Basin Regional Surveillance Network and beyond. The course, hosted by Mahidol University, Bangkok, Thailand focused on design and development of interoperable health information systems for disease surveillance. The course, hosted by Mahidol University (Bangkok, Thailand), focused on design and development of interoperable health information systems for disease surveillance. Students included ministry of health program leaders, university faculty, and nongovernmental organization staff from Southeast Asian countries and beyond, including Vietnam, Laos, Cambodia, China, Thailand, Myanmar, Bangladesh, and Indonesia. Students reported the case on notifiable disease surveillance systems to be extremely useful in thinking about not only the technical strategies for data sharing but also for dealing with the political and social challenges across their country borders as they work together to build regional approaches to data sharing.

The same disease surveillance case was also used in a different international setting for an advanced health informatics course with fellows in the Infectious and Tropical Disease Program, University of Nairobi (Kenya). Students included the fellows, University of Nairobi faculty, graduate students, nongovernmental organization staff, and faculty from the Kigali Institute of Science and Technology in Rwanda. A second case, developed by Fuller on the basis of an anonymized description of an actual HIV/AIDS facility in Kenya, provided complex but realistic challenges for students to work through and develop a strategic health information system plan for the clinic and affiliated hospital.

Appropriate Style and Cases

Case teaching is unique in that no right answer exists; it is experiential. Both student and teacher assume responsibility for student learning. The teacher serves as a facilitator and is responsible for mastering the facts, issues, and materials of the case, anticipating questions, and preparing for the discussion, how it might progress, and how it should conclude. The teacher also develops plans for the after-action review of the discussion and identifies take-home lessons and points of view that might have been previously overlooked.

The case method requires the teacher to transform into a discussion leader and to get to know each of the students and their differing perspectives. To teach cases, the teacher must listen with discipline and sensitivity, and respond to students in constructive and respectful ways to build trust and community. Case teaching requires giving extra attention to students and the learning process.

The first step in case planning is finding an appropriate case for the desired teaching points, student level, and time frame available. Three types of cases of varying length and complexity are available. Comprehensive analyses are 20 or more pages in length and require a significant time commitment. Focused issues cases are five to fifteen pages long, and feature select issues and concerns but are less comprehensive. Cases that contain simpler lessons or nuggets are less than three pages long, and highlight a simple or short objective.

Useful cases have several common elements. They have an issue as well as tell a good story. They depict a real world challenge with some facts altered to simplify the story or names changed to maintain anonymity (Abell, 1997). Useful cases include supporting data, documents, or other real world artifacts like data tables or possible sources of additional information. Complex cases can evolve in real time, with new facts presented over time, simulating a realistic emerging situation (Naumes & Naumes, 2006). Cases most beneficial to student learning contain an open-ended problem with multiple potential solutions; potential end products could range from a single paragraph response to fully developed actions plans, proposals, or decisions. Time devoted to a case could range from a single class period for simple cases to an entire quarter for more complex cases.

Three primary styles of case teaching are available:

- Research cases allow students to interpret the case by using only the information contained within, and find lessons learned by the case actors. They are on the outside looking in and reacting to what they have read. The teacher guides the discussion, ensuring that important points are identified and discussed.
- Simulation cases involve role-playing that allows students to step into the main actor's shoes and discussion can develop organically without teacher interference or guidance. At the case conclusion, the teacher and students can together debrief and identify actors' motivations for actions taken.
- Analytic frameworks can be applied to a case in either the research or simulation approach. These frameworks can provide different overlays or foci, possibly including a legal, social, or political perspective. These frameworks can be used to interpret what happens in the case and prepare a recommendation for what the case actor should do in differing situations (Boehrer, 1995; Naumes & Naumes, 2006).

The teaching style to be adopted can depend on a variety of factors. First, the development and use of case studies are driven by the learning needs of the participants.

The ADDIE (Assessment, Design, Development, Implementation, and Evaluation) model of instructional design begins with assessment of participant learning needs. For example, a particular topic of discussion might need development of the ability to analyze multiple perspectives to a problem (Gustafson & Branch, 2002). Moreover, the learning outcomes to be evaluated might dictate use of a certain style of case teaching. For example, if a desired learning outcome includes the ability to step into a stakeholder's role to examine motivation for positive or negative action, a simulation might elicit learning behaviors aligned with those learning outcomes. Second, the competency requirements defined for a particular domain drive the development of training program curricula and consequently learning activities that support didactic learning, including case studies. For example, as public health informatics is a discipline that borrows concepts, principles, and methods from contributing disciplines, case studies might emphasize use of borrowed analytic frameworks from the social sciences, information and computer sciences, management science, and other related domains. In addition, the level of learning required might include multiple cognitive domains (e.g., knowledge, synthesis, and evaluation) as presented in Bloom's Taxonomy of Learning (Naumes & Naumes, 2006). Lastly, the topics to be emphasized in a case study to support achievement of the learning objectives of a course can dictate the style to be adopted in the implementation of a case study.

Pedagogy might be best understood through exemplification and application. Therefore, we invite you to experience the process in the next section of this chapter.

EXPERIENCE THE PROCESS

Utilizing cases in teaching requires careful planning in advance. We will use a case that all three authors have used to help you experience parts of the process. We ask you first to step into the role of the student and then to take the role of a case facilitator to enrich your understanding of pedagogy and process.

Student Perspective

Facilitators might want to first put themselves in a student role in approaching a case. During the first class session dedicated to a case, the facilitator should set the stage for the class. This includes explaining why a case is being used and its benefits to the students. The facilitator should clarify that no right or wrong answers are available. The case analysis process should be clearly outlined for students, and they should be told what to expect and what is expected of them. The difference between student contribution and participation throughout the case analysis process should be made clear. The facilitator should remind students to listen to others' input, keep their own comments short, simple and frequent, and remember that they will improve with practice. Students should also be advised to avoid jargon, vague generalities, and trying to say it all as they share their perspectives.

Students should be directed to ask themselves questions in preparation for the case analysis process. These questions allow students to identify the main actors, their motives, concerns and objectives, and the central issues and constraints facing actors in the case. The following are some questions students should pose to themselves initially.

- Who is the decision maker? What decision(s) need to be made?
- What are the decision maker's objectives?
- Are there other important actors? What are their goals or agenda?
- What are the key issues? That is, what questions must be addressed and points resolved to reach a decision?
- What are the constraints and opportunities affecting the decision? What is the environmental context?
- What alternative actions can the decision-maker take? What would I (the student) do? Why? (Randrup, 2007)

Task 1: Student Assessment

You are a student in the graduate health informatics class. You next class meeting will focus on the topic of change management. The facilitator has reviewed the dynamics of the case method and provided guidance on how to approach cases.

1. Read the Challenges in Implementing Electronic Laboratory Reporting in State Oz case (hereafter referred to as the State Oz case) provided in Appendix A. Do not read the case questions.
2. How would you answer the aforementioned bulleted questions for the State Oz case?

You are the Facilitator

Assume that you are assigned to teach a health informatics session for graduate students in a health informatics course on change management in health care settings. The case approach is particularly suited to this topic because the complexities of both managing and participating in the change management process require a variety of analytical and management skills best learned from participation in a realistic case. You will need to identify your learning goals for the case experience, which can be different, and in addition to the learning goals contained in the case itself.

Candidate cases are based on alignment with learning goals and stellar case characteristics. The State Oz case supports our learning goals by engaging students in the change management process and by exploring how the recommendations that Julia (main character in the State Oz case) prepares will be adopted by the stakeholders. Table 1 lists features that a case used in the classroom should have, as identified by Linda Swayne (2009), and demonstrates which of these features are present in the State Oz case. State Oz is an excellent example of a complex case with data that can be taught over time and new information provided to students to simulate a realistic, evolving situation that requires adaptation and rethinking strategies. Additionally, the case can provide an opportunity for assigned role-play with students engaging in discussions and meetings to discuss or debate facts.

After the case has been selected, important considerations are required to be defined. The realities are that case teaching and research require more preclass preparation than traditional lecture-style teaching. Your role as facilitator requires you to do substantial planning so that students acquire the experience and skills that you expect.

Planning begins with deciding what students will do before the actual class meeting. An initial consideration is whether you want to students to read the case in advance. Some cases best come alive in the moment after reading. Other cases require preparation and analysis. If preparation and analysis are preferable, you need to ensure that students read and analyze the case, particularly when no written work is assigned to students. To accomplish this goal, you can instruct students to be prepared to lead a discussion or preassign an active role in the analysis. Student groups could be assigned in advance to encourage preclass discussion amongst students. You must also strategically decide whether or not to provide questions in advance to the students. Preparing questions encourages students to find solutions and a teacher might prefer the students find questions themselves.

Task 2: Designing the Student Homework Assignment

1. Given the setting of the health informatics graduate course, the learning goals associated with change management, and the State Oz case characteristics, would you require students read the case in advance?
2. If you did require students to read the case in advance, how would you encourage students to prepare for case discussion?

The State Oz case has been used in situations without advanced preparation for the purpose of evaluating candidates' teamwork skills and analytical abilities when challenged with an ambiguous task requiring immediate attention. The case has also been used with advanced reading (including additional materials related to change

Table 1. Characteristics of a stellar case

Characteristics	Characteristics as Demonstrated in State Oz Case (Appendix A)
Sets the hook in the introduction by including elements as follows: • Industry. • Key players. • Decision situation. • Answers the question, 'Why am I reading this'? • Attention is achieved or lost during the introduction.	•Attention is achieved through the descriptive opening with vivid imagery; the reader can figuratively put himself in Julia's shoes. •The case's key player is introduced immediately. •Julia is in a decision situation. She has a problem to solve; electronic lab reporting must be implemented for the State of Oz. •The industry and Julia's relevant background are introduced on the first page.
Introduces relevant and interesting characters • Has a decision maker with a personality. • Involves key players in the case. Size of the organization and complexity of the situation will determine how many key players are included. • Provides different perspectives. • Characters have opinions.	•Key players are introduced; their roles and viewpoints are explained. •Julia's thoughts are clearly depicted throughout the case, demonstrating her personality and opinions. •Debra Moore's perspective is included. •Each laboratory is a player and each has a unique set of circumstances and perspectives regarding the implementation of standardized electronic reporting.
Provides analytical stimulation and challenge • Provide an important problem and decision situation. • Provide sufficient data to thoroughly analyze the case and develop solutions. • The context for making a decision is clear. • Provides 'red herrings.' • Provides no obvious correct answer. • Challenges the analytical and logical thinking of the reader.	•An issue about proliferation of local coding standards is brought up by Debra Moore (see excerpt from one conversation). •No single, obvious solution for Julia's problem. Different solutions offer benefits to different stakeholders. The need for a solution is clear. •The context for decision-making is muddled with problems at the organizational and technical levels. •Data tables and conversations highlighting situational undertones are provided to distract the students from the real issues and challenge their analytical, logical, and systems thinking.
Provides appropriate context • Is timely. Current problems are more interesting, but classic problems have no time boundaries. • Provide decision orientation versus description of an event. • Deals with changing policy. • Deals with changing technology. • Different problems capture attention and interest, but avoid truly unique problems that cannot be applied to other contexts.	• The time span of the case, 1997–2010, highlights ELR as a classic public health problem and ties it to the historical context, where a 2010 survey reveals increasing adoption of ELR indicates this classical problem has no time boundaries and becomes more important as more electronic systems are adopted. • Julia faces attention-grabbing issues that are general and universal, including engaging stakeholders that can have conflicting motives to participate in ELR; developing a systematic approach for implementing an ELR solution while weighing the pros and cons of the different approaches, resource constraints, and balancing the demands of the policy and information security environment with the need to facilitate efficient and effective health information exchange. • Julia is dealing with policy and technology problems involving the changing policies surrounding ELR.

continued on following page

Table 1. Continued

Characteristics	Characteristics as Demonstrated in State Oz Case (Appendix A)
Is well written • Clear and easy to understand. • Avoids embellishments to create a better case (fiction). • Does not draw conclusions (belongs in the instructor manual). • Does not include everything the case-writer knows. • Avoids duplication of material. • Makes every word count. • Keeps the case-writer out of the story. • Facilitates reading (headings and subheadings). • Avoids acronyms. • Explains technical terms. • Avoids excessive use of footnotes or endnotes. • Uses exhibits to present data (numbered sequentially). • Makes each exhibit material to the discussion. • Has consistent financial data (inconsistency of data years confuses the reader). • Is meticulous in making numbers match. • Does not repeat exhibit data in text. • Uses past tense (except direct quotes). • Avoid use of terms 'currently,' 'recently,' and 'now.' • Identify the time frame.	• This case is divided into sections with subheadings, making it easier to read. • Charts are used to clearly present data. • The case is comprehensive enough to present all necessary information and perspectives but does not present an unmanageable amount of information or include everything the author knows about the topic. • Technical terminology is explained and used only when necessary. • Opens with a flashback and subsequently uses past tense to tell Julia's story. • The case writer is not part of the story. • Does not duplicate facts or material. •The relevant time frame is identified (1997–2010).
Have a great information manual that includes the following: • Overview of the case. • Key problems. • Learning or teaching objectives. • Suggestions for effective teaching. • Strengths, Weaknesses, Opportunities and Threats (SWOT). • Discussion of crucial issues. • Questions and answers. • Epilogue.	An information manual for this case might include the following: • Advantages and disadvantages to stakeholders of various solutions. • Recommendations for introducing the case and the process. • Questions to ask students and crucial discussion points. • Brief descriptions of the reading materials and logistical considerations. • Unmasking of the real characters in the case study.

management) and homework question response required when the learning objective is to develop skills on change management to allow students to consider various theories and dynamics of change management in the health informatics context.

Advanced staging is required for the classroom process. Figure 2 depicts the planning steps of the case delivery process to be considered by the facilitator (Barnes, et al., 1994). This case delivery road map provides a useful tool guiding you through the planning process.

Beginning a case discussion with a class can be difficult; thus, the introduction requires consideration. Initiating the discussion can be accomplished in different ways. Goals and values testing can be utilized to begin the discussion. This involves asking students why they believe this case was selected for their benefit and why the timing was appropriate. A single concrete image, event, or moment from the case could be chosen to initiate case discussion. The teacher could generate a truth statement to present to students and seek their responses. For example, a facilitator could begin a conversation with, "True statements regarding health information exchanges include…" and wait for students' replies. The scene could set by the facilitator's selection of music, quotations, or speech to invite student responses. Rather than the facilitator beginning the discussion in an intentional way, s/he could instead require that students prepare a discussion question in advance to begin the case discussion on a topic of interest to students.

Different question types are appropriate for use when engaging in a case analysis and discussion. Factual questions, or a review of the main case facts, are important for clarification purposes and are typically used first. Application and interpretation questions require students to apply knowledge and demonstrate comprehension. Connection and cause-and-effect questions force students to think about the relationships between events and decisions. Evaluation questions prompt students to synthesize information, make a judgment, or assess a situation. The instructor could prompt students to consider how a change in context could influence the crucial decisions made throughout the case. For example, the facilitator could ask how a situation might change if it took place in Europe rather than in the United States, or if the main actor were a nurse instead of a doctor.

While considering process, one must remember that case teaching should be a discussion rather than a lecture. To create this dynamic in a classroom traditionally used for lecture-format courses, the chairs can be moved to facilitate conversations. Cases can be role-played to increase each student's involvement. Different perspectives can be discussed and students can debate different actors' actions and decisions.

Task 3: Case Delivery Planning

By using the Case Delivery Planning Process presented in Figure 2 as a guide, plan the delivery of the "State Oz" course to the health informatics graduate student class by addressing the following questions:

1. **Introduction:** What broad overview will you present?
2. **Initiating or Priming:** Do you want to set-up a part of the discussion with an exercise?

Figure 2. Case Delivery Planning Process

Introduction
What broad overview will you present?
You may decide to provide no introduction to the content of the case and let the case speak for itself. You do need to provide an introduction to the process for the students, especially if it is their first experience with case-based teaching.

Initiating
Do you want to set up a part of the discussion with an exercise?
You might, for instance, provide an overview of the actors' qualifications as context for the case. These facts can provide a useful context for students during role-play.

Opening
What perspectives do you want students to adopt first in the case analysis -- actor or group observer? Will different students be assigned different roles?
Depending on the nature of the learning objectives in the case, students could play the roles of different stakeholders with differing opinions about the nature of and solutions to the problem.

Questions
What responses do you expect from students? Which questions are most important for thorough discussion?

Display Plan
How will you display or organize the students' analysis visually in order to prompt further analyses of points that were missed?

Process
Small groups or as a whole?
In a large class, you may want to break into several groups. Each group captures their discussion and outcomes and then shares the results with the entire class. This is a particularly effective way of demonstrating different approaches and strategies for dealing with the change management issues. Time management is a critical issue with small groups as some groups get hung up early in the case and never complete the case. You need to serve as a facilitator and make sure the discussion and role-play progress.

Closure
How will you conclude discussion? What question(s) will you present for further reflection?
How will you pull the key take-aways and lessons learned regarding change management?

Case Debrief
What might you want to discuss about the case discussion process itself (content, learning, approach)?
For example, you may point to particular points where the role-play may have broken down and ask the class how this might be addressed in future case discussions.

3. **Opening:** What perspective do you want students to adopt first, an actor or group observer in case? Will different students be assigned different roles?

4. **Questions:** What responses do you expect from students? Which questions are most important for thorough discussion? Appendix A contains some questions and responses for the State Oz case. Would you use all of these questions? What questions would you add?

5. **Display Plan:** How will you display or organize the students' analysis visually, in an effort to prompt further analysis of points that were missed?

6. **Process:** Divide into small groups or group as whole? Role play?

7. **Closure:** How will you conclude discussion? What question(s) will you present for further reflection?

8. **Case Debrief:** What might you want to discuss about the case discussion process itself (e.g., content, learning, and approach)?

During reflection on our experiences with the State Oz case, the choices indicated in Table 2 provides some of the most effective choices we have made in case delivery towards health informatics change management learning goals.

RECOGNIZING THE CHALLENGES

Initially, a novice case-teaching instructor can expect to struggle with challenges that are unique to the case-teaching methodology. Several reactions are common among students as they begin the case analysis process. Students tend to seek the right answer from the facilitator rather than freely exploring various options. Some students do not enjoy speaking in class and struggle with this type of exercise. Students might desire constant feedback on their performance or insights from the instructor, or reluctant to participate if they feel they lack the expertise of other students or cannot relate to the case's main actors. Lack of new insight can prompt a student to 'beat a dead horse' to fulfill participation requirements or prompt a response such as, "He said what I was going to say." These common responses are only a few of the barriers that instructors should prepare to respond and strive to overcome.

An important lesson for the facilitator is to familiarize her/himself with his students' backgrounds, including their professions, previous experience, or culture. This will acquaint the instructor with what students might already know and assumptions students might have as they begin to analyze a new situation. Developing a personal relationship with students will drive their contributions to the process. Knowledge of students individually will help an instructor determine when it is appropriate to call on a student or when to assign which portion of the assignment.

Table 2. Effective choices made for "State Oz" case from author experience

Case Delivery Planning Process Step	Choices Made for Use of the State Oz Case from Author Experiences that Resulted in Effective Learning
Introduction What broad overview will you present?	Example Overview Electronic laboratory reporting is next level of improvement for standards-based health information exchange coming from nonautomated paper and electronic recording, and exchange of laboratory data to support public health surveillance functions. We have been implementing electronic laboratory reporting in the United States during the previous 15 years. Why does it take so long?
Initiating or Priming Do you want to set-up a part of the discussion with an exercise?	Example Priming Each student comes from a different country and in various stages of setting up nationwide health information systems, use of electronic medical records and health information exchange. Does anyone have similar experiences as described in the case today?
Opening What perspective do you want students to adopt first, actor or group observer in case? Will different students be assigned different roles?	Example Opening As you will be filling Julia's shoes later when you lead your own InfoAids, examine Julia's capacity as a problem solver for electronic laboratory reporting in State Oz.
Questions What responses do you expect from students? Which questions are most important for thorough discussion?	Example Questions that Fueled Discussion Why cannot states mandate electronic laboratory reporting for all public health partners? Differences among state and laboratory perspectives on information security, coding standards, and message formats. Are there differences between small and big laboratories? Who maintains coding standards? What happens during version changes?
Display plan How will you display and organize the students' analysis visually, to prompt further analysis of points that were missed?	Example Displayed Information Enumerate and describe stakeholders in electronic laboratory reporting at the federal, state, and local (county or city) levels. Describe the types of data standards used in electronic laboratory reporting.
Process Divide into small groups or group as whole? Role play?	Divide the class into two groups and have them discuss answers to the questions and generate questions for the other group to answer. Answer questions individually and generate questions for the class to discuss. In the role-play, you could ask different students to take particular stands for, against, and neutral related to the changes in a meeting to discuss adoption. You could ask students what Julia could do at each step in her analysis to ensure buy-in and participation not just from the leadership but from the other stakeholders in the process.
Closure How will you conclude the discussion? What question(s) will you present for further reflection?	Example Closing Statement Determining solutions for informatics problems related to electronic laboratory reporting require an understanding of the problem at different levels.
Case Debrief What might you want to discuss about the case discussion process itself (e.g., content, learning, and approach)?	Debrief questions that can be used after the case study session. What do you think went well in the case study? Were the reading materials and assignments too much, too little, or the right amount? Which parts of the case study were not clear to you? Why? Would you recommend that we include this case study for the next orientation? If not, what case study would you like to use?

Personal, open relationships can be built through e-mail or telephone, and through individual attention including personal comments on written work.

Case-based teaching with professionals is different than with traditional students. Typically, limited time is available for preparation. Similarly, time limitations for teaching and discussion is common; however, given their extensive experience, professionals have a lot to say and are often eager to share. Participants should be encouraged to compare case situations with their experiences but be sure to relate these comparisons to the case in a clearly defined manner. Because of this time constraint, the facilitator will need to be selective in the questions chosen for discussion and timing and priorities will need to be predetermined. After the teaching session, these students should be encouraged to teach this case back to their coworkers, employees, or supervisors as an added benefit of the case analysis process.

Numerous questions about challenges are presented at case writing workshops and have been posed to the authors in collegial sharing. Table 3 includes questions that case-facilitators are likely to face, particularly during initial phases of the learning process as well as insights from the authors' experience with reference to addressing these common challenges.

Table 3. Addressing common challenges

Challenge	Insights from leading health informatics cases
How should I evaluate student participation?	Like any training activity, learning outcomes from participation in case studies can be measured by using existing evaluation frameworks. One such framework is the 4-level model developed by Donald Kirkpatrick (Kirkpatrick, 1998) that examines learning outcomes at 4 levels. Level 1 (Reaction) – how the learners react to the learning process. In the PHIFP setting, a postcase-study debrief session enables staff to capture feedback. Level 2 (Learning) – the extent to which the learners acquire relevant skills and knowledge. This can involve implementing pretest and posttest activities to measure change in skills and knowledge. Level 3 (Performance) – the extent to which learner behavior leads to intended consequences (consequential learning), usually measured at 60-90 days after the training activity. Level 4 (Results) – can include collection of hard and soft metrics involving increased efficiency, lowered costs, increased production, or customer satisfaction that accrue to the organization providing resources for the training.
How long should I wait for a response from students to a question?	The time between asking the class a question and getting a student to raise his or her hand in response can feel like an eternity. This time is often around one second, but the facilitator should aim for five seconds between asking the question and selecting a student to first respond.

continued on following page

Table 3. Continued

Challenge	Insights from leading health informatics cases
How do I get students to talk or discuss with each other (not to me)?	PHIFP staff frame case studies (and any problem-solving activity) to fellows as a problem solving activity within another problem solving activity. In the conduct of the case study, the problem solvers may become obstacles in collaborative problem solving and making learners aware of this possible situation enables them to become more self-aware of their impact on others (emotional intelligence). As not all students may be native English speakers, prompting and assistance is essential to get non-English speakers a moment to speak and providing them with clear-cut opportunities to communicate to a technical audience. Providing learners with a schedule for group discussion also helps the process.
How do I get students to use course concepts?	Occasional interruption of a potentially wayward discussion by the case study facilitator to remind students about concepts revealed in theoretical readings and other learning materials helps students use course concepts. This requires that the case study facilitator has access to all prior learning materials and is oriented to how the concepts in reading materials align to the case.
Should I assign discussion questions in advance?	If you want to ensure students read a case and think about it, it is best to assign questions in advance. Questions that involve calculations or the need to research information can be particularly thought provoking. If a collaborative problem solving exercise is part of the case objective, then the case might not be assigned in advance. Instances occur when you want to see the group problem solving based situation in a time-constrained context.
What question or introduction do I use to start discussion?	What are the key facts of the case? You might be faced with this problem one day. Who has experienced this type of problem? Give introductions indicating situations that you know the persons involved in the case (if true) or someone like them. Portray the writer of the case as an expert here to inform us.
How do I use the white board or PPT?	Document key facts, figures, and graphs for reference during the discussion. Instead of using the whiteboard yourself, turn note-taking over to the students to actually write down what they see as important.
Do I tell them the facts of what actually happened?	In the PHIFP setting, as most case studies were developed out of actual projects, fellows assume that PHIFP staff has detailed background knowledge of both anonymized and nonanonymized cases. Fortunately, for most case studies, the fellow involved in the underlying project is among the case study faculty assigned to the particular case.
Is it best to use a published teaching note or to develop one?	The decision to use published teaching cases versus developing one usually depends on whether the published teaching note can adequately support the learning objectives of the orientation modules. In addition, if the benefits of developing a case for a particular module outweigh the logistical resources (usually extensive time spent involving planning, staff discussion and stakeholder meetings and validation).
How many cases should I use?	The decision regarding how many cases to use depends not only on the flow of content but on the amount of time that can be provided to learners to meaningfully process the content provided. Reducing the number of case studies to a limited number strategically situated across a program to provide better mapping of cases might be the best course.
Is it better to go deep or broad?	Consider the audience as well the learning objectives. For example, there is no point in going into great detail on a technical issue if this is not suited to the audience or the learning objectives to the class. Mapping the learning objectives to Bloom's taxonomy will help to guide whether to go broad or deep.

NEXT STEPS

This book addresses an important next step, which is locating relevant cases for health informatics courses that can be a challenge. This book will be a valuable contribution to those involved in the teaching of health informatics. Cases developed in a variety of domains could be adapted for use in the health informatics classroom.

Because case-teaching is so different than traditional lecturing, a steep learning curve for teachers new to using cases in the classroom is often involved. Even when someone is a veteran case facilitator, the use of a new case can present a learning curve. Moving through the learning curve is best accomplished through practice in the classroom. Participants' feedback and ideas from debriefing should be utilized in future case-teaching sessions, especially in situations of a new case. The facilitator should try to work with different groups of students to see what works best when teaching cases in various contexts; the same case could be used with graduate students, undergraduate students, and professionals, for example. Keeping a log about what works and what does not will facilitate improvement. This is an iterative process; those new to case-teaching will improve with practice and experience, and veterans will only get better. Cases involve engagement and provide an experience. Our association with those who have adopted the case method have indicated their practice yields both a rewarding and enjoyable learning experience for the facilitator as well as the students.

REFERENCES

Abell, D. (1997, Autumn/Fall). What makes a good case?. *European Case Clearing House*, 4-7.

Barnes, L. B., Christensen, C. R., & Hansen, A. J. (1994). *Teaching and the case method* (3rd ed.). Boston, MA: Harvard Business School Press.

Boehrer, J. (1995). *How to teach a case*. Boston, MA: Harvard.

Elwyn, G., Greenhalgh, T., & Macfarlane, F. (2001). *Groups: A guide to small group work in healthcare, management, education and research*. Abingdon, UK: Radcliffe Publishing.

Gustafson, K. L., & Branch, R. M. (2002). What is instructional design? In Reiser, R. A., & Dempsey, J. V. (Eds.), *Trends and Issues in Instructional Design and Technology*. Columbus, OH: Merrill Prentice Hall.

Naumes, W., & Naumes, M. (2006). *The art & craft of case writing*. Armonk, NY: M.E. Sharpe.

Randrup, N. (2007). *The case method: Road map for how best to study, analyze and present cases*. Rodovre, Denmark: International Management Press.

Schneider, D. K. (2006). *Case-based learning*. Retrieved October 31, 2010, from http://edutechwiki.unige.ch/en/Case-based_learning

Swayne, L. (2009). *Case writers newcomers 'workshop*. Paper presented at the North American Case Research Association Conference. Santa Cruz, CA.

ADDITIONAL READING

Atkins, C., & Sampson, J. (2002). Critical appraisal guidelines for single case study research. In *Proceedings of ECIS 2002*. Gdańsk, Poland: ECIS.

Benbasat, I., Goldstein, D., & Mead, M. (1987). The case research strategy in studies of information systems. *Management Information Systems Quarterly, 11*(3), 369–386. doi:10.2307/248684

Chelvarajah, R., & Bycroft, J. (2004). Writing and publishing case reports: The road to success. *Acta Neurochirurgica, 146*, 313–316. doi:10.1007/s00701-003-0203-2

Darke, P., Shanks, G., & Broadbent, M. (1998). Successfully completing case study research: Combining rigour, relevance and pragmatism. *Information Systems Journal, 8*, 273–289. doi:10.1046/j.1365-2575.1998.00040.x

David, F. (2003). Strategic management case writing: Suggestions after 20 years of experience. *SAM Advanced Management Journal, 68*, 36–43.

Davis, C., & Wilcock, E. (2003). *Teaching materials using case studies*. London, UK: The UK Centre for Materials Education.

Farhoomand, A. (2004). Writing teaching cases: A reference guide. *Communications of the Association for Information Systems, 13*.

Gibson, C. K., & Cochran, D. S. (1982). Case writing: An acceptable professional activity or an exercise in futility? *Journal of Business Education, 57*(8), 308–310.

Graham, P. T., & Cline, P. C. (1980). The case method: A basic teaching approach. *Theory into Practice, 19*(2), 112–116. doi:10.1080/00405848009542883

Hackney, R. A., McMaster, T., & Harris, A. (2003). Using cases as a teaching tool in IS education. *Journal of Information Systems Education, 14*(3), 229–234.

Harling, K. F., & Akridge, J. (1998). Using the case method of reaching. *Agribusiness, 14*(1), 1–14. doi:10.1002/(SICI)1520-6297(199801/02)14:1<1::AID-AGR1>3.0.CO;2-8

Hassall, T., Lewis, S., & Broadbent, M. (1998). Teaching and learning using case studies: A teaching note. *Accounting Education: An International Journal, 7*(4), 325–334. doi:10.1080/096392898331108

Herreid, C. (1994). *Case studies in science: A novel method of science education.* Retrieved from http://sciencecases.lib.buffalo.edu/cs/pdfs/Novel_Method.pdf

Kim, S., Phillips, W. R., Pinsky, L., Brock, D., & Keary, J. (2006). A conceptual framework for developing teaching cases: A review and synthesis of the literature across disciplines. *Medical Education, 40*, 867–876. doi:10.1111/j.1365-2929.2006.02544.x

Kirkpatrick, D. L. (1959). Techniques for evaluating training programs. *Journal of the American Society of Training Directors, 13*, 3-9, 21-22.

Lee, A. S. (1989). A scientific methodology for MIS case studies. *Management Information Systems Quarterly, 13*(1), 33–50. doi:10.2307/248698

Lundberg, C. C., Rainsford, P., Shay, J. F., & Young, C. A. (2001). Case writing reconsidered. *Journal of Management Education, 25*(4), 450–463. doi:10.1177/105256290102500409

Mostert, M. P., & Sudzina, M. R. (1996). Undergraduate case method teaching: Pedagogical assumptions vs. the real world. In *Proceedings of the Annual Meeting of the Association of Teacher Educators.* Association of Teacher Educators.

Paterson, G. I., Abidi, S. S., & Soroka, S. D. (2005). HealthInfoCDA: Case composition using electronic health record data sources. *Studies in Health Information Technology, 116*, 137–142.

Raju, P., & Sankar, C. (1999). Teaching real-world issues through case studies. *Journal of Engineering Education, 88*(4), 501–508.

Rippin, A., Booth, C., Bowie, S., & Jordan, J. (2002). A complex case: Using the case study method to explore uncertainty and ambiguity in undergraduate business education. *Teaching in Higher Education, 7*(4), 429–441. doi:10.1080/135625102760553928

Shanks, G. (2002). Guidelines for conducting positivist case study research in information systems. *Australasian Journal of Information Systems, 10*(1), 76–85.

van der Blonk, H. (2003). Writing case studies in information systems research. *Journal of Information Technology, 18*(1), 45–52. doi:10.1080/0268396031000077440

Wasserman, S. (1994). Using cases to study teaching. *Phi Delta Kappan, 75*(8), 610–611.

Webb, H. W., Gill, G., & Poe, G. (2005). Teaching with the case method online: Pure versus hybrid approaches. *Decision Sciences Journal of Innovative Education, 3*, 223–250. doi:10.1111/j.1540-4609.2005.00068.x

Yin, R. (1981). The case study crisis: Some answers. *Administrative Science Quarterly, 26*(1), 58–65. doi:10.2307/2392599

APPENDIX

Case Study: Challenges in Implementing Electronic Laboratory Reporting in State Oz

Herman Tolentino
Centers of Disease Control and Prevention, USA
J.A. Magnuson
Oregon Health Authority, USA
Arunkumar Srinivasan
Centers of Disease Control and Prevention, USA

Student Guide

Learning Objectives
By the end of this session, the participant should be able to

1.   Describe what Electronic Laboratory Reporting (ELR) is, and what it is not.
2.   Describe the scope of ELR solutions.
3.   Describe challenges potentially encountered in implementing ELRs.
4.   Identify sustainability challenges for an ELR project.

The content of this case study is based on experience related to implementation of electronic laboratory reporting at the state level. The mention of brand names of commercial or intellectual property products in this document does not constitute an endorsement and is merely coincidental. The entities alluded to in this document have been altered to protect the identities of persons and organizations involved.

Julia[1] watches the golden west coast sun as it fades away from her office window, taking time to reflect on the long days she has spent writing an implementation plan for Electronic Laboratory Reporting (ELR) for the State of Oz. Tomorrow is among the mandatory unpaid furlough days the state has adopted in response to its budget crisis, but much work remains to be done. The plan was incomplete, as she addresses the complexity of implementing ELR at the state level.

Julia told herself, "Surely, I still have a lot to learn about electronic laboratory reporting. It was not as straightforward as I originally thought."

Julia reminisced about events that had transpired during the previous weeks.

Background

During March 1997, a meeting of experts sponsored by the Centers for Disease Control and Prevention (CDC), the Council of State and Territorial Epidemiologists, and the Association of State and Territorial Public Health Laboratory Directors was held to provide a discussion forum for barriers to creative and practical implementation of effective laboratory reporting standards. The report summarized recommendations in three main areas per guidelines from the CDC (1997):

- Flow: Where, when, and how data should move among users.
- Format: The mechanics of data transfer, including use of Health Level 7 (HL7) messages or other reporting formats and ways to ensure security.
- Content: The determination of which data elements should be included in an electronic system for clinical laboratories.

Table 4 outlines uses of public health surveillance data (specifically laboratory data). Laboratory reports are important to surveillance in public health when they indicate possible occurrence of reportable disease or infectious disease outbreaks. The traditional system of laboratory reporting, however, was slow and incomplete as it often relied on paper reports delivered by mail (Pinner, 2000). During 2008, an evaluation that compared completeness and timeliness of automated, standards-based electronic laboratory reports and spontaneous, paper-based reporting for a

Table 4. Use of public health surveillance data

Public Health Uses of Surveillance Data	Public health system components and emphases (●●● = greatest emphasis)		
	Local	State	Federal
Identification of cases for investigation and follow-up	●●●	●●●	●
Estimate the magnitude of a health problem; follow trends in incidence and distribution	●	●●●	●●●
Detect outbreaks or epidemics to trigger interventions	●●●	●●●	●
Evaluate control and prevention measures	●	●●●	●●●
Monitor changes in infectious agents (e.g., antibiotic resistance, clinical spectrum)		●●	●●●
Facilitate epidemiologic and laboratory research; formulate prevention strategies; formulate hypotheses	●	●●	●●●
Detect changes in health practice (e.g., impact of use of new diagnostic methods on case counts)	●	●	●●
Facilitate planning (e.g., allocation of program resources, policy development)	●	●●●	●●●

Source: Adapted from CDC (1997)

broad spectrum of notifiable diseases in Indiana demonstrated that automated ELR improves the completeness and timeliness of disease surveillance, which will enhance public health awareness and reporting efficiency (Overhage, 2008).

Research Experiment

During March 2002, State Oz received $300,000 grant funding from the federal government to establish Electronic Laboratory Reporting (ELR). As the new CDC PHI Fellow assigned to this state, Julia Martinez was specifically tasked to help develop an implementation plan for ELR at the state level and to develop translations, identify, test and evaluate secure transmission methods, collaborate with local health laboratories, engage local health departments, and involve state program areas to participate in ELR.

The Systems

Julia determined that the state operated the following systems that could potentially benefit from electronic laboratory reporting

1. **HIV/AIDS Monitoring:** Enhanced HIV/AIDS Reporting System is a browser-based application that collects, stores, and retrieves data, through a secure data network that CDC has identified as necessary to monitor the HIV/AIDS epidemic, identify trends in the epidemic, evaluate HIV prevention, care, and treatment planning.
2. **Environmental Monitoring (heavy metal poisoning, air quality, and water quality):** An example is blood lead monitoring which usually comprises a substantial volume of ELR data delivered to public health. The STELLAR (systematic tracking of elevated lead levels and remediation) is a free software application provided by CDC to state and local CLPPPs (childhood lead poisoning prevention programs) with a practical means of tracking medical and environmental activities in lead poisoning cases. Intent of this application is to provide an electronic means of storing childhood lead exposures, medical, and laboratory data that the state program receives from laboratories, providers, clinics, parents, and local health departments.
3. **Other Notifiable Conditions:** The National Electronic Disease Surveillance System (NEDSS) (NEDSS, 2001; CDC, 2005) is an initiative that promotes use of data and information system standards to advance development of efficient, integrated, and interoperable surveillance systems at federal, state, and local levels. A primary goal of NEDSS is the ongoing, automatic capture and analysis of data that are already available electronically. NEDSS system

architecture is designed to integrate and replace a limited number of CDC surveillance systems, including the National Electronic Telecommunications System for Surveillance, HIV/AIDS reporting system, the vaccine preventable diseases, and systems for tuberculosis and infectious diseases (CDC website).

Although she had encountered systems mentioned previously while at CDC, Julia wanted to review examples of data standards used in public health and laboratory reporting. She went to her supervisor, Debra Moore, to learn more information.

Excerpts from their Conversation:

Julia: *"I am just now getting to appreciate the state perspective. Can you please enlighten me on use of standards in laboratory reporting?"*

Debra: *"That's an interesting question. Well, we promote the use of standards but Public Health (PH) departments are just as guilty as anyone else of creating their own local data standards. Because most legacy PH systems have grown organically and are often created by local, state, or federal epidemiologists with no database or data standards background and with an as-needed or as-funded basis, they might have little to no standardization or normalization. So PH data 'standards' (Debra gestures quotes) include a variety of local code systems. Some systems are more formal than others. For example, systems with payer-functions is more likely to include standard codes, such as CPT (current procedural terminology, a billing-code system) or hospital-related diagnostic codes (ICD – International Classification of Disease)."*

Julia: *"That's very enlightening!"*

Debra: *"Oh, it gets better!"*

Julia: *"Tell me!"*

Debra: *"Laboratories have their own coding systems, that allow them to track and bill laboratory work. The coding system in use might be vendor-supplied (built into the Laboratory Information System (LIS)), or might be managed in-house. In any case, use of data standards for PH reporting is not the primary concern of laboratories, as these have only become important to public health with the relatively recent advance of electronic data systems. PH is attempting to get laboratories to use Logical Observation Identifiers, Names and Codes (LOINC) and Systematized Nomenclature of Medicine (SNOMED) coding for their PH reporting, but these practices are still not used by a majority of laboratories. Remember that it is difficult, time-consuming, and expensive for laboratories to incorporate a new coding system into their existing system."*

The Issues

After a limited number of weeks in Oz, the local laboratory environment was beginning to make sense to Julia who enumerated the data partners in Table 5.

Julia showed the table to her supervisor.

After further analysis of information she received from her interviews, casual conversations at work, and site visits, Julia was able to summarize the challenges by the type of laboratory being considered for ELR implementation (see Table 6).

The federal funding that State Oz is receiving comes attached with the following conditions.

Table 5. Laboratory data partners of state oz health department

Laboratory	Type	Population coverage	Cost estimate for implementing lab reporting standards	Level of use of ELR-specific standard test and result codes	Incentive to use standards	Potential return on investment for ELR
National Reference Lab (Hydra Diagnostics)	Commercial	Nationwide	Low	High	PH request	High
Midwest Regional Lab (commercial)	Commercial	Regional (3 states)	Medium	Low	PH request	High
State Hospital Laboratory (Kingston Memorial Hospital)	State Hospital	State	High	Low	PH request	High
Vanguard Laboratory Systems	Commercial	Local	High	Low	PH request	High
Beaumont Integrated Laboratories	Commercial	Local	High	Low	PH request	High
State Oz Public Health Laboratory	Local public health lab	State	Medium	Low	PH need	High
Atlantic City Public Health Laboratory	Local public health lab	City	Low	Low	PH need	High

Table 6. Challenges in implementing ELR for different kinds of laboratories

Type	Challenges or Limitations
National Reference Laboratory	The national laboratory has limitations separating results from notes in their laboratory reporting data. They also have reservations about adopting state-recommended transmission methods and are not willing to spend money to retrofit their Laboratory Information System (LIS) to include standards for public health reporting. Similar to all reference laboratories, they frequently have limited patient demographic data so important to public health (e.g., address or telephone number).
Regional Laboratory	The regional laboratory also has the same limitations above. In addition, LIS limitations yield the inability to generate or extract batch report files. They are unfamiliar with HL7 formatting primarily because they lack capacity to implement it and would need extensive reasons to adopt ELR.
Public Health Laboratory (PHL)	The PHL is working to replace its current LIS but have not decided on a final solution because of challenges in evaluating options, which creates a reluctance to put effort into adopting ELR. The laboratory is looking for an ideal LIS, which is impractical. In addition, they have a lack of sufficient technical knowledge or expertise to make these choices, and will be relying on state public health to assist with the ELR implementation.
Commercial Laboratories	Local laboratories will realize labor cost savings after a paperless reporting system is established, although they find no direct financial benefit from use of standards. They argue that converting systems to use standards will be a drain on resources. These for-profit laboratories insist that they will need more resources available to change their systems to accommodate all ELR requirements.

1. ELR systems adhere to national standards; the funding stipulates use of LOINC and SNOMED data standards, and HL7 formatting standards.
2. ELR systems be PHIN compliant and compatible. This also affects additional characteristics (e.g., transmission security, data storage conditions, and other criteria).

Debra also informed Julia that recent developments have occurred in State Oz that could influence the development of systems and laboratory reporting.

1. Any system to be developed must be compliant with security protocols of the state.
2. Regarding local legislation, the State Oz Senate has proposed an ELR mandate. Debra provided Julia with last week's copy of the Oz *Express* with an article about public health initiatives in Oz legislature, "Senator Rankle Cares for the Public's Health."

Possible Approaches

After weeks of studying the background of laboratory reporting in State Oz, Julia decided to write an initial draft of her project proposal to implement ELR. Numerous potential approaches are apparently possible for implementing ELR in State Oz. Julia began to list the tasks that she had to accomplish (see Table 7 for the Work Breakdown Structure). She will have to consider how to best sequence the tasks to be most effective and efficient.

Table 7. Work breakdown for ELR implementation

ELR Implementation Tasks
A. Inventory of information standards and technologies used by partners.
B. Identify need for electronic information exchange and willingness to provide data.
C. Ensure buy-in.
D. Identify resources (e.g., technical, human, and financial) for project implementation.
E. Develop infrastructure for exchange of electronic messages.
F. Identify stakeholders.
I. Develop a new messaging guide for laboratory reporting in the state.

STUDENT QUESTIONS

Background or Foundational Questions (Might Be Determined on the Basis of Supplemental Text Readings)

1. What is ELR? What is its relationship to Laboratory Information Systems (LIS)?
2. What is HL7?

Case Questions

3. Given this background information, please help Julia systematically develop an initial assessment of the informatics problem in the public health context. You can group statements in your description as follows: PH context, informatics problem, main issues, and possible approaches to meeting challenges.

(Some answers provided. Complete the rest.)

PH context: Laboratory reports are a critical component of public health surveillance.

Informatics Problem

Main Issues

Possible Approaches

4.   Are standards the only way to solve information exchanges among ELRs? Why or why not? If you are advocating for the use of standards, what criteria would you use to determine what are the best standards?

5.   How should Julia sequence the checklist of implementation activities in Column A of Table 8 to ensure that she has an appropriate foundation of information and activities for each additional task? Use Column B to arrange the sequence of Column A items. Be prepared to justify sequencing of items in Column B.

Table 8. Question 5

COLUMN A	COLUMN B
A. Inventory of information standards and technologies used by partners. B. Identify need for electronic information exchange and willingness to provide data. C. Ensure buy-in. D. Identify resources (e.g., technical, human, and financial) for project implementation. E. Develop infrastructure for exchange of electronic messages. F. Identify stakeholders. I. Develop a new messaging guide for laboratory reporting in the state.	*(Starting sequence answers provided below)* *F. Identify stakeholders.* *B. Identify need for electronic information exchange and willingness to send data.* *A. Inventory of information standards and technologies used by partners.* *D. Identify resources (e.g., technical, human, and financial) for project implementation.* *E. Develop infrastructure for exchange of electronic messages.* *(Complete the last two!)*

INSTRUCTOR GUIDE TO ANSWERS

Background or Foundational Questions (Might be Determined on the Basis of Supplemental Text Readings)

1. What is ELR? What is its relationship to LIS?

We define ELR as follows:

- **Electronic:** Requires secure electronic transmission of data, with a limited degree of automation. (Sending a disk through the mail would not qualify.)
- **Laboratory:** Data source includes for-profit laboratories, state public health laboratories, and hospital laboratories.
- **Reporting:** Standards-based notifiable condition data sent to public health organization; legally mandated.

At the public health level, ELR is a separate system that provides data for surveillance and case management.

A laboratory information system is defined as an electronic data processing system designed to automate and expedite the workflow of a general clinical laboratory, and including such functions as patient and specimen identification or login, work flow organization, electronic interfaces among analytical instruments and the system, local and remote result reporting, quality control, security, connections with outside systems (e.g., hospital information systems, electronic medical records, and billing systems) and numerous other features. Specialized versions of LISs serve needs of blood bank or transfusion service, anatomic pathology, molecular pathology and other services.

An LIS should be distinguished from a Laboratory Information Management System (LIMS) (that also deals with clinical aspects), which are typically designed originally to automate a pharmaceutical, research, industrial, or clinical trials laboratory.

Public health partners might require format variations (even when using HL7).

Three different perspectives include laboratories (support PH), health department (carry out PH mission), and CDC (national perspective).

2. What is HL7?

Health Level 7 (HL7) is a standardized format used for electronic health care data interchange. HL7 is a reference to the Open Systems Interconnection (OSI) reference model, which defines the different stages that data must go through to travel over a network. The application level (level 7), includes definition and structure of data.

Benefits of HL7 as a standard are as follows:

- ANSI (American National Standards Institute) approved.
- Already exists in a majority of hospital or clinical information systems.
- Can include recommendations for separate standards (e.g., standardized test and result codes).

HL7 is a complex and flexible set of format protocols encompassing a staggering array of data requirements. The flexibility of HL7 is a good news and bad news attribute, as it can accommodate an enormous variety of data situations, but users can also create an astonishing number of variations upon the standard. HL7 messages are identified by message type and trigger event code. For example, in Oz State, the ELR project uses the ORU R01 message. The message type and trigger event are translated as follows:

- **ORU:** Observation result is unsolicited.
- **R01:** Unsolicited transmission of an observation message.

From Implementation Guide for Transmission of Laboratory-Based Reporting of Public Health Information by Using Version 2.3.1 of the Health Level Seven (HL7) Standard Protocol Implementation Guide Update April 21, 2003 Centers for Disease Control and Prevention:
Example 1: Hepatitis A Virus
MSH|^~\&||MediLabCo-Seattle^45D0470381^CLIA|NEDSS|WA-
DOH|199605171830||ORU^R01|
199605170123|P|2.3.1 <CR>

PID||||10543^^^^^Columbia Valley Memorial Hospital&01D0355944&CL
IA|95101100001^^^^

MediLabCo- Seattle&45D0470381&CLIA||Doe^John^Q^Jr|Clemmons||M||W|
2166 Wells Dr

^AptB^Seattle^WA^98109^USA^^^King||^PRN^PH^^^206^6793240||
|M|||423523049|

DOEJ34556057^WA^19970801||N <CR>

NK1|1|Doe^Jane^Lee^^^^L|SPO^spouse^HL70063|2166 Wells Dr^Apt
B^Seattle^WA^98109^

USA^M^^King^^A|^PRN^PH^^^206^6793240|<CR>

ORC|CN||||||||||||||||||||||||MediLabCo - Northwest Pathology Ltd., Central
Campus^^^45D0470381^^^

CLIA|2217 Rainier Way^^Renton^WA^98002^USA^M^^Black Hawk^^A|
^WPN^PH^helpline@medilab.com^^206^5549097 |115 Pike Plaza^Suite
2100^Seattle^WA^98122^USA^^^^A|<CR>

OBR|1||SER122145|78334^Hepatitis Panel, Measurement^L||||199603210830
||||||||BLDV|

^Welby^M^J^Jr^Dr^MD|^WPN^PH^^^206^4884144||||||||F <CR>

OBX||CE|5182-1^Hepatitis A Virus, Serum Antibody EIA^LN||G-
A200^Positive^SNM||||||F||
|199603241500|45D0480381 <CR>

OBR|2||^Additional patient demographics|<CR>

OBX|1|NM|21612-7^reported patient age^LN||47|yr^year^ANSI+|||<CR>

OBX|2|TX|11294-6^Current employment^LN||food handler||<CR>

Case Questions

3. **Given this background information, please help Julia systematically
   develop an initial assessment of the informatics problem in the public
   health context. You can group statements in your description as follows:
   PH context, informatics problem, main issues, and possible approaches
   to meeting challenges.**

PH context – Laboratory reports are a critical component of public health surveillance.

Informatics problem – Information technology can make laboratory reporting
efficient and effective, but also introduces challenges that include privacy and confidentiality, use of standards, availability of organizational expertise (workforce),
and buy-in from stakeholders.

Main issues

- Tension between a state that needs to receive data from laboratories for public health reporting and lack of incentive for private laboratories to meet this need.
- Information exchange technology has to keep up with evolving standards.
- Sustainability and viability of proposed solutions (workforce and resources).

State of Oz should include

- Check with neighboring regions and try to coordinate ELR requirements when possible.
- Adopt data standards that meet national requirements, but not necessarily the newest version.
- Design a way to assist data senders with technical advice, money, and other problems.
- Determine PHIN compliance needs (e.g., data transmission methodologies and security).

Three possible approaches to implementation

- Charm approach
- Incentive approach (pay laboratories)
- Legislate ELR

4. Are standards the only way to solve information exchange in electronic laboratory reporting? Why or why not? If you are advocating for the use of standards, what criteria would you use to determine what are the best standards?

Standards are the best way to solve the problems, from a PH perspective. However, they are not the only way to consistently transfer information. With considerably more effort, PH could accept any format a laboratory uses, and standardize the data into their own system. Like the saying, 'pay now, or pay later,' someone has to do the work to get the data into a usable form. Requiring laboratories to use established standards helps spread the burden around, giving PH an advantage to cereate their finished product (data); however, it still does not give a finished product to PH.

Best standards would be freely available, easy to understand, easily correlated with current data (e.g., lab tests or results), and easily maintained and updated. Do we have such standards now? Not really.

Note: Instructor can also ask questions regarding

- Experience of fellows in working with standards.
- Alternative to not using standards.

5. **How should Julia sequence the checklist of implementation activities in Column A of Table 9 to ensure that she has an appropriate foundation of information and activities for each additional task? Use Column B to arrange the sequence of Column A items. Be prepared to justify sequencing of items in Column B.**

Table 9. Question 5

COLUMN A	COLUMN B
A. Inventory of information standards and technologies used by partners. B. Identify need for electronic information exchange and willingness to provide data. C. Ensure buy-in. D. Identify resources (e.g., technical, human, and financial) for project implementation. E. Develop infrastructure for exchange of electronic messages. F. Identify stakeholders. I. Develop a new messaging guide for laboratory reporting in the state.	*(Starting sequence answers provided below)* *F. Identify stakeholders.* *B. Identify need for electronic information exchange and willingness to send data.* *A. Inventory of information standards and technologies used by partners.* *D. Identify resources (e.g., technical, human, and financial) for project implementation.* *E. Develop infrastructure for exchange of electronic messages.* *(Complete the last two!)*

ADDITIONAL READING RELATED TO THE STATE OF OZ CASE

Aller, R. D. (2003). The clinical laboratory data warehouse: An overlooked diamond mine. *American Journal of Clinical Pathology*, *120*(6), 817–819. doi:10.1309/TXXABU8MW75L04KF

Centers for Disease Control and Prevention. (1997). *Electronic reporting of laboratory data for public health: Meeting report and recommendations*. Washington, DC: Health Information and Surveillance Systems Board (HISSB).

Centers for Disease Control and Prevention. (1999). *Electronic reporting of laboratory information for public health*. Atlanta, GA: Centers for Disease Control and Prevention.

Centers for Disease Control and Prevention. (2005). *Progress in improving state and local disease surveillance — United States, 2000–2005.* Retrieved from http://www.cdc.gov/mmwr/preview/mmwrhtml/mm5433a3.htm

National Electronic Disease Surveillance System Working Group. (2001). National electronic disease surveillance system (NEDSS): A standards-based approach to connect public health and clinical medicine. *Journal of Public Health Management and Practice,* 7(6), 43-50.

Overhage, J. M., Grannis, S., & McDonald, C. J. (2008). A comparison of the completeness and timeliness of automated electronic laboratory reporting and spontaneous reporting of notifiable conditions. *American Journal of Public Health,*. 98 (2), 344-350.

Pinner, R. W., Jernigan, D. B., & Sutliff, S. M. (2000). Electronic laboratory-based reporting for public health. *Military Medicine, 165*(7Supplement 2), 20–24.

White, M. D., Kolar, L. M., & Steindel, S. J. (1999). Evaluation of vocabularies for electronic laboratory reporting to public health agencies. *Journal of the American Medical Informatics Association, 6*(3), 185–194. doi:10.1136/jamia.1999.0060185

ENDNOTES

[1] JULIA'S BIOSKETCH: Julia Martinez is a microbiologist with 5 years of experience working in a private laboratory before she obtained her Master of Public Health degree at the University of North Carolina and her Ph.D. in Informatics from the Swiss Institute of Technology in Zurich, Switzerland. While a PHIFP two-year fellow, she was assigned to the National Center for Hepatitis, HIV/AIDS, Sexually Transmitted Diseases, Tuberculosis Prevention (NCHHSTP). After graduating from the program, she was accepted into in the third-year PHIFP practicum and was assigned to the State of Oz.

Chapter 2
Individual, Organizational, and Technological Barriers to EHR Implementation

Matthew J. Wills
Indiana University East, USA

EXECUTIVE SUMMARY

This case examines the adoption and implementation of an electronic health record in a regional medical center in Midwest, USA. A background of the organization is provided, including a discussion of the organization's inception, financials, and organizational structure. A brief literature review of technology adoption, use, and performance is presented, followed by a discussion of data analysis techniques and results. A detailed overview of specific technology, management, and organizational concerns is presented along with challenges and solutions. The objective of this case is to highlight the challenges and opportunities during electronic health record adoption and implementation. The hope is that educators and students alike will appreciate the complexity of health information technology adoption and implementation through specific examples of challenges and solutions. While the information contained in this case is indeed specific to one organization in the USA, the lessons learned are broadly applicable to healthcare organizations throughout the world.

DOI: 10.4018/978-1-4666-2671-3.ch002

INTRODUCTION

Electronic Health Records (EHR) are emerging as the foundation of Health Information Technology (HIT), although there is current evidence that fewer than 20% of physician practices have adopted the technology (DesRoches, et al., 2008). Despite this, the current social and political environment appears to favor expansion of EHR adoption and use. As a result of increasing efforts to utilize these and other HIT"s, analysis of user evaluation of and performance with an EHR is an inherently valuable activity.

For more than three decades, Information Systems (IS) research has explored how and why people accept and use technology. IS researchers have also considered how technology impacts individual (Goodhue & Thompson, 1995) and group (Zigurs & Buckland, 1998) performance. IS practitioners who implement technology may benefit from a method of identifying factors that either inhibit, or enhance performance. In business, it is essential that performance impacts are identified, understood, and accordingly planned for. In health care, where the supply chain is replaced with human patients, understanding performance impact is critical to implementation and operational success.

The objective of this case is to describe the evaluation of an electronic health record system in a regional healthcare organization. The case begins by describing the organizational details, which explicate the context in which the study occurred. A brief literature review of adoption, use, and performance research is discussed followed by detail regarding the quantitative and qualitative findings of the study. The specific research questions of interest to the organization are explored in detail. Finally, the case concludes with a discussion of challenges, solutions, and recommendations.

ORGANIZATION BACKGROUND

Like so many others, the genesis of this health care organization arose due to escalating costs and advances in medical technology in the U.S. during the 1970s. In 1973, the region had two competing hospitals and the feasibility of maintaining both came into question. A seven-member Hospital Action Committee was formed to explore the possibility of merging the two hospitals. Incorporated in July of 1973, the organization began with 80 physicians on the Medical Staff and 280 licensed beds.

Since 1973, the organization has in fact evolved into a health system, comprised of many different units and facilities. In 2011, the health system is comprised of five regional hospitals, five specialty care centers (including, hospice, cancer care, behavioral health, rehabilitation, and surgery), thirty-two regional clinics, five regional care centers, home medical equipment and home medical services, and a number of partnerships and management agreements with other regional community care facilities.

The services provided by this organization span three U.S. states. As a whole, the health system demonstrated significant capacity in 2010 with a total of 88,816 inpatient days, 66,014 emergency room visits, and 2597 births. The health system has grown substantially since its beginning and as of 2010 has 4,427 health team members, $246,111,000 in payroll and benefit obligations, $59,796,000 in bad debt, charity care, and unreimbursed Medicaid payments. Table 1 shows the organization's approximate financial summary for the fiscal year 2010 (July1, 2009 – June 30, 2010).

Of the organizations top four executives two are physicians, one is a public health specialist and the fourth is an MBA trained executive. Based on the researchers' personal experience studying the health system, the organizational culture could be classified as Adhocratic; that is, they value flexibility and adaptability, they have an external focus with the goal of differentiation, and they appear to thrive in adverse, challenging technological and economic climates. It should be noted however that the subject of this study was not the organizational culture, and any conclusions noted herein reflect opinion and not tested fact.

Strategic planning has been and continues to be a major business activity for the health system. Since 1973, the organization has experienced continued growth

Table 1. Health system financial summary

Financial Summary (in 2000s)	
Revenue and Expenses	**Fiscal Year 2010**
Net patient services revenue	$466,300
Other operating expenses	25,350
Net Operating Revenues	**$491,800**
Operating Expenses:	
Payroll and Benefits	$246,100
Medical Supplies	63,878
Purchased Services	43,595
Bad Debt	27,518
Other Operating Expenses	35,470
Depreciation	25,676
Interest	3,848
Total Expenses	**$446,097**
Net Revenue	**$45,716**

with acquisition of regional health facilities and it remains active with its regional partnerships and facilities management contracts. Such planning has permitted the organization to remain a leader in the region and financially viable in a difficult economic climate. As a non-profit health system, any net revenues are reinvested into the system and as additional services to the community. Table 2 summarizes the health systems approximate balance sheet for the fiscal year 2010.

In summary, the health system is a dynamic regional leader with reasonably strong financials. Emphasis on long-term strategic planning has yielded good results, while the careful crafting of a flexible, adaptive, and responsive organizational culture has contributed to their success in the region and beyond. The health system is the recipient of a number of major national awards and accreditations, including those by the Joint Commission, the American Diabetes Association, and the American Heart Association, among others.

SETTING THE STAGE

Prior to implementation of the Electronic Health Record (EHR) the organization had a strong record of information technology utilization. Multiple legacy information systems were responsible for managing patient scheduling within each department, laboratory reporting, patient management, staff and facilities scheduling and others. In addition, telemedicine portals provided specialist access to geographically dispersed locations and facilities within the region.

Table 2. Health system balance sheet (July, 1 2009 – June 30, 2010)

Balance Sheet (in 2000s)	
Current Assets	**$128,658**
Funds reserved for buildings, equipment, debt repayment	298,153
Other restricted use investments	14,131
Land, building and equipment	161,019
Other assets	16,353
Total Assets	**$618,314**
Current Liability	$60,167
Long-term debts	134,919
Other liability	36,817
Unrestricted fund balance	375,368
Restricted fund balance	11,043
Total Liabilities and Fund Balance	**$618,314**

One of the last major implementations of information technology prior to EHR implementation was a mobile, bedside tablet pilot program that was later expanded throughout the main medical center. This technology permitted nurses, para-medical and other clinical staff closer contact with patients during the clinical documentation process. From a management perspective, the use of this technology was bold and relatively untested. The concern was voiced by nursing and clinical staff that too much time was allocated for documentation; a process that required staff to be physically separated from patients due to the location of clinical workstations. Management responded by instituting a pilot program to test the device's efficacy for improved patient care.

Following six months of observation and data gathering, the pilot program ended and the device was made available to all departments involved in patient care. As a prelude to EHR adoption and implementation, the use of this device was also considered by key management as a test of technology adoption challenges.

The overarching theme regarding technology adoption has been and continues to be innovation and better service. The key management players—including a senior clinical informatics specialist (RN, Ed.D), chief medical officer (MD) and the chief clinical informatics officer (MD) along with executive management stressed the importance of innovating with new information technologies. The goal was not to implement and adopt technology for technology's sake, rather the operational motive was to improve efficiency, reduce clinical error and enhance patient care.

In-House Development or Vendor?

The organization had developed a strong team of in-house technicians and developers to deal with the challenging task of maintaining legacy systems and development of useful add-ons. The health system carefully considered in-house development of an EHR product. After a 3-month study the organization concluded that in-house development of an EHR was quite simply not feasible. Reasons given for selecting a third-party vendor included cost, legal liability, and regulatory concerns (HIPPA). Another matter of significant concern is the availability of additional Medicare compensation for the use of certified EHR products. Moreover, the organization believed that a tested, flexible system developed by people who had detailed knowledge of EHR product development was the best course of action.

Over a period of 6 months key management personnel evaluated various systems and proposals and invited vendors on-site to demonstrate their products. With vendor and product selection behind them, the goal was to implement the product with a small sample of the health system population, study the impact of system adoption and use, and plan accordingly for broad implementation. It was determined that the organization would concomitantly use paper and electronic medical records during the initial small-scale implementation phase and for a period of one year post-implementation. On April 1, 2009, the organization went "live" with the EHR and the research team was brought in to study adoption, implementation, and technology utilization.

CASE DESCRIPTION

Related Work

Technology acceptance, adoption and performance research have been significantly impacted by theories of human and social behavior emerging from the disciplines of psychology and sociology. With its origin in the area of Social Learning Theory by Miller and Dollard (1941), Social Cognitive Theory is focused on the process of knowledge acquisition through observation (Bandura, 1977). This theory was later expanded, in particular by Bandura (1986) and became known as SET, or Self-Efficacy Theory. In the years prior to Bandura's work on Self-Efficacy, Fishbein and Ajzen (1975) published their research on the Theory of Reasoned Action (TRA). The theoretical basis for TRA lies in the tenets of social psychology, and has been widely accepted as a foundational theory of human behavior.

A product of TRA and SET, the Theory of Planned Behavior (TPB) emerges as an extension of TRA with perceived behavioral control from SET as an additional determinant of intention (Ajzen & Fishbein, 1980). In 1991, Thompson, Higgins, and Howell (1991) published an alternative to TRA and TPB, the Model of PC Utilization. This theory too has its roots in psychology, emanating most distinctly from the Triandis' (1977) work on human behavioral research.

The Technology Acceptance (TAM) model represents the first theory developed specifically for the information systems context, i.e. people in business (Davis, 1989). A few years later, Taylor and Todd (1995) put forth their theory, known as Combined TAM-TPB, or C-TAM-TPB. This theory of technology acceptance combined the predictive elements of TPB with the concept of perceived usefulness from TAM. TAM was further extended to TAM2 (Venkatesh & Davis, 2000), and included subjective norm as a predictor in settings where use is mandatory. The most recent models to emerge from this long line of study are known as the Unified Theory of Acceptance and Use of Technology (Venkatesh, Morris, Davis, & Davis, 2003), and TAM3 (Venkatesh & Bala, 2008).

Central to model predicting acceptance and use is the notion that various situational factors would lead to user intention to utilize the technology resulting in increased actual use. It is often implied that increased use will result in increased performance. However, use of the technology is not always voluntary, e.g., use of EHR systems is usually mandatory. Moreover, increased use is not necessarily positively correlated with increased performance (Goodhue, 1998).

In contrast with models predicting acceptance and use, Task-Technology Fit (TTF) attempts to explain user performance with information systems. The premise of the theory is that individual performance can be enhanced when the functionality provided by the technology meets the user's needs, i.e., fits the task at hand. The original design of TTF was centered on the use of multiple information systems and specifically directed toward managerial decision-making. The theory was first formally proposed by Goodhue (1995), and measures task-technology fit along multiple dimensions. Goodhue also demonstrated the validity of an instrument for information system user evaluation based on TTF (Goodhue, 1998). In 2000, Goodhue established that user evaluations were effective surrogates for objective performance (Goodhue, Klein, & March, 2000).

The TTF model has been used in a variety of ways since originally proposed. It has been studied in group performance situations (Shirani, Tafti, & Affisco, 1999; Zigurs & Buckland, 1998), as intended with the focus on managerial decision-making (Ferratt & Vlahos, 1998), and further examined with an emphasis on ease-of-use (Mathieson & Keil, 1998). TTF has also been extended with the technology acceptance model (Dishaw & Strong, 1999; Klopping & McKinney, 2004; Pagani, 2006). More recently, TTF has been the theoretical basis for a number of studies evaluating user performance with information systems, including Vlahos et al. (2004), Lin and Huang (2008), Teo and Men (2008), Junglas, Abraham, and Watson (2008), and Zigurs and Khazanchi (2008).

More recently, research related to the use of TTF has been conducted in healthcare environments and is specifically oriented toward EHR use (El-Gayar, 2009a, 2009b; Wills, 2009).

Technology Concerns

The research team was contacted by the Director of Clinical Informatics following a prior EHR study at another institution. Concerning EHR technology, the organization expressed interest in conducting a study to assess the following:

1. To what degree does the EHR support clinical task performance?
2. How does the EHR system impact patient care, documentation and workflow?

The research team developed a survey instrument intended to address the organization's questions as outlined above. The instrument gathered demographic information, addressed a number of key questions of importance to the organization, and was based on the Task-Technology Fit (TTF) theory of individual performance.

This study employs a reduced version of the TTF model. The focus is on capturing user evaluation of TTF along various dimensions as identified in Goodhue (1995), impact on individual performance, and the relationship between TTF and individual performance. The TTF dimensions that comprise the model employed in this study include data quality, data locatability, data compatibility, IS relationship to users, ease-of-use and training, correct level of authorization, systems reliability, and IS production timeliness. According to the TTF model, the strength of the link between information systems and performance impacts is a function of the extent to which system functionality responds to task needs (see Figure 1).

The research model shown in Figure 1 hypothesizes the following:

H1: User evaluation of task-technology fit will have explanatory power in predicting perceived performance impact. This can be further divided among the 8 TTF dimensions as follows:

H1a: Data quality will significantly influence user performance. Data quality is evaluated according to the currency of the data, maintenance of the correct data and the appropriate level of detail.

H1b: The locatability of the data will influence user performance. Locatability is assessed by both the ease with which data is located, and the ease with which the meaning of the data can be discovered.

H1c: Data authorization will influence user performance. Authorization measures the degree with which individuals are appropriately authorized to access the data required for the task.

H1d: The compatibility of data from other systems will influence user performance.

H1e: Ease of use and training will significantly influence user performance. The degree to which a person believes a system is easy to use and user training.

H1f: Production timeliness will influence user performance. Production timeliness is evaluated according to the perceived response time for reports and other requested information.

H1g: Systems reliability will influence user performance.

Figure 1. Determinants of performance

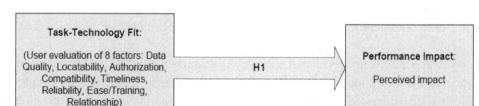

H1h: The IS departments' relationship with users will influence user performance. This factor includes IS understanding of business, IS interest and user support, IS responsiveness, delivery of agreed-upon solutions, and technical and unit planning support.

Data Analysis

Partial Least Squares (PLS) is the analysis technique used in this study. While the utility of PLS is detailed elsewhere (Falk & Miller, 1992), a number of recent technology acceptance studies have used PLS (e.g., Al-Gahtani, 2001; Compeau, 1995a; Venkatesh, 2003). To evaluate the measurement model, PLS estimates the internal consistency for each block of indicators. PLS then evaluates the degree to which a variable measures what it was intended to measure (Cronbach, 1951; Straub, Boudreau, & Gefen, 2004). This evaluation, understood as construct validity, is comprised of convergent and discriminate validity. Following previous work (Gefen & Straub, 2005), convergent validity of the variables is evaluated by examining the t-values of the outer model loadings. Discriminate validity is evaluated by assessing item loadings to variable correlations and by examining the ratio of the square root of the AVE of each variable to the correlations of this construct to all other variables (Chin, 1998a; Gefen & Straub, 2005).

With respect to the structural model, path coefficients are understood as regression coefficients with the t-statistic calculated using a bootstrapping method. 200 samples are generally considered satisfactory (Chin, 1998a). Bootstrapping is a nonparametric technique used to estimate the precision of PLS estimates (Chin, 1998a). To determine how well the model fits the hypothesized relationship, PLS calculates an R^2 for each dependent construct in the model. Similar to regression analysis, R^2 represents the proportion of variance in the endogenous constructs which can be explained by the antecedent constructs (Chin, 1998a).

The study was conducted at a regional health center in the U.S. Midwest. The subjects of the study are registered nurses (RNs) employed in a hospital setting. Surveys were randomly distributed to 100 registered nurses, of which 76 subjects from 12 hospital departments participated in and successfully completed the study. The clinical departments represented include: Emergency department, Pediatrics, Medical/Surgical, Orthopedics/Neurology, Infusion center, PAC (Post-Acute Care), Rehabilitation, Oncology, Pulmonary care, Intensive care, Coronary intensive care, and Home health.

Organization Question 1: To What Degree Does the EHR Support Clinical Task Performance?

To address this question, the research team examined 8 aspects of the EHR technology, including data quality, data locatability, data authorization, data compatibility, data timeliness, data reliability, system ease-of-use and training, and the relationship between clinical staff and the information systems department. Definitions for each term are found in hypotheses H1a-H1h above.

The results for each of the 8 aspects of EHR technology are summarized in Table 3. The results show Composite Reliability (CR) exceeding 0.8 as recommended (Nunnally, 1978). AVE, which can also be considered as a measure of reliability exceeds 0.5 as recommended (Fornell & Larcker, 1981). Together, CR and AVE attest to the reliability of the instrument. The t-values of the outer model loadings exceed 1.96 verifying the convergent validity of the instrument (Gefen & Straub, 2005). Calculating the correlation between variables' component scores and individual items reveal that intra-variable (construct) item correlations are generally high when compared to inter-variable (construct) item correlations. Discriminate validity is confirmed if the diagonal elements (representing the square root of AVE) are significantly higher than the off-diagonal values (representing correlations between constructs) in the corresponding rows and columns (Chin, 1998b).

As shown in Table 4 the instrument demonstrates adequate discriminate validity, as the diagonal values (bold) are greater with respect to the corresponding correlation values in the adjoining columns and rows.

Figure 2 depicts the structural model with path (regression) coefficients and the R^2 for the dependent variable. As shown, the R^2 value for the dependent variable indicates that the model explains 55.2% of the variance for performance. To assess

Table 3. Result summary for the model

Dimension	CR	AVE
Data Quality	0.943	0.738
Data Locatability	0.900	0.693
Data Authorization	0.906	0.829
Data Compatibility	0.936	0.830
Production Timeliness	0.848	0.736
System Reliability	0.879	0.786
System Ease-of-Use/Training	0.962	0.740
IS Relationship to Users	0.944	0.738

Table 4. Square root of the AVE scores and correlation of latent variables

	QUAL	LOCT	AUTH	COMP	PROD	RELY	EOU/ TR	REL/ USR	PERF
QUAL	**0.859**								
LOCT	0.538	**0.832**							
AUTH	-0.148	-0.107	**0.910**						
COMP	-0.028	-0.315	0.460	**0.911**					
PROD	0.492	0.281	0.064	-0.006	**0.858**				
RELY	-0.434	-0.479	0.190	0.531	-0.331	**0.887**			
EOU/TR	0.263	0.444	-0.046	-0.012	0.221	-0.209	**0.860**		
REL/USR	0.426	0.390	-0.134	-0.129	0.666	-0.345	0.342	**0.859**	
PERF	0.563	0.412	-0.194	-0.203	0.468	-0.395	0.510	0.536	**0.869**

the statistical significance of the path coefficients, the bootstrap method was used in PLS-Graph.

With respect to the hypothesized determinants of performance, two constructs significantly influence user performance: data quality ($\beta = 0.393$ p > 0.02) and ease-of-use/training ($\beta = 0.372$ p > 0.0002). These findings are consistent with H1a and H1e respectively. H1h - IS relationship with users ($\beta = 0.200$ p > 0.10) with H4 - data compatibility ($\beta = -0.188$ p > 0.10) are significant at the 10% level. Comparing the results with that reported in Goodhue (Goodhue and Thompson), we find data quality and to a lesser extent the information systems department's relationship with users and data compatibility are significant predictors of performance impact in both studies, while production timeliness is only significant in the (Goodhue & Thompson, 1995) study. Ease-of-use and training while significant in this study was not significant in Goodhue (1995). The remaining TTF dimensions where insignificant predictors for performance in both studies.

In the context of EHR systems, it is no surprise that data quality, i.e., providing access to the right data, at the right level of detail, and currency are significant predictors of performance. Also somewhat consistent with the information systems literature are the significance of the strength of the relationship of the hospital information systems department with users (nurses in this study) and the compatibility of data as predictors of performance. However, the results are particularly surprising with respect to the insignificance of timeliness and data locatability. Normally, one would expect these to be hallmarks for implementing EHR technology.

Figure 2. Model testing results

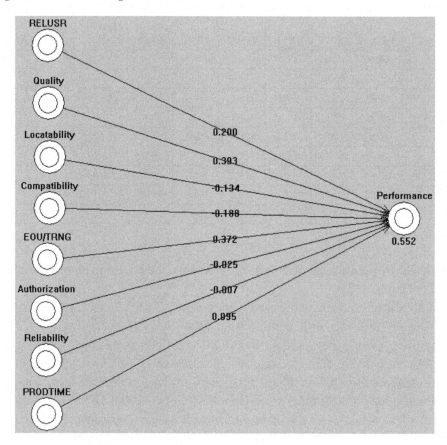

Organization Question 2: How Does the EHR System Impact Patient Care, Documentation, and Workflow?

To address these issues the survey asked a series of questions related to the impact of EHR on patient care, documentation, and workflow. Responses were subjective yet conclusive. More than 60% of respondents indicated that EHR use had a negative impact on patient care. Further investigation of this matter occurred through interviews conducted following the study. It was noted that while the use of mobile tablets brought nursing staff closer to the patient bedside, thereby enhancing the perception of better patient care, implementation of the EHR required accessing a workstation that was physically distant from the bedside.

Similarly, the use of EHR for clinical documentation had a negative perceived impact, resulting in increased time for documenting patient care and progress. Again, nearly 60% of respondents indicated that documentation time increased by more than 10 minutes for each patient. It should be noted that the study occurred within one month of implementation—insufficient time for nursing and clinical staff to adapt to new documentation procedures. Furthermore, the lack of familiarity with the EHR was likely the cause of increased time during documentation. The vendor, along with the organization's management agreed to monitor and assess documentation impact at three, six, and twelve months following implementation.

Workflow impact was another concern identified during the early stages of EHR implementation. 44% of respondents indicated that workflow was "moderately interrupted" as a result of EHR use, while 26% indicated that workflow had been "significantly interrupted" due to EHR use. More than 90% of the nursing staff surveyed believed workflow would return to normal or be improved as user experience with the EHR increased.

Management and Organizational Concerns

In addition to the technology concerns noted above by the organization, management was also interested in gathering information related to EHR training, overall adoption and utilization attitudes, as well as the degree to which EHR adoption and use was enabled or thwarted by social influences within the organization. The two questions addressed in this portion of the study are noted below:

1. How effective is staff training, and are there any subsets of the nursing staff population that require additional training?
2. What aspects of the organization (individuals/organizational culture) enable or thwart use of the EHR?

Question 1: How Effective is Staff Training, and are there any Subsets of the Nursing Staff Population that Require Additional Training?

From the quantitative analysis conducted, the data suggests that training is a significant predictor of perceived performance impact. As noted in Figure 2, the path coefficient for ease-of-use/training was strong, and analysis indicated this construct to be very significant. The results indicate that staff perceived adequate training to be a key indicator of increased performance with respect to EHR use.

While more than 90% of the nursing staff between the ages of 18 and 54 indicated that they had received adequate training on the EHR, more than 80% of nursing staff between the ages of 55 and 65+ believed that training had been "significantly inadequate." Staff between the ages of 18 and 34 rated their ability to learn operation of the EHR higher (5.9 on a scale of 1-7) than their counterparts between the ages of 35 and 54 (4.7) and significantly higher than their colleagues aged 55+ (3.9).

Such findings are not uncommon for technology implementations and clearly represent an opportunity to improve training methods for specific age groups.

Question 2: What Aspects of the Organization (Individuals/ Organizational Culture) Enable or Thwart Use of the EHR?

The research team was approached by top management to conduct this study. This is an important point for two reasons. First, from the perspective of the researchers, conducting a study is always easier with support of top management. This is largely because the directive and rationale for study participation comes from the top of the organization. Second, with the support of top management (who act as champions of the project), researchers know from the beginning that access to resources and study populations is much less likely to be problematic. Even though having a high-level champion does not guarantee research success, the probability of achieving predetermined goals is much more likely.

The culture of this organization, although not specifically studied, was reported by executive management to be highly flexible and adaptive, with a history of overcoming challenges. With previous experience in technology adoption and implementation, extra attention was taken during the adoption process to promote the value of EHR. Value was described by management in terms of increased patient safety and enhanced care.

Less than 5% of the respondents could be classified as "anti-EHR" following implementation. The vast majority of nursing staff had a clear understanding of why EHR was being adopted, and understood the value of using the technology. This is a critical point—knowing the value of a new technology and the advantages (both from nursing and patient perspectives) are key to overcoming the challenges, and sometimes frustrations of learning a new way of doing things.

CURRENT CHALLENGES FACING THE ORGANIZATION

The study highlighted several key challenges that required the attention of the organization. These include inadequate EHR training for some nurses, lack of knowledge regarding documentation and patient information access during EHR outages, increased documentation time, workflow interruptions, and instances of difficult navigation within the EHR during documentation. Solutions to these challenges are discussed in the following section.

80% of nurses in the 55 to 65+ age range surveyed expressed that they had not received adequate training, despite having received the same amount of training as nurses in other age groups. Age can be a factor when considering ease-of-use, primarily due to previous information technology and computer experience.

Respondents were asked to indicate whether or not specific procedures for patient documentation and information access were in place in the event of an EHR outage. 82% of those surveyed indicated that they "don't know" if such procedures existed, 11% indicated that procedures were in place but were not familiar with the specific plans for such an event, and 7% knew of the procedures and where to find them.

As noted in a previous section, nurses reported an average increase of 10 minutes of documentation time for each patient. In intensive care units where each nurse may be responsible for 2-3 patients, increased documentation time resulted in an additional 20-30 minutes of work per shift. In other nursing units such as rehabilitation for example, nurses may be responsible for 4-5 times that number of patients, often resulting in unmanageable increases in documentation workload.

Workflow interruptions were also noted, and were primarily related to increased, redundant documentation with the EHR and paper-based medical records. Nurses reported that increased documentation took time away from patient contact and care. One anonymous respondent commented "Nurses by their very nature are caregivers. Redundant documentation procedures are taking valuable time away from the care of our patients, resulting in less-than-ideal care."

Another problem that surfaced was related to difficult navigation within the EHR during documentation. This problem was not discovered during the survey; rather it was reported to the research team directly from the director of clinical informatics. Details of the user interface issues were not described beyond redundant data entry and cluttered tabs within the software.

SOLUTIONS AND RECOMMENDATIONS

Inadequate EHR training for nurses in the 55 to 65+ age group was immediately met with the development of additional training programs. Although these additional training experiences were developed specifically for persons in this age group, no persons who requested additional training were denied access. The organization promoted these training sessions as "EHR Master Sessions" and participation was voluntary.

A series of four additional training seminars were organized and an outside consultant was brought in to assist training staff with the development of programs specifically aimed at helping persons with less computer experience. The research team received reports of this effort but was not involved in the delivery of training programs. It was reported that persons who completed the training exhibited a greater degree of self-efficacy with respect to EHR use and diminished anxiety regarding its use.

Responding to the lack of awareness regarding documentation and patient information access during planned or unplanned EHR outages, the organization immediately developed a computer-based training program to inform users of the correct procedure during EHR downtimes. Based on the research teams' recommendations, the organization conducted a follow up survey to gauge the success of the training program. Upon completion of training, 98% of EHR users knew that specific procedures existed and were aware of the location of those procedures.

With respect to increased documentation from redundant (electronic and paper-based) EHR data entry, the organization instituted a plan to monitor the issue at three, six, and twelve month increments post-implementation. Such increases to documentation time and workflow interruptions are common when instituting technology and the organization believed that these issues would resolve with time. Specific outcomes related to these issues were not reported to the research team.

The final challenge was related to redundant data entry and "cluttered" user interfaces within the EHR itself. Although the research team was not involved in developing a plan to deal with these challenges, it was reported that the organization worked closely with the EHR vendor to redesign the EHR user interface. Redundancy was reported to be at a minimum and interface problems alleviated following vendor redesign.

REFERENCES

Ajzen, I., & Fishbein, M. (1980). *Understanding attitudes and predicting social behavior*. Englewood Cliffs, NJ: Prentice Hall.

Al-Gahtani, S. S. (2001). The applicability of TAM outside North America: An empirical test in the United Kingdom. *Information Resources Management Journal, 14*(3), 37–46. doi:10.4018/irmj.2001070104

Bandura, A. (1977). Self-efficacy: Toward a unifying theory of behavioral change. *Psychological Review, 84*(2), 191–215. doi:10.1037/0033-295X.84.2.191

Bandura, A. (1986). *Social foundations of thought and action: A social cognitive theory*. Englewood Cliffs, NJ: Prentice Hall.

Chin, W. W. (1998a). Commentary: Issues and opinion on structural equation modeling. *Management Information Systems Quarterly, 22*(1), 7–16.

Chin, W. W. (1998b). The partial least squares approach for structural equation modelling. In Marcoulides, G. A. (Ed.), *Modern Methods for Business Research*. Hillsdale, NJ: Lawrence Erlbaum Associates.

Compeau, D. R., & Higgins, C. A. (1995a). Application of social cognitive theory to training for computer skills. *Information Systems Research, 6*(2), 118–143. doi:10.1287/isre.6.2.118

Compeau, D. R., & Higgins, C. A. (1995b). Computer self-efficacy - Development of a measure and initial test. *Management Information Systems Quarterly, 19*(2), 189–211. doi:10.2307/249688

Cronbach, L. (1951). Coefficient alpha and the internal structure of tests. *Psychometrika, 16*, 297–334. doi:10.1007/BF02310555

Davis, F. D. (1989). Perceived usefulness, perceived ease of use, and user acceptance of information technology. *Management Information Systems Quarterly, 13*(3), 319–340. doi:10.2307/249008

DesRoches, C. M., Campbell, E. G., Rao, S. R., Donelan, K., Ferris, T. G., & Jha, A. (2008). Electronic health records in ambulatory care: A national survey of physicians. *The New England Journal of Medicine, 359*(1), 50–60. doi:10.1056/NEJMsa0802005

Dishaw, M. T., & Strong, D. M. (1999). Extending the technology acceptance model with task-technology fit constructs. *Information & Management, 36*(1), 9. doi:10.1016/S0378-7206(98)00101-3

El-Gayar, O. F., Deokar, A. V., & Wills, M. (2009a). Evaluating task-technology fit for an electronic health record system. *International Journal of Healthcare Technology and Management, 11*(1/2), 50–65. Retrieved from http://www.inderscience.com/search/index.php?action=record&rec_id=33274 doi:10.1504/IJHTM.2010.033274

El-Gayar, O. F., Deokar, A. V., & Wills, M. (2009b). Evaluating task-technology fit for an electronic health record system. In *Proceedings of the 15th Americas Conference on Information Systems*. San Francisco, CA: IEEE.

Falk, R., & Miller, N. E. (1992). *A primer for soft modeling*. Akron, OH: University of Akron Press.

Ferratt, T. W., & Vlahos, G. E. (1998). An investigation of task-technology fit for managers in Greece and the US. *European Journal of Information Systems, 7*(2), 123. doi:10.1057/palgrave.ejis.3000288

Fishbein, M., & Ajzen, I. (1975). *Belief, attitude, intention and behavior: An introduction to theory and research*. Reading, MA: Addison-Wesley.

Fornell, C., & Larcker, D. F. (1981). Structural equation models with unobservable variables and measurement error - Algebra and statistics. *JMR, Journal of Marketing Research, 18*(3), 382–388. doi:10.2307/3150980

Gefen, D., & Straub, D. (2005). A practical guide to factorial validity using PLS-GRAPH: Tutorial and annotated example. *Communication of the AIS, 16*, 91–109.

Goodhue, D. L. (1988). IS attitudes: Toward theoretical and definition clarity. *Database, 19*(3-4), 6–15.

Goodhue, D. L. (1995). Understanding user evaluations of information systems. *Management Science, 41*(12), 1827. doi:10.1287/mnsc.41.12.1827

Goodhue, D. L. (1998). Development and measurement validity of a task-technology fit instrument for user evaluations of information systems. *Decision Sciences, 29*(1), 105. doi:10.1111/j.1540-5915.1998.tb01346.x

Goodhue, D. L., Klein, B. D., & March, S. T. (2000). User evaluations of IS as surrogates for objective performance. *Information & Management, 38*(2), 87. doi:10.1016/S0378-7206(00)00057-4

Goodhue, D. L., & Thompson, R. L. (1995). Task-technology fit and individual performance. *Management Information Systems Quarterly, 19*(2), 213. doi:10.2307/249689

Hair, J. F., Black, B., Babin, B., Anderson, R. E., & Tatham, R. L. (2006). *Multivariate data analysis* (6th ed.). Upper Saddle River, NJ: Prentice Hall.

Junglas, I., Abraham, C., & Watson, R. T. (2008). Task-technology fit for mobile locatable information systems. *Decision Support Systems, 45*(4), 1046. doi:10.1016/j.dss.2008.02.007

Klopping, I., & McKinney, E. (2004). Extending the technology acceptance model and the task-technology fit model to consumer e-commerce. *Information Technology, Learning and Performance Journal, 22*(1), 35.

Lin, T.-C., & Huang, C.-C. (2008). Understanding knowledge management system usage antecedents: An integration of social cognitive theory and task technology fit. *Information & Management, 45*(6), 410. doi:10.1016/j.im.2008.06.004

Mathieson, K., & Keil, M. (1998). Beyond the interface: Ease of use and task/technology fit. *Information & Management, 34*(4), 221. doi:10.1016/S0378-7206(98)00058-5

Miller, N. E., & Dollard. (1941). *Social learning and limitation*. New Haven, CT: Yale University Press.

Nunnally, J. C. (1978). *Psychometric theory* (2nd ed.). New York, NY: McGraw Hill.

Pagani, M. (2006). Determinants of adoption of high speed data services in the business market: Evidence for a combined technology acceptance model with task technology fit model. *Information & Management, 43*(7), 847. doi:10.1016/j.im.2006.08.003

Shirani, A. I., Tafti, M. H. A., & Affisco, J. F. (1999). Task and technology fit: A comparison of two technologies for synchronous and asynchronous group communication. *Information & Management, 36*(3), 139. doi:10.1016/S0378-7206(99)00015-4

Straub, D. W. (1989). Validating instruments in MIS research. *Management Information Systems Quarterly, 13*(2), 147–169. doi:10.2307/248922

Straub, D. W., Boudreau, M.-C., & Gefen, D. (2004). Validation guidelines for IS positivist research. *Communications of the AIS, 13*(24), 380–427.

Taylor, S., & Todd, P. A. (1995). Understanding information technology usage - A test of competing models. *Information Systems Research, 6*(2), 144–176. doi:10.1287/isre.6.2.144

Teo, T. S. H., & Men, B. (2008). Knowledge portals in Chinese consulting firms: A task-technology fit perspective. *European Journal of Information Systems, 17*(6), 557. doi:10.1057/ejis.2008.41

Thompson, R. L., Higgins, C. A., & Howell, J. M. (1991). Personal computing - Toward a conceptual-model of utilization. *Management Information Systems Quarterly, 15*(1), 125–143. doi:10.2307/249443

Triandis, H. C. (1977). *Interpersonal behavior*. Monterey, CA: Brooke Cole.

Venkatesh, V., & Bala, H. (2008). Technology acceptance model 3 and a research agenda on interventions. *Decision Sciences, 39*(2), 273–315. doi:10.1111/j.1540-5915.2008.00192.x

Venkatesh, V., & Davis, F. D. (2000). A theoretical extension of the technology acceptance model: Four longitudinal field studies. *Management Science, 46*(2), 186–204. doi:10.1287/mnsc.46.2.186.11926

Venkatesh, V., Morris, M. G., Davis, G. B., & Davis, F. D. (2003). User acceptance of information technology: Toward a unified view. *Management Information Systems Quarterly, 27*(3), 425–478.

Vlahos, G. E., Ferratt, T. W., & Knoepfle, G. (2004). The use of computer-based information systems by German managers to support decision making. *Information & Management, 41*(6), 763. doi:10.1016/j.im.2003.06.003

Wills, M., El-Gayar, O. F., & Deokar, A. V. (2009). Evaluating the technology acceptance model, task-technology fit and user performance for an electronic health record system. In *Proceedings of the Decision Sciences Institute 40th Annual Conference*. New Orleans, LA: Decision Sciences Institute.

Zigurs, I., & Buckland, B. K. (1998). A theory of task/technology fit and group support systems effectiveness. *Management Information Systems Quarterly, 22*(3), 313. doi:10.2307/249668

Zigurs, I., & Khazanchi, D. (2008). From profiles to patterns: A new view of task-technology fit. *Information Systems Management, 25*(1), 8. doi:10.1080/10580530701777107

Chapter 3
One System of Care, One Electronic Chart

Jennifer Gholson
Regional Health, USA

Heidi Tennyson
Regional Health, USA

EXECUTIVE SUMMARY

Regional Health made a commitment as part of quality and patient safety initiatives to have an electronic health record before the federal government developed the concept of "meaningful use." The "One System of Care, One Electronic Chart" concept was a long-term goal of their organization, accomplished through electronically sharing a patient's medical record among Regional Health's five hospitals and other area health care facilities. Implementing a hybrid electronic record using a scanning and archiving application was the first step toward the long-term goal of an electronic health record. The project was successfully achieved despite many challenges, including some limited resources and physician concerns.

ORGANIZATION BACKGROUND

Regional Health's roots can be traced to a foundation based on communication, cooperation, and collaboration and is a tax-exempt, community-based organization. The original facility, Rapid City Regional Hospital (RCRH), was formed in 1973 by the merger of St. John's McNamara Hospital and Bennett-Clarkson Hospital.

DOI: 10.4018/978-1-4666-2671-3.ch003

The new hospital had 280 licensed beds and approximately 80 physicians on the medical staff. Between the late 1990s and the early 2000s, RCRH purchased four other area hospitals (now known as Custer Regional Hospital, Spearfish Regional Hospital, Sturgis Regional Hospital, and Lead-Deadwood Regional Hospital) in an effort to preserve continuity of care within the Black Hills region. As the health care network continued to grow, the system was renamed Regional Health.

Today, Regional Health provides a continuum of care, which includes Regional Hospitals, Regional Medical Clinics, Regional Senior Care, Regional Cancer Care Institute, Regional Heart Doctors, Regional Rehabilitations Institute, and Regional Behavioral Health Center. The service area extends through western South Dakota, eastern Wyoming, northwestern Nebraska, southwestern North Dakota, and southeastern Montana. RCRH is a regional referral center with 400 licensed beds, operates the busiest emergency room in South Dakota, and is the largest hospital located between Sioux Falls, South Dakota and Billings, Montana. Spearfish Regional Hospital (SPRH) is licensed for 40 beds. Custer Regional Hospital (CURH), Sturgis Regional Hospital (STRH), and Lead/Deadwood Regional Hospital (LDRH) are all critical access hospitals with 11, 25, and 18 licensed beds, respectively. In addition to the hospitals, Regional Health also encompasses over 140 physician practices in the surrounding Black Hills area.

Regional Health has a corporate services division that provides services across the system. In addition, there is collaboration between same-type departments through what is known as Value Analysis Committees (VACs). This design functions well in this region where independence is highly valued. While each hospital has its own CEO, strategic planning is done system-wide using the six pillars philosophy: Patient Safety and Quality, Service, Financial Health, People, Growth/Innovation/Integration, and Community. The One System of Care, One Electronic Chart project was part of the Patient Safety & Quality pillar and the Growth/Innovation/Integration pillar.

SETTING THE STAGE

Prior to the start of the scanning and archiving project, Regional Health's main Health Care Information System (HCIS) was essentially a character-based system that had been in use at RCRH since 1983. By 2006, all five hospitals within Regional Health (RH) had been using this platform in an integrated fashion for at least a year; however, each hospital was in different stages of implementation. Because RCRH had been fully utilizing the new HCIS the longest, they were more proficient and advanced with its functionality.

Prior to the scanning project, each hospital used different methods for medical record retention. Even though state laws allowed for destruction of records (Brodnik,

McCain, Rinehart-Thompson, & Reynolds, 2009), most of the hospitals were either retaining all their paper records or used another method for permanent storage, such as microfilm or standalone document imaging systems. Despite these efforts, the hospitals found they were running out of space for paper chart storage. By 2004, the RCRH Health Information Management Director submitted a formal request to look for an electronic document management solution. A business case was written and originally approved in the fall of 2005 to purchase and implement the scanning and archiving module that was part of the platform being used at the time.

A few months after the project's approval, RH's plans to develop an Electronic Medical Record (EMR) had an impact on the project. A key step in the development of an EMR was the conversions of the core HCIS to a version that had a better (more like Windows) user interface. Because of the large scope of the conversion project, the scanning project was temporarily halted when it was learned that any scanning build done in the old system would have to be completely rebuilt in the new HCIS.

A fundamental element of RH's approach for the scanning project was that the EMR was going to be a system-wide initiative, not just an IT assignment. To reinforce that concept, a project manager from outside the IT department was used when RH converted to the new HCIS. Because that structure was successful, the core team for this project was formed using representatives from various parts of RH. The Health Information Management (HIM) directors from each of the network hospitals (Custer, Spearfish, Sturgis, and Lead/Deadwood) were appointed to the team. The Patient Access (Admissions) Director from RCRH was added to the team and was responsible for communicating project information to the other system Patient Access Directors. In addition, there was an IT Department Lead and the Assistant HIM Director at RCRH was the Project Manager. Regional Health's Chief Information Officer was named the Project Sponsor. In addition, several ad-hoc members were asked to assist at specific points within the project. These included the Regional Health Forms Analyst, various IT Analysts that supported other modules integrating with the scanning and archiving module, as well as HIM and Patient Access staff. The HIM and Patient Access ad hoc team members would specifically be trained as super-users, who would assist IT with front line support and troubleshooting.

Along with advancing the long-range goal of a fully electronic record, there were additional goals established for the scanning project. RH wanted to improve coordination of care between all five hospitals by making available the entire chart (through images) at discharge. The expectation was that making any paper forms from the patient record visible within the EMR would make information sharing easier, cutting down on duplicate testing and faxing of medical information to physicians in the community. Additional goals related more to the operational side of each HIM department. These included increased productivity for HIM staff and decreased costs associated with the storage and retrieval of paper records. Lastly, two regulatory goals were identified. First, various regulatory agencies have requirements for how quickly medical records should be completed and how quickly verbal orders should be signed. RH wanted to improve their already-satisfactory compliance rate with these standards. Second, RH anticipated enhancing the security of electronic medical records. Paper charts are generally secure, but in an electronic environment, a facility can provide extra layers of security and is able to run usage audits that were never possible in a paper environment.

CASE DESCRIPTION

Technology Concerns and Components

Many healthcare facilities use document imaging solutions as an interim step towards a completely electronic medical record. This creates what is known as a hybrid electronic medical record. A hybrid record is defined as one that includes both paper and electronic documents (AHIMA, 2005). In this environment, paper documents are scanned and turned into image files. To create an electronic document, health care workers complete online documentation, containing structured and unstructured data fields. The EMR system gathers the electronic data, formats it into a usable report, and archives the report for future retrieval. Examples of electronic reports include lab results and dictated operative notes (AHIMA, 2003).

The beginning of RH's journey to create a hybrid electronic medical record started with vendor selection. The scanning module offered by RH's main HCIS vendor was specifically chosen because it would have tight integration with the other vendor modules already in use. Despite that, there were several technology concerns. The vendor's release, which RH had just converted to, was relatively new. This was evidenced by the large number of open tickets with the vendor and was identified as a potential concern during a readiness assessment conducted prior to the start of the project (JJ Wild, 2008). Because scanning and archiving was also relativity new in this HCIS version, the project team had to be particularly vigilant with testing and implementing the functionality within the scanning module.

In addition to scanning documents, the application also provided archiving capability. This feature was a key reason why RH selected to purchase the scanning module from the current HCIS vendor. This functionality allowed RH to permanently save any electronic data generated by other modules within the HCIS, such as lab results, to the legal electronic chart. Prior to the implementation of this application, most of the clinical results and documentation were being printed to paper, becoming part of the legal paper medical record. With archiving, this same data is electronically stored and automatically becomes part of the patient's electronic legal record, eliminating the need to print.

The scanning application has two separate workflows associated with it. The more complex workflow was designed for the HIM departments to batch scan discharged patient charts in large volumes. The simpler workflow, called Point-Of-Contact (POC) scanning, was designed for patient registration areas to scan a few key items, such as driver's licenses, insurance cards, and advanced directives, without having to leave their workstation, providing better customer service to the patient. As the team progressed with testing these two workflows, they ran across several technology limitations. The first challenge involved the technology specifications received from the vendor. The specifications were somewhat generic, particularly for barcodes and end user hardware. In 2008, the scanner hardware requirements consisted of having TWAIN compliant scanners. The core team researched scanners and decided on three specific scanners. A decision was made to standardize these choices to help with purchasing power, ease of training and creating training documentation, and ease of troubleshooting problems. Tube scanners were selected for patient access departments that required a smaller scanner footprint because of counter space issues. For patient access areas that had room for a slightly larger scanner, a higher-quality scanner that could handle multiple pages was purchased. For the HIM departments, high-volume scanners with imprinter cartridges were selected.

In addition to scanners, hardware was needed to output documents from the legal electronic chart. High quality color printers were purchased for the HIM departments so staff could print surgical photos or any other items that necessitated a photo-quality color print. PCs for HIM staff were upgraded with CD burners so an electronic copy of a patient's chart could be provided. Inventory throughout the HIM department and physician areas were assessed for all PCs to Windows 2000 or later and video cards that would allow for dual-monitors setup prior to the scanning application going live.

For image storage, the vendor also had general requirements, describing the folder setup on a server, but most of the configuration was left to the customer. Regional Health (RH) chose to purchase three servers for the scanning project: an image server, a cache server, and a background job server. The image server holds the images after being fully indexed. The cache server transfers images between the temporary folder and the permanent folder once the indexing is completed by the user. The background job server runs all the jobs that transfer files. The background job and cache servers assist in retrieving images from the image server and make them available for viewing to an end user. The overall hardware schematic can be seen in Figure 1.

Another reality was checking the new technology to assure compliance with all HIPAA regulations (U.S. Department of Health & Human Services, 2012). Because

Figure 1. Overall hardware schematic

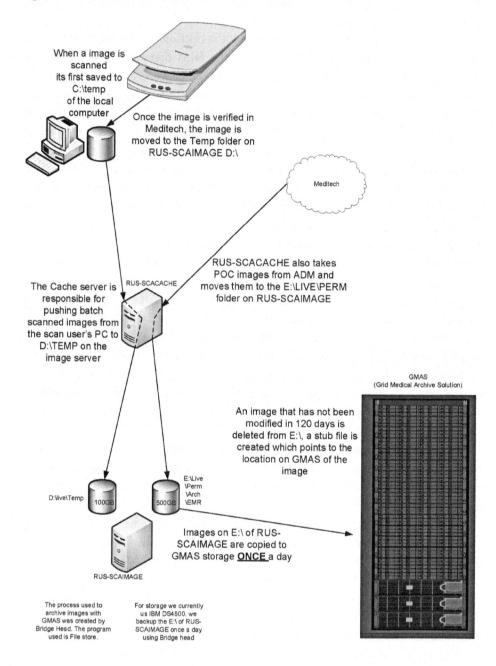

When a image is scanned its first saved to C:\temp of the local computer

Once the image is verified in Meditech, the image is moved to the Temp folder on RUS-SCAIMAGE D:\

Meditech

RUS-SCACACHE also takes POC images from ADM and moves them to the E:\LIVE\PERM folder on RUS-SCAIMAGE

The Cache server is responsible for pushing batch scanned images from the scan user's PC to D:\TEMP on the image server

RUS-SCACACHE

GMAS (Grid Medical Archive Solution)

An image that has not been modified in 120 days is deleted from E:\, a stub file is created which points to the location on GMAS of the image

D:\live\Temp 100GB

E:\Live \Perm \Arch \EMR 500GB

Images on E:\ of RUS-SCAIMAGE are copied to GMAS storage **ONCE** a day

RUS-SCAIMAGE

The process used to archive images with GMAS was created by Bridge Head. The program used is File store.

For storage we currently us IBM DS4800. we backup the E:\ of RUS-SCAIMAGE once a day using Bridge head new technology brings new risks, such as data breaches, the HIM departments needed to have adequate electronic auditing tools to continue to monitor and do their reporting in this new environment (AHIMA, 2010). New workflows had to be designed with the new technology to accommodate outside auditors who have proper authorization to review charts, such as surveyors from the Department of Health or the Joint Commission, researchers, and insurance auditors.

Management and Organizational Concerns

One of the main concerns on the scanning project was that the project team members had other responsibilities and were not dedicated solely to the project. There had not been additional funding budgeted for project staffing, so the team had to be pulled together from existing resources within the HIM departments. Three of the HIM Directors felt it would be more difficult to cope with the lost FTE hours if one of their staff participated on the project so they chose to have their hospitals represented by themselves. The remaining network hospital chose a lead staff member to participate. The Admissions Director from Rapid City was involved in the planning stages but eventually assigned this project to one of his staff. The Project Manager and the IT Lead also had their daily job responsibilities; however, they were both allowed to dedicate more time to the project due to their project roles.

To compensate for limited human resources, a staged rollout of the batch-scanning portion of this application was designed for each facility. Doing so would help prevent an overload on the core team during the first few weeks the system would be live, as well as allowing each facility to tailor its rollout to suit its hospital's best interests. Despite those benefits, there were some unintended consequences. As previously mentioned, the network hospitals had trouble fitting this project in to their daily routine, which extended the rollout plan at each facility. Because of this, staging the rollout necessitated excellent communication insuring that all users of the EMR understood what scanned chart forms would be available and when they would be available for viewing in the EMR.

Outside of project staffing, another concern was the impact this project would have on all users of the main HCIS. One of the challenges to overcome would be assisting all EMR users through this significant change that affected their workflow. Therefore, comprehensive plans on how to best support everyone that might use scanned images had to be developed. This included not only staff employed by RH but any health care physician or facility in the Black Hills area that had HIPAA-compliant access to RH's EMR. Because this user group was large and diverse, the plans would need to be tailored to accommodate different user's needs.

Since the ultimate goal of the project was to promote a system-wide EMR, keeping the team focused on consensus was key. This included standardizing medical record chart forms, HIM process workflows, and the set-up of the scanning functionality and the legal electronic record. Other reasons why it was important to define these processes and procedures for the system included simplified training of all EMR users as well as making it easier to troubleshoot technology-issues.

A final project requirement was the need for a sound legal record. Not only did the transition from a paper medical record to a legal electronic record need to meet state and federal regulations, it also needed to meet Joint Commission standards (AHIMA, 2010) as some of Regional Health's facilities were Joint Commission-accredited. The archived document formats and content were reviewed and approved for legal defensibility.

PROJECT IMPLEMENTATION CHALLENGES AND SOLUTIONS

Regional Health (RH) had been incorporated into one system of care for several years, but it requires continuing effort on the part of many people to insure that all facilities function as a system. Therefore, a lot of effort and energy was spent in keeping the EMR and the processes around it standardized between all facilities. For example, an electrocardiogram should be scanned and indexed the same way, no matter which facility performs the test, so that any physician within RH can find all electrocardiograms in the same area within the EMR. To maintain system standardization within the scanning application, the project team agreed to a process for any changes to the original build based on consensus. If any hospital wanted to make a change, it had to be presented to all the other team members, with the expectation that they would take the proposal to their key stakeholders for feedback. If any facility did not agree with the change, the team would discuss the issue further, sometimes looking for alternate solutions. If no consensus was reached, no change was made. To prevent any one facility from making changes without getting the group's approval, access to the scanning system setup dictionaries was limited to the IT Lead and the Project Manager.

The project team composition and project scope presented challenges as the HIM Directors had several, sometimes higher, responsibilities that they needed to prioritize. The lack of a totally dedicated project resources also made it challenging to keep all the facilities focused on the project. Because the project scope was identified as an HIM project, it was difficult to garner outside interest or participation beyond the HIM staff. To address the challenges associated with project team engagement, a Project Agreement was created in an attempt to prevent a decrease in participation by the network hospitals' HIM Directors. This agreement was designed to give each administrator an estimate of time needed from each HIM Director and define specific project milestones. The intent was that by asking each administrator to commit to the project, the HIM Directors would feel more comfortable spending time on the project. While this resulted in improved communications between the project team members and their respective administrators, it did not have the desired effect on the team members' availability.

Like any new technology, an ongoing issue for the scanning project was assisting physicians to adjust to viewing their patient's chart electronically. Despite having a few physicians involved during the testing phase, it was difficult for them to visualize the scope of the project until it actually affected their day-to-day workflow. Within a few weeks of go-live, the large influx of images into the EMR identified the need for a solution for what they considered "clutter," which slowed them down when viewing an entire chart in the EMR. The project team coordinated with the vendor on better ways to search or filter the EMR. The vendor custom-coded an enhanced filter, enabling the provider to better search for specific documents in the EMR. The Clinical Informatics department provided re-education to the physicians on EMR workflow using the enhanced filter. This training helped some physicians, while others still thought the scanned images should be presented in a more user-friendly way.

Several technical issues arose as the team tested the new scanning application and some continue to this day. Although most of these items were limitations in functionality for HIM staff, they had an effect on the end users of the scanned images. The first example involves the ability of the HIM staff to tag an image with a "best copy attainable" notation. In itself, this is a useful feature; however, the design seems flawed in that it is only viewable in the legal electronic chart (eChart) and the only users that can see it are the HIM staff. This results in physicians calling the HIM departments asking them to rescan a specific document because of the image quality. The vendor has been unable to mitigate this issue in our current version; however, a solution is available in a future release. The only remaining course of action was to train the HIM staff to view the form in the eChart when they received calls before committing to rescan documents or pulling the original document (if still available).

Another feature, that in itself is critical to HIM process, is the ability to redact information from a scanned image. The problem with this feature is that it only applied to the printing or a burned copy of a scanned image. There was no electronic way to redact information from being viewed on the screen. Depending on the circumstances surrounding the need for a redaction, the team developed an alternate process that, while causing extra work for HIM staff, ultimately solved the problem. A form that had information to be redacted was scanned twice: the first scan was the entire form with no redactions and the second scan had the information to be redacted covered. When these were indexed, the form with the redactions was indexed for viewing outside of the HIM department; the form without redactions was indexed to a special category within the eChart that was only viewable by

HIM staff. This process will be long-term as the vendor feels this functionality is working appropriately.

While not directly related to the scanning procedures, one feature that could not fully be taken advantage of related to sending an electronic message to a physician urging them to complete their chart documentation. During the testing phase, the team learned this feature was not programmed correctly resulting in no messages being created. The team worked extensively with the vendor to correct this in the test environment; however, the messaging capability did not complement a typical provider workflow for completing their chart documentation. Along with this challenge, using the messaging feature required a new provider desktop, which, at that time, was used by less than a third of the medical staff. Because of this, as well as the messaging capability being inadequate, HIM staff relied on their existing processes of paper notifications and follow-up telephone calls.

Another component of chart completion in the paper world involved the physician routinely visiting the HIM department to check for charts needing their signature. In the electronic world, the HIM staff wanted to provide the physicians with that same type of visual prompt but the current application was not designed with one in place. The project team requested the vendor develop a custom "pop-up" prompt to remind the physician about chart deficiencies, allowing them to be instantly taken to their e-sign queue. This custom prompt has helped HIM staff reduce the amount of reminder telephone calls as well as improving RH's already satisfactory compliance with CMS regulations for dating and signing all chart entries (Centers for Medicare & Medicaid Services, 2009).

Point-Of-Contact (POC) scanning allows admissions staff the ability to scan documents during the patient registration process without having to leave their workstation. This presented some challenges that weren't discovered during the testing phase. The main issue was that any document, such as a physician's order, could not be electronically tagged for an electronic signature. This delayed implementation in outpatient areas where POC functionality would streamline their daily workflow. The vendor was unable to resolve this in the current version; therefore, the solution involved creating new form identification indexes allowing POC documents to be tracked separately. If, for example, a physician order form needed to be tagged for an electronic signature and it was noted that it was a point-of-contact scan, the HIM staff would print this form, rescan it using the batch scanning method and index and tag it accordingly. Once that was done, the original scan would be deleted. Clearly, this is not an ideal workflow and fortunately, this particular problem is not frequent. A technical solution will be available in the vendor's next version of the application.

One of the productivity-enhancing features of the scanning software involved placement of barcodes on chart forms and printed patient labels. The barcodes represented the patient's account number and the form type. This functionality would dramatically reduce the amount of manual indexing to be performed when batch scanning charts. The vendor's specifications were limited, only giving minimum and maximum sizes for barcodes based on the font used. During the barcode testing phase, the results proved to be inconsistent. After extensive testing achieved a consistent result for the account number, it was discovered that this affected the nursing staff's use of the same account number barcode for bedside glucometer equipment. An additional week of testing brought resolution to this issue; however, in tandem, the inconsistent results when testing barcodes for form type continued to persist. Because this would greatly impact HIM staff productivity, testing continued until a successful result was produced, even though this meant a delay to the project timeline. The delay made it impractical to place form type barcodes on all 5,000 forms, so a decision was made to identify the top 50 high-use forms and barcode these prior to the go-live date. The remaining forms would be barcoded as part of Regional Health's (RH) required bi-annual review process and all new approved forms would have the appropriate form type barcode affixed. This solution prevented further timeline delays.

Additional challenges were identified with the current forms and how hospital staff used them to document the care of the patient. Several facilities still had forms printed on colored paper with some colors drastically affecting the readability of the scanned document. Though most facilities had tried to migrate to all white paper prior to the project starting, there were still departments that had not yet completely converted to white. In addition, the use of highlighters on paper forms sometimes obliterated the highlighted text once it was scanned. Lastly, some departments used colored ink pens, such as green and red that did not read well when the document was scanned. When the project team attempted to address some of these issues, it was discovered that departments would have to redesign their workflow in order to accommodate the requested changes.

To mitigate the problems with colored paper, colored ink, and colored highlighters, additional testing was performed to make sure adjusting scanner settings would not alleviate the poor quality images. When it did not, the actual images were presented to the owners and users of the colored paper, ink, and highlighters. The project manager, with the assistance of the system-wide forms committee, was easily able to eliminate all colored paper with one exception. A compromise was struck with the emergency department at RCRH to allow one color (very light yellow) to maintain efficient workflows. Colored ink and highlighters were not as simple to resolve. While everyone agreed that the image quality was poor, it was difficult developing alternatives. In the instance of highlighters, after numerous meetings, it was agreed that only non-fluorescent yellow highlighters would be used. Red ink pens that were medium point were allowed and all fine point pens were discouraged, regardless of color. These compromises took several months to accomplish and, while they have generally been followed, the HIM staff have learned how to adjust scanner settings to maximize readability when highlighters and colored ink pens are used.

Taking away the paper charts necessitated finding a solution for outside reviewers of medical records, such as Joint Commission or Department of Health surveyors. In the paper world, the HIM departments would receive a list of charts from the requestor, validate the request, and pull the charts so they were ready for their review. In the electronic world, this workflow had to be redesigned to adapt to the new technology. Testing the redesigned process identified several programming errors. The team worked with the vendor to resolve these problems, which took several months to fix. Prior to those fixes, the HIM departments were still able to accommodate outside review requests through extra oversight from the IT department. This feature within the scanning software exceeded RH's expectations. Functionality within the software enables the ability to limit access to accounts and restrict printing or audit what has been printed, and enforce the amount of time the chart stays on the reviewer's worklist.

In a paper environment, when there is legal action involved with a patient, the standard HIM practice involves physically locking up the chart in a special area that requires HIM director approval for access. This process helps preserve the legal integrity as well as maintain the best possible privacy and security of the paper record (Brodnik, McCain, Rinehart-Thompson, & Reynolds, 2009). The scanning application had functionality to mimic the paper process, allowing an HIM director to electronically lock up a medical record, called "sealing a record." The first step in sealing a record involves identifying whether to seal a specific visit, multiple visits, or the entire record (all visits) for a patient. The final step requires listing the users who are allowed to access the sealed portions of the electronic chart. The users granted access to a sealed chart would typically be the HIM management team, the risk manager, and the staff attorney. The process of sealing a record was tested and appeared to work well. The project manager worked with key RH officials to determine how best to use this functionality, develop the new workflows, and draft appropriate usage policies. Because sealing a record is not a frequent occurrence, it is difficult to train every user of the EMR for a situation they might rarely encounter. Currently, the message that displays to an end user simply states that the patient has no accessible visits. This can be confusing to the physician trying to treat the patient who knows the patient has past medical charts. A request has been submitted to the vendor for a more descriptive message; however, the short-term solution was educating the HIM staff on how sealing a record appears to end users so they can take appropriate action.

CONCLUSION

Part of the success of the scanning and archiving project is due to the substantial amount of collaboration and communication between the various stakeholders involved, including the vendor, to maximize functionality and make the product more user-friendly for the physicians. The team also worked closely with many end user groups, including physicians, nurses, HIM staff, and admissions staff, to review existing workflows and incorporate this new technology in their daily routines. There were many efficiencies gained by involving departments that were not originally anticipated by the project team. Some areas have reported timesavings by having the complete chart available in the computer. Other areas have been able to eliminate steps in their daily processes, such as faxing reports and delivering paper copies of chart documents. The Patient Access (Admissions) Department and the Patient Financial Services Department have been able to streamline their processes through the ability to scan and view insurance cards.

While implementing new technology can be a painful process, Regional Health's scanning project successfully achieved its goal of developing a hybrid electronic medical record that would be used by all five hospitals in a standardized fashion. Having a system-wide electronic medical record enables information sharing that contributes to better patient care throughout the Regional Health continuum of care. The careful planning for education and extra support of all the end users has, over time, helped Regional Health embrace this new technology. This project brings Regional Health one step closer to a fully electronic medical record, promoting the new normal of using an electronic medical record in a "meaningful use" environment.

REFERENCES

AHIMA. (2005). Update: Maintaining a legally sound health record – Paper and electronic. *Journal of American Health Information Management Association, 76*(10), 64A–L.

AHIMA. (2010a). *Managing the transition from paper to EHRs*. Retrieved October 31, 2011, from http://library.ahima.org/xpedio/groups/public/documents/ahima/bok1_048418.hcsp?dDocName=bok1_048418

AHIMA. (2010b). *Information security—An overview*. Retrieved October 31, 2011, from http://library.ahima.org/xpedio/groups/public/documents/ahima/bok1_048962.hcsp?dDocName=bok1_048962

Brodnik, M., McCain, M., Rinehart-Thompson, L., & Reynolds, R. (Eds.). (2009). *Fundamentals of law for health informatics and information management.* Chicago, IL: American Health Information Management Association.

Centers for Medicare & Medicaid Services. (2009). *Revised appendix A: Interpretive guidelines for hospital.* Pub. 100-07 State Operations Provider Certification, Transmittal 47. Washington, DC: Centers for Medicare & Medicaid Services. Retrieved November 26, 2011, from https://www.cms.gov/transmittals/downloads/R47SOMA.pdf

U.S. Department of Health & Human Services. (2011). *Summary of the HIPAA privacy rule.* Retrieved October 22, 2011, from http://www.hhs.gov/ocr/privacy/hipaa/understanding/summary/index.html

Wild, J. J. (2008). *Scanning and archiving assessment/implementation strategy for regional health.* Unpublished manuscript.

ADDITIONAL READING

AHIMA EHR Practice Council. (2007). Developing a legal health record policy. *Journal of American Health Information Management Association, 78*(9), 93–97.

Amatayakul, M. (2009). *Electronic health records: A practice guide for professionals and organizations* (4th ed.). Chicago, IL: American Health Information Management Association.

Burrington-Brown, J. (2008). In search of document imaging best practices. *Journal of American Health Information Management Association, 79*(9), 60–61.

Clark, J. (2009). Using document imaging to strengthen revenue cycle. *Journal of American Health Information Management Association, 80*(4), 54–55.

Dinh, A. (2009). Dealing with paper post–document imaging. *Journal of American Health Information Management Association, 80*(5), 54–55.

HIMSS. (2012) *EHR adoption resources.* Retrieved from http://www.himss.org/ASP/topics_FocusDynamic.asp?faid=198

Strong, K. (2008). Enterprise content and records management. *Journal of American Health Information Management Association, 80*(2), 38–42.

KEY TERMS AND DEFINITIONS

Archiving: To copy data from a live disk to a long-term storage medium. In this project, the long-term storage is the legal electronic chart.

Centers for Medicare and Medicaid Services (CMS): Part of the U.S. Department of Health & Human Services that is responsible for various federally-funded insurance programs.

Electronic Medical Record (EMR): The electronic version of a patient record that is used by physicians and other health care staff caring for a patient.

Health Care Information System (HCIS): A comprehensive suite of integrated applications, usually from a single vendor, providing both clinical and administrative functionality for a healthcare organization.

Health Insurance Portability and Accountability Act (HIPAA): A federal regulation that provides privacy and security requirements for patient information as well as health care information systems.

Joint Commission: An accrediting agency for health care organizations.

Legal Electronic Chart: A healthcare organization's legal record of business and contains both the archived data and scanned images, typically maintained by the health information management department.

Redaction: Restricting specific information within the medical record to meet legal requirements or to protect a patient's privacy in specific disclosure situations.

Scanning: The process of taking paper documents and creating digital images for storage within the electronic medical record.

Structured Data: Data that resides in fixed fields within a record using standard data attributes. This makes data analysis possible. Examples include ICD-9 codes, lab results, and vital signs data.

TWAIN Scanning Interface: A common image capture interface for operating systems, typically used as an interface between image processing software and a scan device or digital camera so that the system can understand the scan.

Unstructured Data: Data that does not reside in fixed fields. The most common example of unstructured data is free-form text.

Chapter 4
Big Information Technology Bet of a Small Community Hospital

Sergey P. Motorny
Dakota State University, USA

EXECUTIVE SUMMARY

Broadlawns Medical Center (BMC) is a teaching acute care community hospital of 200 beds located in Des Moines, Iowa. As other safety net providers across the nation, the hospital operates in a difficult environment with a growing number of uninsured patients and simultaneously dwindling tax support. By 2005, George Washington University and several Joint Commission reports had publicly highlighted the hospital's challenges of financial sustainability and the provided quality of care. The hospital's senior management team decided to adopt an Electronic Health Record (EHR) system in an attempt to gain access to real-time performance data. The EHR adoption project posed many organizational, managerial, and technological challenges but also provided numerous eventual benefits. BMC had not only successfully resolved the stated problems of healthcare quality, financial stability, and patient satisfaction scores, but also became one of the national leaders in healthcare information technology.

DOI: 10.4018/978-1-4666-2671-3.ch004

BACKGROUND

The case study takes place at Broadlawns Medical Center, which is a teaching acute care community hospital in the state of Iowa. The hospital combines multiple clinics, which offer a wide spectrum of traditional and specialty services in such areas as emergency, primary care, pediatric, internal medicine, surgical, foot and ankle, and mental health. BMC was recently recognized as one of the nation's "Most Wired – Small and Rural Hospitals" by Hospitals & Health Networks magazine (Weinstock & Hoppszallern, 2011). The hospital's mission statement is based on the premise of providing high quality healthcare regardless of the patients' ability to pay.

Broadlawns Medical Center values such strategic business priorities as continuous improvement of healthcare quality, commitment to patient satisfaction, development of motivated professionals, and advancing of nursing, dental, and medical student education (Broadlawns, 2011). The hospital has been providing health care to the residents of Polk County for over 85 years with the increasing emphasis on high quality and high value services (Stier, 2011). BMC continues to serve nearly 40,000 people with almost $70 million in uncompensated care on a yearly basis (Stier, 2011). Taxes, which partly support Broadlawns Medical Center, have stayed unchanged since year 2000, but the hospital has experienced a notable 15 percent increase in the number of uninsured patients in 2010 alone (Stier, 2011).

INTRODUCTION

The Joint Commission (TJC) is a not-for-profit health care quality accreditation organization based out of the United States. Many state governments recognize TJC accreditation as a prerequisite to Medicaid reimbursement. Healthcare providers participating in the TJC accreditation program are subjects to triennial accreditation cycles. TJC accreditation hinges on surveys, which are conducted impromptu 18 to 39 months apart. Hospital accreditation decisions and potential Requirements for Improvement (RFIs) are made public with the date accreditation is awarded. TJC updates the standards it uses on a yearly basis and posts them on its website. Broadlawns Medical Center surveys of 1998, 2001, and 2004 did not result in TJC delivering full three-year accreditations due to quality problems. Instead, The Joint Commission issued RFIs with tentative follow-up focus surveys meant to correct the revealed quality deficiencies.

In June 2005, George Washington University released a comprehensive study, which raised doubts about "the continued viability of Broadlawns Medical Center (Jenner, 2011)." The study highlighted such problems as the increasing numbers of uninsured patients, insufficiency of funding sources, and absence of a clear sustainable model for delivering safety net services to the uninsured patients of Polk County, Iowa (Nolan, et al., 2005). University researchers interviewed more than thirty area informants and drew secondary data from a variety of official sources. The study stated that Des Moines healthcare safety net offered few specialty services, which were highly fragmented and poorly coordinated when matched with the national statistics. The study mentioned several failed attempts to create an electronic collaboration system, which would assist the uninsured patients in navigating the highly fragmented and increasingly complex healthcare environment. Broadlawns Medical Center learned from the report that it was considered the county's core safety net healthcare provider. The hospital also gathered that even though the community wanted BMC to survive, taxpayers and officials were reluctant to guarantee the hospital's future financial stability. Broadlawns needed to act quickly by raising the focus on healthcare quality, reducing fragmentation of the specialty services, strengthening partnerships with other healthcare providers, promoting the positive image of the hospital, and increasing public support.

Until recently, the hospital's information systems solution was Siemens software suite originally implemented in 1984. By 2004, the software lacked many of the needed updates and was a significant impediment to the future operations of the medical center. The same year, BMC senior management decided that a technological transformation was necessary.

The Healthcare Information and Management Systems Society (HIMSS) is a United States (US) organization striving to improve such areas of healthcare as quality, safety, cost-effectiveness, and access via utilization of information technology and management systems (wikipedia.org, 2009). HIMSS Analytics is a HIMSS division responsible for collecting and distributing analytical data of healthcare. HIMSS Analytics admits that hospital Electronic Medical Record (EMR) systems are of variable capabilities, which in turn poses significant challenges to their comparison. HIMSS Analytics has formulated an EMR Adoption Model with seven distinct stages intended to simplify peer comparisons of hospital organizations and assist in the EMR adoption strategies (himssanalytics.org, 2011).

Some of the HIMSS Analytics Stage 6 requirements include having physician templates (documentation and charting) for at least one patient care service area, basic decision support in the form of compliance and variance alerts, and the displacement of film-based imaging by an integrated Picture Archiving and Communication System (PACS). According to the most recent survey (himssanalytics.org, 2011), fewer than five percent of all US hospitals have achieved HIMSS Analytics Stage 6 of cumulative EMR capabilities.

By 2010, Broadlawns Medical Center was already one of the few hospitals across the nation to become Stage 6 certified (Stier, 2010). BMC senior management adopted an EHR system and led the hospital through an extraordinary transformation, which improved healthcare quality, financial sustainability, and patient satisfaction scores. Project leaders encountered many organizational, managerial, and technological challenges along the way. The leaders had to find resolutions for such obstacles as stringent budget constraints, general end-user resistance, inadequacy of physician templates, and simultaneous evolution of government requirements. BMC senior management developed a comprehensive EHR adoption plan, which collected the necessary funding, evaluated software alternatives, involved and educated hospital associates, established new partnerships, and utilized the system's real time data to better prepare the medical center for its role as a core safety net provider. Table 1 contains a comprehensive list of important dates mentioned throughout this case study.

MAIN FOCUS OF THE CHAPTER

Assembly of Business Criteria

BMC senior management decided to consider the adoption of an electronic health record system as a way of mitigating and resolving some of the existing problems. The hospital solicited departmental input to create a comprehensive business criteria document, which the future EHR system was to address. The document was called Physician Practice Management and HIS System Selection Business Criteria, and it was distributed to all of the potential vendors together with the Request for Proposal (RFP) worksheets.

The Business Criteria document contained five types of various corporate objectives deemed vital to the hospital's future operations. There were three clinical objectives, one decision support system objective, four financial objectives, three patient management objectives, and one physician practice objective. Each of the defined objectives was further divided into three subcomponents: metric, method, and output. For example, a metric of a clinical objective may have been "decrease medication errors," a corresponding method could have stated, "using bar code technology to match patient, drug, and employee," and, finally, the outcome of such objective could have said, "increase of medication knowledge for Registered Nurses (RNs)."

Broadlawns Medical Center has spent a lot of time and effort laboriously assembling a broad, albeit, very specific lists of business objectives, their metrics, methods, and the subsequently desired outputs. It was not uncommon to see an objective containing ten various metrics, over thirty methods, and over twenty anticipated outcomes. BMC has put a significant energy into developing business criteria meant to assist the hospital's turnaround from the quality of care and financial standpoints.

Table 1. Listing of important dates

1984	Siemens software is installed
1998	First partial TJC accreditation
2000	Taxes revenue freeze
2001	Second partial TJC accreditation
Jun-03	Six Days Cash on Hand available
Jun-04	Nine Days Cash on Hand available
15-Dec-04	BMC issues RFPs to eight potential EHR vendors
29-Dec-04	BMC holds Optional Bidders' Conference
2004	Third partial TJC accreditation
21-Jan-05	RFP response cut-off time
Feb 1, 2005 - Feb 18, 2005	BMC schedules on-site evaluations
Feb 28, 2005 - Mar 18, 2005	BMC visits vendor sites
25-Mar-05	MEDITECH selection announcement
Jun-05	George Washington University study released
31-Jul-05	Expiration of vendor price quotes
Sep-05	MEDITECH implementation begins
Jan-06	Empower Ed installation
Feb-06	MEDITECH financial modules go-live: General Ledger, Fixed Assets, Accounts Payable
Nov-06	MEDITECH administrative modules go-live: Admissions, Discharges, Transfers, Billing
Nov-06	MEDITECH rudimentary electronic medical record (EMR) go-live
2006	MEDITECH pharmacy replaces Cerner
2007	MEDITECH in-patient nursing go-live
2007	MEDITECH radiology replaces Cerner
2007	First full three-year TJC accreditation
Dec-08	MEDITECH first ambulatory clinic (Family Health Center) go-live
Dec-08	HIMSS Analytics Stage 6 certification eligibility mentioned
2008	MEDITECH laboratory replaces Cerner
17-Feb-09	HITECH Act signed into law
30-Dec-09	Meaningful use Interim Final Rule released by CMS
2009	Press Ganey officially records an increase in patient satisfaction scores
13-Jul-10	Meaningful use Final Rule released by CMS
Oct-10	State launches IowaCare Medical Home project
Dec-10	MEDITECH meaningful use certification announced
2010	HIMSS Analytics Stage 6 certification achieved
2010	Second full three-year TJC accreditation

continued on following page

Table 1. Continued

2010	15% jump in uninsured patients
2010	BMC posts $4 million in profits on $100 million in revenue
Feb-11	HIMSS Analytics Stage 6 certification is officially awarded
Mar-11	BMC achieves meaningful use Stage 1 certification
Jun-11	One hundred and seven Days Cash on Hand
2011	MEDITECH replaces Empower ED
2011	BMC Primary Care Group clinic is first to implement electronic prescribing
2011	BMC Patient Identity Security System (35 palm scanners) implemented
2011	BMC recognized as "Most Wired - Small and Rural Hospitals"
2012 (pending)	Last ambulatory clinic expected to join EHR
2013 - 2014 (pending)	Complete electronic prescribing, advanced health maintenance module, patient health records, meaningful use Stage 2, HIMSS Analytics Stage 7 certification
2016	CMS begins reimbursement reductions for providers without meaningful use

Assembly of RFP Requirements

During the RFP composition time, Broadlawns Medical Center pharmacy, radiology, and laboratory applications were already provided and serviced by Cerner Corporation. The RFP stated that Broadlawns would still seek information on pharmacy, radiology, and laboratory modules but only for the purpose of considering their future replacement possibilities. Pricing for the three modules was to stay separated from the remainder of the quote. Similarly, Broadlawns Medical Center had already committed to an electronic management system for the hospital's Emergency Department (ED). The RFP document still sought information on the alternative ED application but without an intention of the immediate software purchase.

Original RFP issue date was December 15, 2004, and the official cut-off time to deliver the RFP response was stated to be noon on Friday, January 21, 2005. On December 29, 2004, BMC held an optional Bidders' Conference where software vendors were given an opportunity to gain clear understandings of the hospital's goals and objectives, ask RFP-related questions, meet BMC senior management, and tour the facilities.

Broadlawns leaders decided to use help in mapping the identified business criteria to the corresponding technical specifications and matching those with the available EHR vendors. Senior management invited Beacon Partners to assist in translating the provider's business criteria into technical requirements as well as compiling the initial list of potential EHR vendors. Beacon Partners is a United States consulting firm specializing in healthcare management. Beacon proposed using KLAS Data to gain useful insights of experiences from other comparable hospitals. KLAS is a company, which conducts healthcare provider interviews on over 250 healthcare technology vendors and 900 existing products (klasresearch.com, 1996). KLAS reports to be interviewing over 1,900 healthcare providers on a monthly basis (klas-research.com, 1996). The company's mission statement is to continuously update an impartial database to help measure vendor performance and product quality. A combined effort of Beacon Partners, Broadlawns, and KLAS Data had helped select eight potential vendors for the initial RFP distribution.

Senior management had hired another external consultant to help commence the EHR system selection process. Superior Consulting was the firm, which distributed the RFPs, responded to the letters of intent, and coordinated vendor presentations. Superior Consulting agreed that careful consideration of all of the hospital's business and vendor requirement criteria should have yielded a comparatively short list of the initial vendor alternatives. The consultant had sent an official Letter of Intent to respond to the eight selected EHR vendors, which stated that all contact during the vendor selection process had to be made through Superior Consulting. Vendors failing to abide by this request were going to be automatically disqualified from further consideration.

The distributed RFP document stipulated that all vendor responses and the included price quotes had to stay valid for a period of six months until July 31, 2005. The response of the selected vendor was going to automatically become part of the final contract. The RFP document contained four major sections, which were business and clinical requirements, technical requirements, pricing information, and vendor and product history. BMC was especially concerned with the total cost of ownership of the potential EHR system including such items as required hardware, installation costs, and future costs of vendor support contracts. The RFP stated that Broadlawns Medical Center reserved the right to request a complete previous client list from any of the participating vendors. The document also said that Broadlawns Medical Center might have asked for either all or any of the following documents: vendor's previous five year financial history, copy of a standard contract, vendor's future strategic and software development plans, and class syllabuses with dates and available training locations. Finally, the hospital might have requested software documentation samples, previous implementation templates, and official course materials for user and system administration classes.

Potential EHR vendors were expected to submit cost and technical evaluation worksheets. Technical evaluation contained twelve pages of open-ended questions divided into several sections: data extraction and report production, client/server processing, interfaces, graphical user interface, use of technology, implementation planning, technical training, end-user training, and technical documentation. The total number of technical evaluation questions was sixty-three. Many of the questions were directly related to the hospital's desire to obtain real-time reporting capabilities for all of its departments and clinics. The worksheets also had many questions particularly technical in nature and meant to be evaluated by someone with prior knowledge of healthcare information technology.

Cost evaluation worksheets contained six pages of preformatted tables meant to draw cost and financial conclusions about the vendor, software suite, and pricing models. Potential vendors had to summarize hardware and software costs and explicate product and company information. Hardware, software, and summary cost tables contained the columns visibly separating EHR purchase fees, software installation fees, and ongoing maintenance fees. Product and vendor information tables were meant to evaluate the firm's past experience as well as its future prospects. Broadlawns Medical Center wanted to learn about the number of healthcare providers already utilizing the software, the original year of the application development, and the date of the most recent version update. BMC had also inquired about the vendor's total number of full-time employees, yearly budget allocated to research and development plans, and geographical location of the main technical support center.

Broadlawns and Superior Consulting had proposed an aggressive timetable, so that vendor selection and contract negotiation stages could be completed expeditiously. On-site evaluations lasted from February 1, 2005 to February 18, 2005. The on-site evaluation process was structured as a conference, where vendors presented their cases and demonstrated abilities to address the hospital's business criteria requirements. Broadlawns associates had received open invitations to participate whether they were able to join for the entire day or just a few minutes. Based on the on-site evaluations, four potential EHR vendors were identified: Cerner, CPSI, Keane, and Medical Information Technology (MEDITECH). Epic software also had a high selection opportunity, but the vendor's own site qualification requirements were a challenge to meet for a hospital the size of Broadlawns. The date of the final vendor selection announcement was March 25, 2005 (see Table 1).

Vendor Selection

BMC was interested in assessing the EHR system of Cerner Corporation because of the existing investment in the vendor's pharmacy, radiology, and laboratory applications. However, a closer evaluation revealed several limiting factors. First, the already installed software was considered a legacy system reaching its end of life cycle. All three applications would have had to be reinstalled and reconfigured if the medical center was to proceed with the vendor. Second, Cerner EHR suite lacked some of the desired functionalities such as human resources and materials management modules. Finally, the hospital found the cost of Cerner EHR to be prohibitive given the project's allocated budget.

CPSI was another system to fail a closer assessment. Adoption stakeholders visited a comparable Iowa hospital with CPSI in place and found that it did not satisfy their template flexibility requirements.

Keane software suite seemed to fulfill both business criteria and pricing requirements. However, the stakeholders noted that Keane's market share penetration did not adequately address the predetermined vendor selection criterion. In the end, Broadlawns management decided to designate MEDITECH as the future EHR vendor. Table 2 summarizes vendor selection process for the four potential EHR vendors.

MEDITECH is a Massachusetts-based privately held company founded in 1969 by its current Chairman A. Neil Pappalardo (wikipedia.org, 2011). Broadlawns Request for Proposal document identified two tiers of potential vendor evaluation criteria (Staurovsky, 2004). Some of the vendor-specific line items of the documented tiers included the alignment of the vendor's mission and business objectives with those of Broadlawns, the firm's proven financial viability, and longevity track record of the considered software.

MEDITECH mission statement emphasizes effective patient management by providing an integrated software suite to optimize the financial and business potential of health care providers (meditech.com, 2012). The company has established relationships with over 2,300 customers operating in United States, Canada,

Table 2. BMC vendor selection process

Criteria/ Vendor	Business and Clinical Requirements	Technical Requirements	Pricing Requirements	Vendor and Product History Requirements
Cerner	Failed selection: absent human resources and materials management modules.	Failed selection: legacy software end of life cycle.	Failed selection: over the allocated budget limit.	Passed selection.
CPSI	Passed selection.	Failed selection: lack of desired template flexibility.	Passed selection.	Passed selection.
Keane	Passed selection.	Passed selection.	Passed selection.	Failed selection: existing market penetration criterion.
MEDITECH	Passed selection.	Passed selection.	Passed selection.	Passed selection.

Note. EPIC presented BMC with own site qualification requirements, which were considered difficult to meet.

United Kingdom, Ireland, South Africa, Latin America, and Spain. According to the corporate website, MEDITECH has been developing and supporting health care software solutions around the world for over forty-one years (meditech.com, 2012). MEDITECH software revenues were $459 million in 2010.

Broadlawns stressed the importance of the proposed EHR system to contain both Physician Practice Management (PPM) and Hospital Information System (HIS) components. The PPM requirement, albeit non-traditional for a public hospital, was meant to represent the specialty clinics, which were stated to be the future business driver for the medical center. BMC unequivocally stated that it would not sacrifice the PPM functionality. Also, one of the hospital's early strategic objectives was to acquire both HIS and PPM components from a single software vendor to ensure long-term interoperability.

MEDITECH software suite contains both HIS and PPM functionalities. Moreover, MEDITECH's own organizational structure consists of two distinct entities, which are the corporate headquarters developing and supporting the Hospital Information System portion and the acquired subsidiary, LSS Data Systems, which builds and services the Physician Practice Management solution. Originally, LSS was a separate Minnesota-based medical software and service company founded in 1982 (wikipedia.org, 2011). In 2001, MEDITECH and LSS joined forces to offer health care providers a complete suite of Hospital Information System, Physician Practice Management, and integrated financial software.

Broadlawns vendor site visits were scheduled to take place during the time window of February 28 through March 18, 2005. While considering MEDITECH, a large group of Broadlawns representatives visited Citizens Memorial Hospital in Bolivar, MO, which was willing to demonstrate its EHR utilization and overall system capabilities. Broadlawns team regarded Citizens Memorial Hospital as one of the health information technology leaders, and no further client site visits were deemed necessary to demonstrate the successful practical utilization of MEDITECH.

Vendor Implementation

The EHR selection and vendor site visit stages were meant to consider each of the following software modules: inpatient, outpatient, and billing support, clinic and physician practice management support, patient accounting and accounts receivable, scheduling, ADT (Admission, Discharge, and Transfer), medical records, order processing, general ledger, accounts payable, payroll, materials management, decision support, clinical documentation, and, finally, pharmacy, radiology, and laboratory. Presently, Broadlawns Medical Center owns all of the available MEDITECH modules including the ones for pharmacy, radiology, and laboratory, which were previously managed by Cerner software and the one for the emergency department, which was preceded by the Empower ED application.

BMC had established several core implementation teams for the EHR adoption project: Selection Oversight team, Clinical Management team, Financial Management team, and Patient Management team. Other project stakeholders were involved at different times, but the composition of the core teams stayed constant and intact throughout the duration of the project. Selection Oversight team was the most multidisciplinary group consisting of twelve members from various hospital departments. Clinical Management team had the highest number of three assigned physicians and totaled eleven members. Patient Management team was the largest core group with fifteen assigned associates. Finally, a Financial Management team was comprised of thirteen hospital employees with the vast majority of players possessing some kind of financial background. BMC deemed important the assignment of Information Technology (IT) associates as well as hospital physicians to every core team.

MEDITECH actively participated in the initial stages of the EHR adoption project management. The vendor introduced a Project Tracking System (PTS), assisted in creating Gantt charts of timelines and dependencies, gave recommendations on the minimum number of core team members, and proposed the members' involvement and necessary training. Figure 1 and Table 3 provide samples of the MEDITECH modules implementation Gantt chart and their corresponding dependencies.

It was decided that communication among the core team participants was important, and, thus, internal weekly meetings were scheduled early in the implementation stage. Typical MEDITECH involvement in the core team meetings was on a monthly basis unless either a go-live date approached or was specified otherwise

Figure 1. Sample of the MEDITECH modules implementation Gantt chart

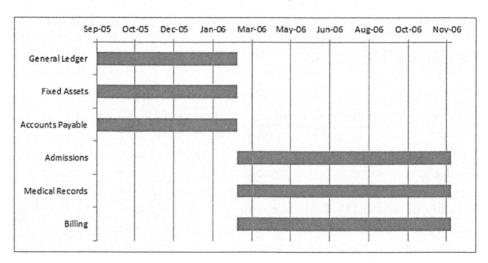

Table 3. Sample of the MEDITECH modules Gantt chart dependencies

Module Name	Start Date	End Date	Event	Priority	Status	Responsibility
General Ledger	9/1/2005	9/1/2005	First Conference Call	Important	Completed	Vendor & BMC
Fixed Assets	9/1/2005	9/1/2005	First Conference Call	Important	Completed	Vendor & BMC
Accounts Payable	9/1/2005	9/1/2005	First Conference Call	Important	Completed	Vendor & BMC
General Ledger	10/3/2005	10/7/2005	Finalize Selection Choices	Important	Pending	BMC
Fixed Assets	10/3/2005	10/3/2005	Software Delivery	Important	Pending	Vendor
Accounts Payable	10/3/2005	10/7/2005	Begin Selection Input	Critical	Pending	BMC

by the hospital's management. The meetings would discuss approaching deadlines, present obstacles, go-live date preparations, and overall project progress.

MEDITECH financial modules were the first to be brought online at the beginning of 2006. Fixed assets, general ledger, and accounts payable were considered vital given the hospital's desire for financial stability. Many of the following EHR implementation phases required approximately nine months of planning and preparation prior to the official go-live dates.

In November 2006, MEDITECH administrative applications became functional, which were the modules responsible for admissions, discharges, transfers, and billing services. Rudimentary Electronic Medical Record (EMR) system was also brought online at that time but in a form of a mere data repository. Initially, Broadlawns physicians still relied on handwriting their orders and submitting them to the designated entry system specialists. Physician documentation and ordering functions were part of a separate installation phase.

MEDITECH in-patient nursing module was activated in 2007. Then, in December 2008, Family Health Center was the first ambulatory clinic to begin using the software. Also in 2008, the medical center's potential eligibility for the HIMSS Analytics Stage 6 certification was first mentioned. Legacy Cerner applications were migrated in three separate phases. Pharmacy software made the switch in 2006, while radiology and laboratory systems were replaced in 2007 and 2008 respectively. In February 2011, BMC was officially awarded the HIMSS Stage 6 certification, and March 2011 signified the achievement of meaningful use Stage 1. Also in 2011, MEDITECH finally replaced Empower ED, and the hospital's emergency department became electronically integrated.

Adoption Challenges and Resolutions

Broadlawns stakeholders admitted that one of the biggest project challenges was the absence of adequate physician templates. Template development was a tedious process, which often took as many as six weeks per specialty physician. Even though the process of template creation was somewhat less complicated during the more recent adoption of MEDITECH Emergency Department Management system, many challenges still remained. Generic templates provided by the vendor had to be modified based on the unique workflow requirements of specialty physicians. It was important to foster the collaboration of the eventual EHR users and hospital IT personnel in order to define template specifications in a timely manner.

General end-user resistance posed another significant obstacle to the EHR adoption project. Early in the process, end users challenged the management's decision to go with the hospital-wide EHR system. After the system's implementation, vendor choice and software usefulness were often questioned. Broadlawns key stakeholders viewed end-user resistance as a normal reaction to change. However, they knew that the resistance should not be simply ignored but rather addressed in an orderly, strategic fashion. Senior managers had sent clear messages attesting their unanimous support for the project. As a result, many hospital associates understood that the implementation of an EHR system was not optional. Core team members were selected to represent the vast majority of the future end-user groups. Broadlawns associates were encouraged to participate in the product selection process, and the potential EHR vendors were invited to publicly address the hospital's RFP and business criteria requirements. End-users were intimately involved in the template creation processes, which consequently fostered the feelings of system co-ownership. Training and educational opportunities abounded and were provided on an ongoing basis. Project stakeholders suggested organizing early training opportunities for the physician support staff in order to maximize the availability of technical assistance after each go-live date. EHR adoption stakeholders developed a plan to identify and educate end-user champions who would then assist in promoting the system's usefulness and utility throughout the organization.

Broadlawns IT support staff was often reminded that the first three weeks of the most recent go-live date would routinely prove to be the most difficult. System novelty, ongoing template modifications, and temporary loss of productivity would often be mixed with feelings of end-user frustration. The stakeholders recommend following a phased EHR adoption approach in order to stay cognizant of the reported issues and capable of addressing the problems quickly. The decision to connect all medical center departments with the software of the same vendor created a desirable organizational unity in the system's educational and promotional efforts.

The next EHR adoption challenge lay within the hospital's lack of information technology experience and the obvious shortage of resources to undertake a massive systems implementation project affecting every department. BMC IT associates had always been a small and efficient group. In 2004, there were only nine IT staff members for the entire hospital, and there were only thirteen IT associates employed by the medical center in 2011. Strong support of the senior management ensured that the medical center's shortage of information technology staff and the existing knowledge gaps could be effectively closed by the experience of external consultants. BMC recruited outside help whenever it was needed. Broadlawns Medical Center had either formed contractual relationships or accessed knowledge of such consultants as Beacon Partners, KLAS, Superior Consulting, and Morgan Hunter. Beacon Partners had helped gather the list of the initial vendors for consideration, and KLAS data were referred for that purpose. Superior Consulting assisted in writing the RFPs, sending official invitations, and leading the first round of vendor selection process. Morgan Hunter was hired to oversee the project and provide valuable input based on its past systems implementation experiences. Finally, BMC ensured that technical resources of MEDITECH, LSS Data Systems, and Vital Support Systems were always available to participate in problem resolutions, core team meetings, and preparations for the official go-live dates.

According to the latest Report to The Community, Centers for Medicare and Medicaid Services (CMS) are the biggest insurance reimbursement payers of BMC (Jenner, 2011). The Health Information Technology of Economic and Clinical Health (HITECH) Act defined the meaningful use concept, which manifested itself through the CMS incentive programs. The definition of meaningful use encouraged healthcare providers to prove their utilizations of the certified EHR systems in ways, which increased quality, efficiency, and patient safety (cms.gov, 2010). CMS outlined three stages of meaningful use. For Stage 1, the centers proposed over 24 objectives for eligible hospitals. The objectives were then divided into the mandatory core and optional menu sets. For Stage 2, some of the optional objectives became mandatory, and other criteria were added in the areas of disease and medication management, decision support, and patient access integration. Stage 3 expanded the baseline even further with a focus on the high-priority national conditions and treatment outcomes. In order to receive the maximum incentive payment, program participation must begin by 2012 (cms.gov, 2011). Moreover, CMS will start penalizing providers failing to adopt an EHR suite by 2015 with the tiered reimbursement adjustment of up to 3 percent.

Even though the arrival of meaningful use requirements allowed BMC to accelerate the Return On Investment (ROI), achieving Stage 1 presented a challenge. Meaningful use requirements did not exist when MEDITECH was initially installed and configured. HITECH Act was signed into law on February 17, 2009 (hhs.gov,

2009). Vendors and healthcare providers witnessed a major revision of the meaningful use requirements before the final rule took effect on July 13, 2010 (hhs.gov, 2010). EHR firms, including MEDITECH, had to certify their products with CMS. Certification process was laborious and time-consuming. Broadlawns Medical Center first heard about the official certification of its vendor in December 2010. Following the certification, MEDITECH had to release the updates, assist installing the software, and help reconfiguring the templates to satisfy the final rule requirements of meaningful use. For Broadlawns, it was important to stay in close contact with the vendor, patiently wait for the completion of its certification process, and then actively engage during the times of software patching and template reconfigurations.

Financial Analysis

Prior to the adoption project, Broadlawns experienced significant financial difficulties. Days Cash on Hand is an accounting metric indicating the amount of cash, which a business possesses to cover outstanding obligations. Finance Committee Memos reveal that back in 2003 and 2004 Broadlawns Medical Center had as few as six Days Cash on Hand.

BMC senior management had to make a series of necessary financial decisions prior to commencing with the selection of an EHR system. The system required a large up-front capital investment, and the hospital needed to seek a special tax levy in the amount of $3.4 million. Meanwhile, there was a noticeable increase in the numbers of self-pay and underinsured patients resulting in a further reduction of finances available for investing in the expensive information technology.

Broadlawns Medical Center leadership developed a business plan in an attempt to estimate the future return on investment and highlight other potential benefits of adopting an electronic health record system. The hospital projected significant future savings from embracing a single information technology vendor and scrapping the expensive and outdated Siemens technology. At the time, Siemens software was hosted by an external provider located in Pennsylvania. Therefore, the hospital had to pay for maintaining costly Wide Area Network (WAN) connections and third-party data center fees. BMC had calculated that it could potentially save over $50,000 per month by eliminating Siemens software and maintaining its own data center.

Centers for Medicare and Medicaid Services require that providers submit CMS-1500 forms for reimbursement purposes. Broadlawns Medical Center typically submitted 180,000 bills per year. The hospital used to outsource the CMS-1500 service bearing the cost of $1.25 per every processed bill. Replacing the outsourced CMS-1500 billing service with MEDITECH was going to result in $125,000 of recurring savings for Broadlawns.

BMC sought and received a special $3.4 million tax levy and significantly increased the budget of the IT department. Broadlawns Medical Center Foundation, which is the entity devoted to supporting the image and financial viability of the hospital, performed additional fundraising, which was fully devoted to the EHR adoption project. BMC also asked its working associates to contribute to the upcoming project through the internal campaign of combined giving.

The highest EHR system bills were the original software and hardware quotes of $3,283,000 and $1,026,583 respectively. Thus, the total amount of the initial software and hardware investment was $4,309,583 dated September 2005. New provider LSS Data System support costs were $794,182. After the initial software and hardware investment, Broadlawns Medical Center had to continue its operations with the legacy technology still in place. Thus, the hospital incurred ongoing Siemens and Cerner System Software Support costs in the amount of $204,512 ($81,012 for Siemens and $123,500 for Cerner). Previous hospital leadership adopted Empower ED suite for the emergency department. Empower ED software and system support costs resulted in the eventual expenditure of $630,000. Superior Consulting fee was $30,000. Project oversight consultant, Morgan Hunter Healthcare, billed a single charge of $12,464. Official BMC staff training trips over a period of three years totaled $125,000. MEDITECH modules support fees over a period of five years were $380,000. In the end, all of the direct return on investment calculation costs amounted to $6,503,741 (see Table 4).

Table 4. Project's direct costs from the return on investment calculations

Type	Amount
Original Sofware Quotes	$ 3,283,000
Original Hardware Quotes	$ 1,026,583
Initial Purchase	$ 4,309,583
LSS Provider System Support	$ 794,182
Staff Training Trips (3 years)	$ 125,000
Siemens System Support	$ 81,012
Cerner System Support	$ 123,500
Cisco Support	$ 18,000
Morgan Hunter Project Oversight	$ 12,464
Superior Consulting	$ 30,000
ED System Support	$ 200,000
Empower ED System with Interface	$ 430,000
MEDITECH Modules Support	$ 380,000
Total Direct System Costs	$ 6,503,741

Even though staff implementation time for IT and other user areas was not included in the ROI calculations, Broadlawns Finance Committee Memos mentioned that a conservative estimate of 40 Full-Time Equivalents (FTEs) over a period of three years yielded an internal project adoption cost of $2.5 million. Participation in the CMS EHR incentive programs had greatly accelerated the medical center's ROI schedule. The incentive payments under the programs were broken down into several portions. The grand total of Medicaid reimbursement equaled $5,433,846 to be paid to Broadlawns over a period of three years with 40 percent in years one and two and 20 percent in the final following year. Medicare reimbursement payment was estimated to be $800,000.

In the end, BMC replaced its expensive and disconnected emergency department Empower ED system and cut the maintenance costs by additional $34,000 per year. The hospital's replacement of Cerner pharmacy, radiology, and laboratory software with MEDITECH resulted in a 50 percent reduction of yearly maintenance costs. In 2010, BMC demonstrated over $4 million in net profits on the total revenue of only $100 million (Jenner, 2011).

Adoption Benefits

After the successful assimilation of MEDITECH, Broadlawns discovered numerous improvement and evolvement opportunities. The medical center had strengthened its professional partnership with the University of Iowa Hospitals and Clinics by establishing electronic collaboration. As a result, the fragmentation problem of the safety net specialty care, previously stated by the George Washington University study (Nolan, et al., 2005), was substantially alleviated. University of Iowa Health Care physicians could now access the medical histories of their referred patients prior to their effective arrivals (Broadlawns, 2010). Seamless information sharing between the two hospital systems started to deliver noticeable benefits to the quality of patient care and provider operating efficiencies.

Broadlawns senior management had an early vision to utilize the EHR system in improving the provider's financial stability and decreasing dependence on tax revenue. Successful EHR adoption and the subsequent analysis of real-time financial data allowed streamlining internal processes and workflows to increase the accuracy and timeliness of patient billing. Based on the data, the hospital's management decided to change its billing structure to the split model, which clearly separated billable services into professional and technical. Professional services were provided by the physicians of BMC clinics while technical services were rendered in the hospital setting.

Recent Finance Committee Memos further revealed the medical center's focus on collecting performance data and measuring financial vital signs. Some of the typical financial vital signs of BMC included Non-billable Service, No Authorization, Exceeds Timely Filing, Non-payable Diagnosis, Not Medically Necessary, and Non-covered Provider. One of the hospital's latest goals was to reduce the number of such financially destabilizing services by 0.5 percent from the last year's total of 3 percent.

Medical Group Management Association (MGMA) is an organization, which delivers comparable performance metrics for hospitals of various sizes and with different business objectives. At Broadlawns, MGMA metrics in combination with an encompassing EHR system have simplified and facilitated the pursuit of healthcare quality and financial sustainability. BMC senior leaders successfully increased the number of Days Cash on Hand to over one hundred and seven by June 2011. According to Finance Committee Memos, one day of the hospital's operating cash presently stands at $256,200 (Broadlawns, 2011).

Broadlawns senior leaders agree that even though medical centers are beginning to understand the requirements for achieving meaningful use, the expectations of data sharing and interoperability standards across providers are still rather vague. Positioning itself as an early technology leader, Broadlawns Medical Center has gained a unique opportunity in establishing new partnerships while developing statewide interoperability standards and shaping the future of Iowa Health Information Exchange.

IowaCare is a healthcare program designed by the state of Iowa for adults ages 19 through 64 who would not be covered by Medicaid under the normal circumstances (iowa.gov, 2011). The initial intention of the program was to provide healthcare to approximately 14,000 uncovered Iowa residents, but it quickly grew to serve over 72,000 people since its inception in 2005 (iowa.gov, 2011). According to the hospital's senior management, 15,000 of the uncovered Iowa residents live in Polk County, which is the provider's direct area of responsibility. Recent Report to the Community stated that BMC rendered over $43 million in various medical services for IowaCare patients in 2010 alone (Jenner, 2011).

IowaCare Medical Home is a state project of IowaCare providers started in October 2010. IowaCare Medical Home is a collaborative effort of four hospital systems including Broadlawns Medical Center, which focuses on preventative services, long-term disease management, and continuity of care of IowaCare patients. IowaCare Medical Home project proposed additional compensation for the providers, which could prove their effectiveness in managing chronic conditions. Participation in IowaCare Medical Home is preceded by the requirements to adopt an Electronic Health Record (EHR) system, establish meaningful use, and report chronic conditions registry data (iowa.gov, 2010). Having adopted an EHR system and achieved HIMSS Analytics Stage 6 as well as meaningful use Stage 1 certifications, Broadlawns Medical Center quickly grew as a key player in the IowaCare Medical Home project.

Once BMC matured in its use of information technology, it became more eager to maximize its potential. The hospital recently invested in one of the latest video technologies, which help analyzing and diagnosing true causes of patient seizures. Dr. Waldman, who is a staff neurologist and epileptologist at Broadlawns, had found that numerous epilepsy diagnoses were often misrepresentations of spells caused by other problems, such as metabolic imbalances or migraines (Stier, 2008). Quick and accurate diagnoses may not only reduce the number of acute care episodes and the ensuing expensive hospitalizations but also accelerate the patients' returns to normal productive lives.

BMC continuously serves almost 40,000 patients who speak in excess of 40 different languages (Stier, 2011). Recently, BMC became the first healthcare provider in Iowa to implement a novel technological solution to assist with patient registration and admission procedures. The hospital installed thirty-five palm scanners as a part of the new Patient Identity Security System (Stier, 2011). The scanners use near-infrared light to identify a patient's vein pattern and match it biometrically to the image stored in the corresponding medical record. The technology is considered to be one hundred times more accurate than fingerprinting, and it effortlessly distinguishes even between identical twins (Stier, 2011). Broadlawns Medical Center had reportedly enrolled over 1,000 patients with the palm scanner technology by the end of the first week (Broadlawns, 2011). The system is anticipated to improve security, quicken registration and admission processes, increase efficiency, and decrease language translation errors.

Jody Jenner joined the hospital's senior leadership team as the new Chief Operating Officer (CEO) in 2006. Jody Jenner continuously stressed the importance of the hospital's commitment to measuring and improving quality of care. Broadlawns patients began recognizing positive quality of care changes by 2009 (Stier, 2009). Press Ganey Associates, Inc. conducted a survey, which officially recorded an increase in patient satisfaction scores. Press Ganey collected customer feedback and returned actionable data, which were especially useful to BMC as a provider interested in continuous performance improvements. One of the recorded positive effects of the EHR adoption was the reduction of overall wait times through better access to pertinent clinical information (lssdata.com, 2010). Patient wait times noticeably improved at all Broadlawns clinics.

The Joint Commission organization also acknowledged the improvements in the quality of care and granted the medical center two full three-year accreditations in the 2007 and 2010 healthcare surveys, which subsequently secured Broadlawns Medicaid reimbursements.

Past Errors

BMC system adoption stakeholders suggested that the hospital could have benefited from having the clinics elect dedicated physicians to test the software during their regular work hours for at least a week prior to every anticipated go-live date. Workplace EHR testing would had allowed for an early system treatment meant to begin the laborious process of programming and personalization of physician templates.

BMC stakeholders also mentioned that it could have been useful to do additional investigative work before commencing to design their first system template. The stakeholders were aware of the existence of external consultants specializing in template recommendations and design. Given the time length and the involved complexity of designing a new template, it could have been helpful to contract one of such consulting firms during the early configuration stage. BMC information technology team had briefly considered modifying the existing third-party templates provided by the company Zynx Health but found the templates to be too vast and generic.

Admittedly, physician participation was somewhat lackluster during the on-site evaluation process with the vast majority of invitees staying busy with their daily responsibilities. Physician absence created noticeable difficulties during the software implementation stage because of some questions remaining unanswered even after the product selection process was completed.

One of the final noted errors was the decision of the previous chief executive officer to allow the purchase and installation of the Empower ED application in the emergency department without stressing the need to carefully consider the hospital's business, strategic, and interoperability requirements. New senior management team emphasized that for a successful EHR assimilation, all of the hospital departments must be interoperable, and the future EHR system should be selected following the best-of-fit rather than the best-of-breed approach. Eventually, Empower ED software had to be replaced by a better fitting MEDITECH module but not before costing the hospital over half a million dollars and requiring over nine months of meticulous planning for the system migration.

FUTURE DIRECTIONS

Currently, full electronic prescribing is only available at one of the hospital's clinics. Primary Care Group became the first Broadlawns clinic to communicate with pharmacies electronically. Even though physicians already issue electronic scripts at other hospital clinics, they still have to perform a manual step of faxing their refill requests. BMC stakeholders are arranging to enable full electronic prescribing in the remaining clinics, but the process is notably slow due to the shortage of information technology associates.

BMC is preparing to use its EHR system to focus on promoting continuity of care. When the medical center enables the advanced health maintenance module, it will be capable of proactive patient management. Physicians will be prompted on overdue tests and check-ups based on the patients' previous histories and regardless of the presently exhibited complaints and conditions. Advanced health maintenance module is expected to pave the way for the hospital's successful participation in IowaCare Medical Home Model where effective continuity of care is expected of all providers.

BMC has already integrated all but one of its clinics with the EHR suite. Physicians of the last full-time clinic are remaining skeptical and exhibiting a degree of end-user resistance. The stakeholders are diligently working toward the goal of connecting the last clinic in the spring of 2012.

The hospital is planning to further increase efficiency by joining its electronic health record system with a Patient Health Record (PHR) website. PHR portal will enable secure messaging between the hospital's patients and their physicians. Secure online messaging is anticipated to replace many unnecessary phone calls and even some office visits.

CONCLUSION

Broadlawns EHR adoption project is an inspiring story of a transformation of a small community hospital fostered by the successful utilization of modern healthcare information technology. BMC senior management is dedicated to continue finding new ways to benefit from its EHR investment. The hospital is already planning to reach CMS meaningful use Stage 2 and HIMSS Analytics Stage 7 certifications.

BMC stakeholders stated that following a phased approach to the EHR adoption was one of the major contributing factors to the system's eventual success. First, the hospital's scarce technical resources were able to focus their efforts on each of the individual EHR modules and specialty clinics. Second, the medical center was capable of minimizing its exposure to the risk of encountering unexpected problems. Third, the hospital's technical team could effectively address the challenge of end-user resistance by having the time to listen and personalize software interfaces and templates. Finally, the positive experience of one EHR module and medical clinic fostered internal collegial communication and served as an encouragement to other hospital departments.

The last stakeholder recommendation positively highlighted the strategic objective to join the entire hospital with the software from a single vendor. The single-vendor solution had benefited the project in many ways. BMC was able to significantly cut costs by replacing multiple vendor support contracts. End-user resistance was alleviated by centralizing educational, promotional, and support efforts. Finally, organizational interoperability guaranteed the integrity and availability of real-time performance metrics, which the hospital's senior management successfully turned into an eventual competitive advantage.

REFERENCES

Broadlawns. (2010). *Broadlawns, UI hospitals and clinics share records electronically.* Retrieved July 20, 2011, from http://www.broadlawns.org/news.cfm?article=139

Broadlawns. (2011a). *Broadlawns medical center: Strategic business priorities.* Retrieved November 3, 2011, from http://www.broadlawns.org/pdfs/priorities2011.pdf

Broadlawns. (2011b). *Business service update to the finance committee.* Retrieved from http://www.broadlawns.org

cms.gov. (2010). *CMD finalizes definition of meaningful use of certified electronic health records (EHR) technology.* Retrieved November 2, 2011, from https://www.cms.gov/apps/media/press/factsheet.asp?Counter=3794

cms.gov. (2011). *Overview EHR incentive programs.* Retrieved from https://www.cms.gov/ehrincentiveprograms/

hhs.gov. (2009). *HITECH act enforcement interim final rule.* Retrieved November 7, 2011, from http://www.hhs.gov/ocr/privacy/hipaa/administrative/enforcementrule/hitechenforcementifr.html

hhs.gov. (2010). *Secretary Sebelius announces final rules to support 'meaningful use' of electronic health records.* Retrieved November 7, 2011, from http://www.hhs.gov/news/press/2010pres/07/20100713a.html

himssanalytics.org. (2011a). *U.S. EMR adoption model trends.* Retrieved October 25, 2011, from http://www.himssanalytics.org/docs/HA_EMRAM_Overview_ENG.pdf

himssanalytics.org. (2011b). *US EMR adoption model.* Retrieved October 25, 2011, from http://www.himssanalytics.org/stagesGraph.asp

iowa.gov. (2010). *Iowacare medical home model.* Retrieved November 1, 2011, from http://www.idph.state.ia.us/hcr_committees/common/pdf/prevention_chronic_care_mgmt/082710_model.pdf iowa.gov. (2011). *IowaCare - Medicaid reform.* Retrieved October 25, 2011, from http://www.ime.state.ia.us/IowaCare/

Jenner, J. (2011). *Report to the community.* Retrieved November 2, 2001, from http://www.broadlawns.org/pdfs/REPORT_TO_COMMUNITY_09_10.pdf

klasresearch.com. (1996). *Company - KLAS helps healthcare providers by measuring vendor performance.* Retrieved November 4, 2011, from http://www.klasresearch.com/About/Company.aspx

lssdata.com. (2010). *Broadlawns medical center emerges as a health IT leader in Iowa.* Retrieved September 18, 2011, from http://www.lssdata.com/news/viewnews.php?n=146

meditech.com. (2011a). *MEDITECH at a glance.* Retrieved October 30, 2011, from http://www.meditech.com/AboutMeditech/pages/ataglance.htm

meditech.com. (2011b). *MEDITECH mission statement.* Retrieved October 30, 2011, from http://www.meditech.com/AboutMeditech/pages/mission.htm

Nolan, L., et al. (2005). *An assessment of hospital-sponsored health care for the uninsured in Polk County/Des Moines, Iowa.* Unpublished.

Staurovsky, R. (2004). *Broadlawns medical center hospital information system and physician practive management system selection. Request for Proposal.* Southfield, MI: Superior Consultant Company, Inc.

Stier, M. (2008). *Polk county residents gain access to latest seizure diagnosis video technology.* Community News From Broadlawns Medical Center.

Stier, M. (2009). *Patients give Broadlawns medical center higher satisfaction scores.* Community News From Broadlawns Medical Center.

Stier, M. (2010). *Broadlawns earns HIMSS EMR certification.* Community News From Broadlawns Medical Center.

Stier, M. (2011a). *Broadlawns by the numbers.* Des Moines, IA: Broadlawns Medical Center.

Stier, M. (2011b). *Broadlawns installs first-in-Iowa patient identity security system.* Des Moines, IA: Broadlawns Medical Center.

Stier, M. (2011c). *Economic impact.* Des Moines, IA: Broadlawns Medical Center.

Stier, M. (2011d). *Mission.* Des Moines, IA: Broadlawns Medical Center.

Weinstock, M., & Hoppszallern, S. (2011, July). Most wired 2011. *Hospitals and Health Networks.*

wikipedia.org. (2009). *Healthcare information and management systems society.* Retrieved November 3, 2011, from http://en.wikipedia.org/wiki/HIMSS

wikipedia.org. (2011a). *LSS data systems.* Retrieved October 28, 2011, from http://en.wikipedia.org/wiki/LSS_Data_Systems

wikipedia.org. (2011b). *MEDITECH.* Retrieved from http://en.wikipedia.org/wiki/MEDITECH

ADDITIONAL READING

Agarwal, R. (2010). Research commentary - The digital transformation of healthcare: Current status and the road ahead. *Information Systems Research, 21*(4), 796–809. doi:10.1287/isre.1100.0327

Fichman, R. G. (2011). Editorial overview - The role of information systems in healthcare: Current research and future trends. *Information Systems Research, 22*(3), 419–428. doi:10.1287/isre.1110.0382

Holroyd-Leduc, J. M. (2011). The impact of the electronic medical record on structure, process, and outcomes within primary care: A systematic review of the evidence. *Journal of the American Medical Informatics Association, 18*(6), 732–737. doi:10.1136/amiajnl-2010-000019

Kane, G. C., & Labianca, G. (2011). IS avoidance in health-care groups: A multi-level investigation. *Information Systems Research, 22*(3), 504–522. doi:10.1287/isre.1100.0314

McAlearney, A. S. (2010). Perceived efficiency impacts following electronic health record implementation: An exploratory study of an urban community health center network. *International Journal of Medical Informatics, 79*(12), 807–816. doi:10.1016/j.ijmedinf.2010.09.002

Peterson, L. T. (2011). Assessing differences between physicians' realized and anticipated gains from electronic health record adoption. *Journal of Medical Systems, 35*(2), 151–161. doi:10.1007/s10916-009-9352-z

Russ, A. L. (2010). Electronic health information in use: Characteristics that support employee workflow and patient care. *Health Informatics Journal, 16*(4), 287–305. doi:10.1177/1460458210365981

Saleem, J. J. (2011). Paper persistence, workarounds, and communication break-downs in computerized consultation management. *International Journal of Medical Informatics, 80*(7), 466–479. doi:10.1016/j.ijmedinf.2011.03.016

Sittig, D. F., & Singh, H. (2009). Eight rights of safe electronic health record use. *Journal of the American Medical Association, 302*(10), 1111–1113. doi:10.1001/jama.2009.1311

Venkatesh, V. (2011). Doctors do too little technology: A longitudinal field study of an electronic healthcare system implementation. *Information Systems Research, 22*(3), 523–546. doi:10.1287/isre.1110.0383

Chapter 5
Physician Interaction with EHR:
The Importance of Stakeholder Identification and Change Management

Cherie Noteboom
Dakota State University, USA

EXECUTIVE SUMMARY

Research Medical Center is a regional medical center that meets the needs of residents of a rural area in the Midwest. It is part of a large healthcare system. The primary care hospital implemented the Electronic Health Record (EHR). The endeavor to implement Health IT applications including Computerized Physician Order Entry (CPOE), EHRs, nursing documentation, and paperless charts, adverse drug reaction alerts, and more were introduced with the corporate initiative. The core applications were clinical and revenue cycle systems, including CPOE. The planning, implementation, and training was developed by the parent operating company and efforts to engage the local physicians were minimal. There were over 300 physicians involved. The physicians were primarily not hospital employees. They had the ability to choose to adopt the EHR and adapt their social, work, and technology practices, or to avoid usage. Follow up research indicated the change management and support efforts were not successful for the physician stakeholder.

DOI: 10.4018/978-1-4666-2671-3.ch005

ORGANIZATION BACKGROUND

Living the traditions, visions and values of healthcare, Research Medical Center is a regional medical center that meets the needs of residents in a rural area of the Midwest. Research Medical Center partners with other community healthcare providers to sponsor a regional cancer center, paramedic services, hospice services, a freestanding surgery center and a variety of other health services.

Research Medical Center has earned more national recognition for quality patient outcomes than any other hospital in the region. The medical center has earned multiple honors for its leadership and excellence in several clinical areas including cardiac care, orthopedic services, vascular surgery, stroke care, and cancer care. The organization is home to the only Level II Trauma Center in the area, and provides a vital, lifesaving link to rural areas via Air Care, the hospital's helicopter ambulance service.

Research Medical Center is a member of a large healthcare system. The parent company's vision is to be a leader in improving health care delivery with technology initiatives. They became an industry leader, embracing leading leading-edge technology and implemented an Electronic Health Record (EHR). The record is supported by Cerner, and the hospital went live with several Cerner modules to support patient care, including FirstNet, INet, physician computerized order entry. The EHR goal was to reduce errors, streamline documentation, improve clinical quality, and create a more efficient process. The planning and implementation was created from with a centralized, corporate perspective. To provide consistency and achieve the goals of integrated systems, the implementations for all parent company hospitals were achieved with the same goals, objectives, and project plan.

SETTING THE STAGE

Research has shown that the healthcare industry is plagued by rapidly increasing costs, poor quality of service, lack of integration of patient care, and lack of information access to EHR. According to the Institute of Medicine (IOM, 2001), medical errors are a major problem that decreases the quality and increases the costs of the U.S. healthcare system. Medical errors result in 98,000 deaths a year and many more injuries, and as a result, patient safety has become a top priority in U.S. healthcare.

The use of Information Technology (IT) has the potential to help healthcare organizations improve quality of service while reducing costs. The Institute of Medicine (IOM, 2001) reported that the U.S. healthcare system is "fundamentally broken" and called on the federal government to make a major investment in information technology in order to achieve the changes, such as the "commitment to technology to manage the knowledge bases and process of care" (p. 178), needed to repair the broken healthcare system.

During the past 25 years, many medical records have been converted from a handwritten record format to an EHR format, and studies have indicated that EHR is complicated and requires a serious, sustained commitment to human resources, process re-engineering, technology, and funding. The healthcare system has been slow to take advantage of EHR and realize the benefits of computerization (McDonald, 1997): that is, improved access to and records of patient data, enhanced ability to make better and more-timely decisions, and improved quality and reduced errors.

It is commonly assumed that U.S. healthcare services organizations are approximately 10 years behind the Information Systems (IS) curve when compared to organizations from other industries of comparable size and complexity. According to IOM (2001), "healthcare delivery has been relatively untouched by the revolution in information technology that has been transforming nearly every other aspect of society" (p. 15). This inability to take full advantage of computerization is unfortunate because EHR has the potential to improve patient care and patient safety. In 2007, however, the American Hospital Association reported that only 11% of hospitals had fully implemented EHR, and these hospitals were likely to be large, urban, and/or teaching hospitals. Vishwanath and Scamurra (2007) reported less than 10% of physicians in different practices and settings in the US use EHR, whereas more than half of the physicians in countries like Sweden, Netherlands and Australia have adopted EHR. Blumenthal (2009) cites only 1.5% of US hospitals have comprehensive EHR systems. A similar 2009 study by the American Hospital Association shows less than 2% of hospitals use comprehensive EHR and about 8% use a basic EHR in at least one care unit. According to a study published in the New England Journal of Medicine, United States patients get appropriate medical care only 55 percent of the time. Greater use of EHRs could improve care by tracking patients' medical history and providing electronic reminders about needed test and treatments.

At Research Medical Center's parent company, the member hospital teams and clinical operations improvement and information systems have set the goal to enable the organization to extract full value from its technology investments while positioning it to take advantage of future quality improvement and cost saving opportunities. The clinical components are to increase patient safety and quality of care with evidence based, decision making tools and standardized best practices. The revenue management components contribute by improving financial performance, securing revenue more effectively by enabling insurance verification at time of registration and improving claims editing.

There is increasing pressure to operate efficiently in health care. Costs are spiraling out of control, due in part to huge amounts of redundancy and waste. Medical errors arise because of process failures and ineffective communication. Prior to the implementation of the electronic medical record, the hospital used a paper medical record for documentation.

CASE DESCRIPTION

Technology Concerns

Electronic Health Records (EHRs) and Computerized Physician Order Entry (CPOE) are revolutionary technologies that transform the way medicine is being practiced, taught, and advanced. However, these are merely technology tools. The tools are only as good as the process behind them. True quality care through health IT is achieved by automating processes based on evidence in order to provide better outcomes and safer care. At the same time, automation can eliminate unnecessary steps in order to increase clinicians' productivity and efficiency.

The enterprise change and transition from departmental 'silo' systems to the integrated system is relatively simple from a technology perspective, but difficult from a people perspective.

Typical allocation of cost for these large IT endeavors is 12% for hardware, 15% for software, 15% for data conversions, 43% for developing work processes (reengineering), and 15% for preparing employees for the new system (training and change management).

Technology Components

Health IT applications including CPOE, EHRs, nursing documentation, and paperless charts, adverse drug reaction alerts, and more were introduced with the corporate initiative. The core applications were clinical and revenue cycle systems, including Computerized Physician Order Entry (CPOE).

The clinical components were expected to increase patient safety and quality of care with evidence based, decision making tools and standardized best practices to support the transformation of patient care delivery. The vendor, Cerner, provided pharmacy, emergency department clinical documentation, CPOE and medical records modules. A clinical data repository is developed and utilizes "expert rules" functionality to leverage the value of turning data into information.

Goals of the revenue management components were to improve financial performance, secure revenue more effectively by verifying insurance and improved claims editing.

Systems are designed with full redundancy to hold downtime and failure to a minimum. In event of a disaster, it is estimated only 60 seconds of clinical data will be lost. Historical tape backup systems risked loss of 24 hours of data.

Management and Organizational Concerns

There is increasing pressure to operate efficiently in healthcare. Costs are spiraling out of control, due in part to huge amounts of redundancy and waste. Medical errors arise because of process failures, ineffective communication, and lack of information. It is time to make the best use of new technology in every phase of a patient's experience to drive out efficiencies, eliminate errors, and enhance communication. Capturing the benefits from EHRs is the next step in the journey to make hospital care better and safer for everyone. However, the required process changes for the implementation of systems of this magnitude cause management concern. Losses in revenue, profits, and market share results when core business processes and IT systems fail or do not work properly.

The organization will undergo changes in communication, process, and teamwork. "Implementing CPOE is very much not an IT project, this is a clinical project that has huge IT aspects to it" (Chessen, 2005). It will transform the way the medical staff and all hospital staff do their work. One obvious change is the way nurses and physicians will communicate. Physicians are able to access patient information far beyond the hospital walls. Clinicians have access to the electronic record. They can review the information together. On the process side, hospitals are better able to measure true clinical improvement in various activities.

Teams to define improved care processes and how to integrate the processes into the electronic health care record system are centralized. The success will be measured by the ability to improve core clinical indicators, productivity measures, patient satisfaction, and financial performance.

In a CPOE environment, the number of physicians who utilize the application and the percentage of orders made via computer gauge success. However, few healthcare providers boast 100 percent utilization. For one, introducing CPOE into daily workflow and patient care flows is no easy feat. CPOE is all about a change in the practice of medicine. The cultural changes posed by CPOE, plus the idea that physicians can be resilient to computer technology, the limited amount of CPOE products on the market and the complexity of implementation has hindered adoption.

CPOE represents a huge change in operations for the hospital. It involves a change in physician practice. Not only because the physician is being asked to enter orders on the computer rather than scribble them on a chart or call them in on the phone, but the whole value of this is in the decision support and the standardization of care. Order sets are being developed for certain diagnoses and the doctor is expected to use them. Other staff members affected because some of the task used to be done by the unit clerks, some of is used to done in pharmacy and nursing.

Probably the biggest barrier to CPOE adoption is the cultural one. It is difficult for physicians who have been in practice for a decade or two to adopt computers in medicine. Information technology has been used by many organizations for the past 40 years. Manufacturing, banking, finance, and other industries have capitalized on new technology and experienced increased quality, lower costs, and a competitive advantage. There are many examples of IT's benefits: (a) improved customer relationship management and knowledge management, (b) cost reductions, and (c) improved quality. IT, however, has produced less significant results in the healthcare system. It is routinely possible to access bank accounts electronically from anywhere in the world, but it is often impossible to access medical information from an office next door. IOM (2001) claimed that the healthcare system needs to join the IT revolution, and improved information systems may be a critical factor for improving the healthcare system because of the pervasive need to access, record, and share information in order to provide high-quality medical care (Thrall, 2004). EHR is a journey that has just started (Ondo, Wagner, & Gale, 2002).

Knowledge and learning play important roles in the use of IT, and researchers have developed the diffusion, adoption, and acceptance theories to explain how people adopt, accept, and use complex organizational technologies. Attewell (1992) defined complex organizational technologies as "technologies that, when first introduced, impose a substantial burden on would-be users in terms of the knowledge needed to use these technologies effectively" (Fichman & Kemerer, 1997, p. 1346). From an organizational learning perspective, Attewell defined technology assimilation as "a process of organizational learning in which individuals and an organization as a whole acquire the knowledge and skills necessary to effectively apply the technology" (Fichman & Kemerer, 1997, p. 1345). The burden of learning creates a knowledge barrier that inhibits the diffusion of IT. In these cases, the use of IT can be inhibited as much by the ability to adopt IT systems as the desire to adopt these systems. Consequently, IT penetration into the market from which the stakeholders could benefit is seriously affected and the benefit undermined.

The healthcare system is a complex organization characterized by knowledge workers working as independent professionals. The ability for these knowledge workers to access data effectively and efficiently would improve the quality of work processes and patient care. However, EHR, which enable people to work effectively and efficiently access data, have been underused by U.S healthcare professionals such as physicians. In order to improve the use of IT in the U.S. healthcare system, it is necessary to understand what healthcare professionals, especially physicians, think about the use of EHR.

"To be a professional includes three ideals: 1) that one has skill acquired through specialized training; 2) that one can have a rational account of one's own activities, explaining the 'whys'; 3) that one is dedicated to using one's skills for the well-being of others" (Benveniste, 1987; Weick & McDaniel, 1989). Professional organizations are created to apply professional values and expertise to the resolution of difficult, often ambiguous problems. One can view a professional organization as a strategy for reducing uncertainty about what can be done using professional expertise and should be done using professional values (Anderson & McDaniel, 2000). Often the physicians' expertise is based on specialized cognitive knowledge and specialized skills. Healthcare organizations are "unique among professional organizations in that rather than one profession occupying all the major professional roles, there are several different professions that are central to the organizations success. Historically, physicians have a dominant role in the medical model of healthcare" (Anderson & McDaniel, 2000). Physicians have experienced highly demanding educational and specialized training and are experts in their own profession and accustomed to practicing in a particular way or style similar to which they were trained. Findings from prior research suggest physicians are reluctant to give a positive response to implementation of an IS that interferes with their traditional routines (Chau & Hu, 2002). A key element in understanding physician use of EHR is the critical role played by expertise and values in their work processes. Anderson and McDaniel feel professional expertise and values can be powerful inhibitors of innovation.

In addition, when the implementation of information systems interferes with physicians' traditional practice routines, they are not likely to be accepted by physicians (Anderson & Aydin, 1997). According to Anderson, physicians will oppose any systems that impose major limitation on how clinical data is recorded and how the medical record is organized. Physicians feel it interferes with the way they organize their thought processes in caring for patients. A key element in understanding physician perspective of EHR is the critical role played by expertise and values in their work processes. Understanding how physicians work with knowledge in the healthcare domain and the knowledge identities they utilize is an important step in understanding the physicians' perspective on EHR usage.

The physician perspective reflects the unique role and responsibilities of the physician. The physician role is characterized with professional autonomy, status role, expertise, experience, and intuition. The ability to incorporate technology into physician practice based on specialized training, experience and intuition is a challenge that requires more than merely providing the opportunity of technology.

The physicians are asked to adopt order sets. Most physicians recognize that medicine is a combination of science and art. As you go to order sets, you are taking out a bit of the art and that is another barrier (physicians) have to overcome. Thirdly, these are not out-of-the-box applications that hospitals can just use intuitively. It takes a bit of learning, which has been a significant challenge for clinicians. The systems were not written for the way clinicians work. It has been a growing process and we are constantly working to improve the application.

In this case, the physicians identified organizational process categories providing challenges to them. These are the organizational processes that were obtained from analyzing their responses. These categories illustrate the bundles of meaning relating to how physicians perceive the support or lack of support in their adaptation of EHR. The data indicates the physicians feel the EHR decision was made without their input and buy-in. They feel they were 'mandated' to adapt to the EHR and were not considered as primary users. They felt they were left out of key decision-making processes, yet were required to adjust to the EHR functions by 'becoming the highest paid user doing the lowest paid work.' These are further analyzed in Table 1 with the categories, number of positive instances, number of negative instances and total number of instances in each category.

The physician communication and change management category explains the physician perspective of the communication and change management efforts directed towards physician engagement. All of the physician coded instances in this category were negative. This indicates an area of failure for this implementation. Future implementations would benefit from attention to the influence of physician communication and change management.

Table 1. Influence of administration on physician adaptation of EHR

Administration	Description	Positive (n)	Negative (n)	Total
Physician Communication and Change Management	The physician perspective of physician communication and change management	0	39	39
Value Perception of Administration	The physician perspective of the value perception of administration related to EHR. Physician perspective of administrations view on HER	0	22	22
System Changes	The physician perception of lack response, delivery and communication on issues where opinion was requested	2	7	11
Physician Input and Buy	The physician perspective of the importance of inclusion of physician in planning, input and buy-in phase.	4	35	39
Total		6	86	92

Value perception of administration is the physician perspective of the administration valuation of EHR and the physician value related to EHR. It primarily describes the lack of value associated with the increased amount of physician efforts and the perceived administrative stance of 'rosy view of EHR.' All of the physician instances in this category were negative. The importance of value of physician effort cannot be ignored.

System change is the physician perspective of response, delivery, and communication on issues of system changes, fixes, and enhancements. The data indicates the physician requests for system changes and modifications are not met. They suggest their work processes are made less efficient and their productivity declines as a result of the slow response to requests.

Physician input and buy-in is the physician perspective of the importance of inclusion of physician in planning, input and buy-in phases. As physicians feel they were not included in the planning, input and buy-in phases, the physicians feel this contributed to the lack of support provided by the EHR for their work practice needs.

Therefore, this case specifically focuses on the physician aspect of the system implementation and the physician perspective. Physicians are key stakeholder in the EHR efforts. Their professional work and knowledge process requires attention to the integration of EHR into their work.

CURRENT CHALLENGES FACING THE ORGANIZATION

There is increasing pressure to operate efficiently in health care. Costs are spiraling out of control, due in part to huge amounts of redundancy and waste. Medical errors arise because of process failures and ineffective communication. Changes in billing, quality, and reimbursement strategies continue to impact healthcare.

After the implementation of the system, the hospital experienced a drop in census. There was a shift in admissions to the other healthcare alternatives in the community. Physicians were dissatisfied with the approach to organizational change, lack of acknowledgement of increased physician work and the resulting decrease in physician productivity levels. The lack of effective training and change management for physicians became apparent. In the competitive healthcare environment, the physicians had choice of hospital and choice of adoption of the technology and choice of adaptation of technology into their work requirements.

The biggest barrier is the hospital first encountered CPOE was that it took to long to use and was not intuitive for physicians. The system was originally built for ward clerks and pharmacy clerks, not for physicians. After major renovation, the current limiting factor is the resources to train doctors on how to properly use the system. Initial CPOE usage rates failed to meet the target goals. Eventually, the CPOE usage rate struggled to 50 percent.

A second significant barrier was the manner in which the system functionality and the order set use was introduced. Physicians had developed unrealistic expectation regarding the system. The introduction and use of enterprise systems requires relatively consistent usage by the end users. This was the first exposure to standardized order sets.

Overall, the clinical staff worked significantly more hours during the preparation and Go-Live time period. The continued stress of the implementation resulted in low staff morale (see Table 2).

The process and infrastructure issues are IT context issues. They primarily deal with the physician perspective of how the system was developed and implemented, training, support and functionalities of the system. IT context issues have the potential power to influence IT Adaptation (Beaudry & Pinsonneault, 2005, p. 505). The following data instances are examples of IT context issues identified by physicians. They are:

What is currently happening is the clinicians are being asked to pay for it, especially the ones that are on productivity, are being asked to pay for it out of their productivity dollars and they are not going to make a return from it.

I think that one concern is that you actually spend less face-to-face time with people whether it is personal family/friend time or patient care, too.

Education, the education process I think was too compact. I think over time the process could have been a little bit more user friendly.

One of the things we hear with the Computerized Physician Order Entry system we have here, CPOE, is that most providers will tell us that it costs them time.

Overall, the data indicates the physician perspective does not find the influence of processes and infrastructure as a positive influence on adaptation. The above analysis suggests that the technological difficulties surrounding EHR have affected the physician adaptation and their level of comfort with the technology. The technological adaptation of EHR by physicians is negatively affected as a result of these technical difficulties described above.

Further analysis of this case suggests that technological adaptation comprises of additional characteristics that are unique to the ways in which physicians perceive technology and its usefulness to them. In particular, the case indicates value in

Table 2. Influence of processes and infrastructure on physician adaptation of EHR

Processes and Infrastructure	Description	Positive (n)	Negative (n)	Total
Systems Development	The physician perspective on the development aspects of the EHR specific to their functionality.	0	29	29
Hardware & Configuration	The Physician perspective on the hardware and configuration aspects of the EHR	0	10	10
Training	The physician perspective on the training aspects of the EHR specific to their functionality	6	41	47
Documentation	The physician perspective on the documentation aspects of the EHR specific to their functionality	0	17	17
Knowledge & Learning	The physician perspective on the knowledge and learning environment (e.g. barriers, difficulties, positive impacts).	3	31	34
Desire Integrated Systems	The physician perspective on the desire to have integrated systems across functions and organizations specific to their functionality – actual request for integration	31	5	36
Duplicate System Difficulties	The physician perspective on the difficulties encountered due to duplicate systems.	0	21	21
Downtime Concern	The physician perspective on the issues related to EHR usage and downtime	0	28	28
Total		40	182	222

consideration for digital native and digital immigrant difference (Prensky, 2001) and diffusion theory influences.

It is possible that physician interaction with EHR is affected by generational differences: That is, some physicians may be digital natives, and some of them may be digital immigrants. According to Prensky (2001), digital natives are people who have "spent their entire lives surrounded by and using computers, video games, digital music players, video cams, cell phones and all the other toys and tools of the digital age" (p. 1). Digital natives are used to receiving information quickly, like to parallel process and multitask, prefer their graphics before their text, prefer random access, perform best when networked, and thrive on instant gratification and frequent rewards. Digital immigrants tend to adopt and use technology, but they retain their digital immigrant accent, which can be seen in such things as turning to the Internet for information second rather than first, reading the manual for computer use rather than assuming the program will teach them how to use it, or printing their email. The differences between digital natives and digital immigrant are frequently a focus of training and education efforts, and these two groups of IT users tend to favor learning in different environments and learn effectively from different methods.

Diffusion theory provides insight on the use and adoption in organizations. It provides insight into one of the most challenging topics in the IT field: that is, how to improve technology assessment and adoption. Diffusion theory provides tools for assessing the likely rate of technology use in an organization and identifies factors that facilitate or hinder technology adoption. These factors include the characteristics of the technology, characteristics of adopters, and the means by which adopters learn about and are persuaded to adopt the technology (Rogers, 2003).

Diffusion is defined as "the process by which an innovation is communicated through certain channels over time among the members of a social system" (Rogers, 2003, p. 5). Rogers claimed that individuals move through five stages when making a decision about whether to adopt or reject an innovation: (a) awareness, (b) interest, (c) evaluation, (d) trial, and (e) adoption. Rogers synthesized the results from more than 3,000 studies that examined adoption and diffusion and made several generalizations about innovation diffusion: (a) Innovations possess certain characteristics (i.e., relative advantage, compatibility, complexity, trialability, and observability), which, as perceived by adopters, determine the ultimate rate and pattern of adoption; (b) some potential adopters are more innovative than other adopters and can be identified by their personal characteristics (e.g., cosmopolitanism or level of education); (c) the adoption decision unfolds as a series of stages (i.e., flowing from knowledge of the innovation through persuasion, decision, implementation, and confirmation), and adopters are predisposed to different types of influence (e.g., mass market communication versus word of mouth) at different stages; (d) the actions of certain types of individuals (e.g., opinion leaders and change agents) can accelerate adoption, especially when potential adopters consider these individuals to be similar to themselves; and (e) the diffusion process usually starts out slowly among pioneering adopters, reaches a take-off point as a growing community of adopters is established and the results of peer influence take effect, and levels off as the population of potential adopters becomes exhausted, which leads to an S-shaped cumulative adoption curve (Fichman, 1992, p. 196).

The above analysis suggests that the technological difficulties surrounding EHR have affected the physician adaptation and their level of comfort with the technology. The technological adaptation of EHR by physicians is negatively affected as a result of these technical difficulties described above. Further analysis of this data suggests that technological adaptation comprises of additional characteristics that are unique to the ways in which physicians perceive technology and its usefulness to them. Table 3 illustrates the sub-categories discovered through open coding and the perceptions of physicians within those categories.

Table 3. Technological adaptation

Tech Adaptation	Positive	Negative	Total
Diffusion (Rogers)	28	30	58
Digital Native Digital Immigrant– Generational Age Difference	21	9	21
Total	40	39	79

Diffusion is defined as "the process by which an innovation is communicated through certain channels over time among the members of a social system" (Rogers, 2003, p. 5). Rogers claimed that individuals move through five stages when making a decision about whether to adopt or reject an innovation: (a) awareness, (b) interest, (c) evaluation, (d) trial, and (e) adoption. Open coding of the data revealed the physician perspective on EHR. The diffusion does appear to be influenced by digital immigrant/digital native or generational influence.

Technological adaptation amongst physicians appears to be influenced by their level of comfort and experience with technology. While older physicians are opinion leaders with respect to clinical decisions, younger physicians are frequently leaders in using information technology (Anderson, 1997). This is supported by this research as indicated by the data, such as:

rather than sitting down and thinking "could this be something else, what am I missing, what else could it be?" and we don't have time to that anymore, you don't have time to use our clinical skills to take care of our patient. Now, with that being said, we have a whole generation of physicians coming up that are not as good at their clinical skills. I am not as good at my clinical skills as my elder colleagues. They can walk into a room and diagnose something because they were good clinicians.

Now, with that being said, we have a whole generation of physicians coming up that are not as good at their clinical skills. I am not as good at my clinical skills as my elder colleagues. They can walk into a room and diagnose something because they were good clinicians. Now we look at a patient and say what do they have and then we look at the data and make the data fit what we want it to. Does the data fit what it could possibly be rather than I think it's this, what do I need data-wise to confer? And so I think with EHR we are doing a lot of it, we are spending more time trying to find out what it could be with data rather than talking to a patient.

I think that people that are coming out of training in the last 5 years would have similar thought processes to me on use and benefits of technology. I think that every

10 years you are going to see a generation of different people that even it's just more of who they are and what they do.

I think that the exact opposite...the people that have been here for 20 years and have had a little tough time adapting to, not just new technology, but how fast new technology is updated. The change process and the changes continue to happen... it's a logarithmic progression. Every 5 years the change, I mean, the change we have seen in the last 5 years is exponentially greater than the change we saw in the 5 year period 10-15 years ago. You have to learn to use a new phone and computer every couple of years now.

As the case indicates, there are challenges to resolve related to physician interaction with EHRs.

SOLUTIONS AND RECOMMENDATIONS

It is recommended to have a physician system interface that allows doctor to enter orders as quickly or faster than they can hand write them or else the chances of success will be slim. If the system can be made faster than on paper, all you have to do is incentivize the doctors through the learning curve.

Working with professionals requires understanding their work requirements. Recommendations for influencing physician interaction with EHR: 1) Emphasize clinical value; 2) Don't waste physician time; 3) Provide easy access login and sequence; 4) Provide tools for physicians to find their patients information; 5) Focus on streamlining the interface between the physician and the computer; 6) Identify medical staff needs; 7) Build a system that addresses the medical staff's needs (that is different than understanding what your hospital needs are and addressing your hospital needs); 8) Engage clinical leadership; 9) Prepare for culture shock. EHR and CPOE can improve patient safety. It must be a component with a larger culture of patient safety and it is a component that must be used carefully.

"To be a professional includes three ideals: 1) that one has skill acquired through specialized training; 2) that one can have a rational account of one's own activities, explaining the 'whys'; 3) that one is dedicated to using one's skills for the well-being of others" (Benveniste, 1987; Weick & McDaniel, 1989). Professional organizations are created to apply professional values and expertise to the resolution of difficult, often ambiguous problems. One can view a professional organization as a strategy for reducing uncertainty about what can be done using professional expertise and should be done using professional values (Anderson & McDaniel, 2000). Often the physicians' expertise is based on specialized cognitive knowledge and specialized skills. Healthcare organizations are "unique among professional organizations in that rather than one profession occupying all the major professional roles, there are several different professions that are central to the organizations success. Historically, physicians have a dominant role in the medical model of healthcare" (Anderson & McDaniel, 2000). Physicians have experienced highly demanding educational and specialized training and are experts in their own profession and accustomed to practicing in a particular way or style similar to which they were trained. Findings from prior research suggest physicians are reluctant to give a positive response to implementation of an IS that interferes with their traditional routines (Chau & Hu, 2002). A key element in understanding physician use of EHR is the critical role played by expertise and values in their work processes. Anderson and McDaniel feel professional expertise and values can be powerful inhibitors of innovation.

In addition, when the implementation of information systems interferes with physicians' traditional practice routines, they are not likely to be accepted by physicians (Anderson & Aydin, 1997). According to Anderson, physicians will oppose any systems that impose major limitation on how clinical data is recorded and how the medical record is organized. Physicians feel it interferes with the way they organize their thought processes in caring for patients. A key element in understanding physician perspective of EHR is the critical role played by expertise and values in their work processes. Understanding how physicians work with knowledge in the healthcare domain and the knowledge identities they utilize is an important step in understanding the physicians' perspective on EHR usage.

Often new technologies fail to produce the benefits expected by an organization. A new technology is introduced, and the focus moves to other priorities. The diffusion of IT use, however, requires additional attention because IT has a history of following the 80/20 rule: 80% of the time, only 20% of the capability is utilized. According to Boynton, Zmud, and Jacobs (1994), absorptive capacity theory, when applied to the domain of IT use, suggests that an organization's development of a mosaic of IT-related knowledge and processes binds together the firm's IT managers and line managers: "An organization's absorptive capacity reflects its ability to 'absorb,' through internal knowledge structures, information regarding appropriate innovations so that these innovations can be applied in support of operational or strategic activities" (p. 300).

The physician perspective reflects the unique role and responsibilities of the physician. The physician role is characterized with professional autonomy, status role, expertise, experience, and intuition. The ability to incorporate technology into physician practice based on specialized training, experience and intuition is a challenge that requires more than merely providing the opportunity of technology. As innovative and exciting IT applications target individual 'professionals,' it has been important to investigate the perspectives of professionals (e.g. physicians) in their professional settings.

REFERENCES

Attewell, P. (1992). Technology diffusion and organizational learning: The case of business computing. *Organization Science, 3*(1), 1–19. doi:10.1287/orsc.3.1.1

Benveniste, G. (1987). *Professionalizing the organization.* San Francisco, CA: Jossey-Bass.

Blumenthal, D. (2009). Stimulating the adoption of health information technology. *The New England Journal of Medicine, 360*(15), 1477–1479. doi:10.1056/NEJMp0901592

Fichman, R., & Kemerer, C. (1997). The assimilation of software process innovations: An organizational learning perspective. *Management Science, 43*(10), 1345–1363. doi:10.1287/mnsc.43.10.1345

Greenhalgh, T., Potts, H. W. W., Wong, G., Bark, P., & Swinglehurst, D. (2009). Tensions and paradoxes in electronic patient record research: A systematic literature review using the meta-narrative method. *The Milbank Quarterly, 87*(4), 729–788. doi:10.1111/j.1468-0009.2009.00578.x

Institute of Medicine. (2001). *Crossing the quality chasm: A new health system for the 21st century.* Washington, DC: National Academy Press.

Lewin, K., & Minton, J. (1986). Determining organization effectiveness: Another look and an agenda for research. *Management Science, 32*(5). doi:10.1287/mnsc.32.5.514

Manos, D. (2009, March 25). New study shows few hospitals have comprehensive EHR. *Healthcare IT News.*

Markus, L., & Robey, D. (1988). Information technology and organizational change: Causal structure in theory and research. *Management Science, 34*(5), 583–598. doi:10.1287/mnsc.34.5.583

McDonald, C. J. (1997). The barriers to electronic medical record systems and how to overcome them. *Journal of the American Medical Informatics Association, 4*(3), 213–221. doi:10.1136/jamia.1997.0040213

Niazkhani, Z., Pirnejad, H., Berg, M., & Aarts, J. (2009). The impact of computerized provider order entry systems on inpatient clinical workflow: A literature review. *Journal of the American Medical Informatics Association, 16*(4), 539–549. doi:10.1197/jamia.M2419

Noteboom, C., & Qureshi, S. (2011). Physician interaction with electronic health records: The influences of digital natives and digital immigrants. In R. Sprague & J. Nunamaker (Eds.), *The Forty-Fourth Annual Hawaii International Conference on System Sciences*. Washington, DC: IEEE Computer Society Press.

Ondo, K. J., Wagner, J., & Gale, K. L. (2002). The electronic medical record (EMR): Hype or reality? *HIMSS Proceedings, 63*, 1–12.

Prensky, M. (2001). Digital natives, digital immigrants. *Horizon, 9*(5). doi:10.1108/10748120110424816

Rogers, E. M. (2003). *Diffusion of innovations* (5th ed.). New York, NY: Free Press.

Simon, H. (1997). *Models of bounded rationality*. Cambridge, MA: The MIT Press.

Thrall, J. (2004). Quality and safety revolution in health care. *Radiology, 233*, 3–6. doi:10.1148/radiol.2331041059

Vishwanath, A., & Scarmurra, T. (2007). Barriers to the adoption of electronic health records: Using concept mapping to develop a comprehensive empirical model. *Health Informatics Journal, 13*(2), 119–134. doi:10.1177/1460458207076468

Weick, K., & McDaniel, R. R. (1989). How professional organizations work: Implications for school organization and management. In Sergiovanni, T., & Moore, J. H. (Eds.), *Schooling for Tomorrow Directing Future Reforms to Issues that Count* (pp. 330–355). Boston, MA: Allyn and Bacon.

ADDITIONAL READING

Blumenthal, D. (2009). Stimulating the adoption of health information technology. *The New England Journal of Medicine, 360*(15), 1477–1479. doi:10.1056/NEJMp0901592

Greenhalgh, T., Potts, H. W. W., Wong, G., Bark, P., & Swinglehurst, D. (2009). Tensions and paradoxes in electronic patient record research: A systematic literature review using the meta-narrative method. *The Milbank Quarterly, 87*(4), 729–788. doi:10.1111/j.1468-0009.2009.00578.x

Institute of Medicine. (2001). *Crossing the quality chasm: A new health system for the 21st century*. Washington, DC: National Academy Press.

Lewin, K., & Minton, J. (1986). Determining organization effectiveness: Another look and an agenda for research. *Management Science, 32*(5). doi:10.1287/mnsc.32.5.514

Manos, D. (2009, March 25). New study shows few hospitals have comprehensive EHR. *Healthcare IT News*.

Markus, M., & Robey, D. (1988). Information technology and organizational change: Causal structure in theory and research. *Management Science, 34*(5), 583–598. doi:10.1287/mnsc.34.5.583

Niazkhani, Z., Pirnejad, H., Berg, M., & Aarts, J. (2009). The impact of computerized provider order entry systems on inpatient clinical workflow: A literature review. *Journal of the American Medical Informatics Association, 16*(4), 539–549. doi:10.1197/jamia.M2419

Noteboom, C., & Qureshi, S. (2011). Physician interaction with electronic health records: The influences of digital natives and digital immigrants. In R. Sprague & J. Nunamaker (Eds.), *The Forty-Fourth Annual Hawaii International Conference on System Sciences*. Washington, DC: IEEE Computer Society Press.

Simon, H. (1997). *Models of bounded rationality*. Cambridge, MA: The MIT Press.

Chapter 6
Primary Care Patient Management and Health Information Technology

Nina Multak
Drexel University, USA

EXECUTIVE SUMMARY

Electronic Health Records (EHR) are a system of Health Information Technology (HIT) components including clinical documentation, medication orders, laboratory and diagnostic study results, management, and evidence based clinical decision support. In this case, a patient's care is compromised because of incomplete documentation of medical information and lack of integration among data collection systems. The patient has had over fifty years of medical care in a U.S. government health system followed by care in a private primary care setting. Effective implementation and utilization of EHRs in primary care settings, will positively affect patient safety and quality of care. Appropriate use of EHR provides challenges to clinicians, HIT developers, and healthcare administrators. Provision of quality patient care utilizing HIT is challenging to use and implement, but when patients receive healthcare from multiple sources, the challenge becomes even greater. The need for integrated EHR systems is evident in the geriatric population (Ash, et al., 2009), where the ability to provide data to new clinicians may be affected by cognitive decline in this population. Management of health and chronic conditions in the geriatric population requires an ongoing commitment to HIT implementation for safer and more effective care.

DOI: 10.4018/978-1-4666-2671-3.ch006

CASE DESCRIPTION

A 70-year old man with multiple chronic medical problems relocates to a new community and seeks medical care from a local primary care provider. As a retired military officer, he has previously received care in a government health care facility. He has recently retired to Florida with his wife and seeks care in the civilian sector due to its proximity to his new home. His primary health care needs are for diabetes and cardiac disease as well as communication with an ophthalmologist, and podiatrist. Monitoring for colon cancer is needed due to a positive family history.

Following the initiation of healthcare in the private sector, the patients' medical records are requested. This patient is in need of care before the records become available and the clinician must rely on the patient to provide all necessary information about his medical history. The patient's medical condition is stable initially and the primary care physician is able to help the patient keep all medical conditions under control. After the medical records are received, data obtained from them is incorporated in to the primary care office electronic medical record system.

After becoming an established patient in the primary care practice, one of the medical conditions becomes unstable, requiring the patient to be hospitalized at the local community hospital. During the hospitalization, the patient receives a medication, which had previously caused him to have an allergic response.

This medication caused the patient to have difficulty breathing resulting in the placement of an endotracheal tube to provide him with respiratory support. Monitoring needs of the endotracheal breathing tube required the patient to be cared for in the intensive care unit. This patient required care in the intensive care unit for two weeks.

When the inpatient medical records of this patient were reviewed, there was no visible documentation of an allergy in the hospital record. Clinicians at the hospital reported that a patient history was not obtained from this patient orally because medical records from the primary care provider office had been provided. Further medical record evaluation revealed that there was documentation of the allergy in the record from the previous health care system. The inability to obtain information from medical records in an efficient manner caused a medical error, which was preventable. Providing rapid access to medical information through integrated systems would support the provision of patient safety measures.

A well trained health IT champion for this small primary care practice would support the clinicians and office staff to use electronic health records for quality patient care by: providing and documenting routine health visits, ordering and monitoring lab work and diagnostic tests, implementing standing orders for cardiac and diabetes care: annual referral to an ophthalmologist and podiatrist, order screening tests: colon cancer, prostate cancer, provide medication list and prescriptions as well as immunization needs: influenza and pneumonia vaccinations.

INTRODUCTION

Outpatient ambulatory care providers need HIT to improve outcomes and assist in the provision of effective healthcare. The exchange of information between users and collaborative decision-making about patient care using HIT systems will contribute to the development of healthcare safety protocols and enable an effective flow of information between providers and among healthcare systems. The cooperation of multiple health professionals and institutions will contribute to the development of effective systems, which meet the needs of the users and provide safer healthcare.

In this chapter, the reader will identify and describe methods of electronic data exchange utilized in the primary care setting including common challenges, identify and describe features of electronic health records which support quality care measurement (flags, alarms, charts), review the use of templates in electronic health records which provide clinician support for specific medical conditions, identify effective electronic patient education services including telemedicine and patient portals, and to identify and review issues affecting geriatric health literacy and strategies to assist these patients with health care navigation.

BACKGROUND

This case is based on healthcare received in a primary care practice in Florida. In this privately owned group practice, there are three physicians, two nurses, and two office staff workers employed full time. The age range of the patients is between 58-99 years of age. Most patients have Medicare coverage, while a small percent have insurance through private carriers. Portable tablet computers are carried between patient rooms by the physicians to document results of medical histories, physical exams, and treatment plans. Nurses enter vital signs and the reason for the office visit in a designated area on an electronic encounter form. At the completion of the office visit, patients are provided with a print out which includes the date and time of the next office visit, but no summary of medical conditions, prescription summary or recommended screening or diagnostic tests. Patients are provided a written prescription for lab work and other diagnostic studies as well as for medications as many patient use remote pharmacies for economic reasons.

Expectations for HIT suggest that it will improve patient safety. In institutions with well-developed, longstanding HIT, evidence suggests that in fact, improvements have been made (Niazkhani, et al., 2009). Electronic clinical documentation systems in the primary care setting enhances the value of EHR's by providing electronic capture of clinical notes and data exchange. Incentives have been put in place to encourage clinicians to use EHRs to improve the safety, quality, and efficiency of healthcare. An essential component of an EMR is the use and customization of templates in the documentation system. A template is a tool that organizes, presents, and captures clinical data an EHR system. The majority of certified EMRs allow for customized templates, permitting practices to gather relevant information for their work conveniently on a single screen, while populating the information into the patients' medical record. Most information in a patients chart, such as scans, x-rays, lab results, etc., require careful organization for ease of data and content retrieval.

Sophisticated Computerized Physician Order Entry (CPOE) enable clinicians to electronically order laboratory, pharmacy, and radiology services. CPOE systems offer a range of functionality, from pharmacy ordering capabilities alone to more sophisticated systems such as complete ancillary service ordering, alerting, customized order sets, and result reporting. Closing the data loop by obtaining information about results and sharing these with the patient and other providers is a needed to provide safe patient care (Poon, 2004).

Electronic prescribing using computerized provider order entry has been studied extensively in the inpatient setting, but outpatient analysis has been less extensively evaluated (Nanji, et al., 2011). Nanji et al. found that while medication and adverse medication related events were common and preventable in the ambulatory setting, using new technologies was identified as a frequent source of unintended consequences.

Clinicians have access to other automated information features, which support healthcare quality including improved organization tools, and alert screens. Alerts are an important component of EHRs because they identify medication allergies and other needed reminders. For clinical researchers, alerts can be established to assist with recruitment efforts by identifying eligible research participants. Clinician response to alerts has been studied in the inpatient setting and additional studies are needed in the outpatient setting to further evaluate.

Challenges that EHRs may present to workflow processes include: increased documentation time (slow system response, system crashes, multiple screens, etc.), decreased interdisciplinary communication, and impaired critical thinking through the overuse of checkboxes and other automated documentation. EHR implementations must coincide with workflow patterns to ensure increased efficiencies, to generate improvements in quality of care, and to realize the maximum benefits of an automated environment.

Telemedicine provides interactive healthcare utilizing technology and telecommunications. It allows patients to visit with clinicians live over video for immediate care. Capture video, still images and patient data are stored and sent to physicians for diagnosis and follow-up treatment. With appropriate training of the clinicians and patients, telemedicine could provide chronic disease management for the geriatric population who may have transportation issues.

Patients are often faced with complex medical information and treatment decisions. They must be able to locate health information, evaluate information for validity, analyze risks and benefits, and calculate medication doses. In order to accomplish these tasks, patients must be literate, able to operate a computer, able to obtain relevant information from documents, and have basic quantitative abilities. Health literacy requires individuals to have a level of ability that enables them to manage their health and the health of those in their care (Schillinger, 2002). Patient portals can be utilized to support patient communication with primary care practices.

Health literacy affects all citizens; however, there are discrepancies in prevalence and severity. Groups which are more likely to experience limited health literacy include: adults over the age of 65 years old, non-white racial and ethnic groups, immigrants, non-native speakers of English, individuals with less than a high school degree and people who are economically disadvantaged. Low levels of health literacy adversely affects management of chronic disease (Schillinger, 2002) and community health clinicians are well suited to support these populations in managing their health.

MAIN FOCUS OF THE CHAPTER

Issues, Controversies, Problems

Documentation

The impact of safer patient care using HIT involves the individuals using it, implementation, as well as the technology. Evidence in the literature identifies success, but most studies have occurred in inpatient settings (Niazkhani, 2009). Studies that evaluated outpatient settings have noted limitations, sometimes due to partial utilization of the EHR. Data is needed to analyze the safety of implementing healthcare technology. The inability to acquire this information prevents safety data from being shared. There are no reporting requirements for adverse effects. In some instances, confidentiality measures prohibit the reporting of unsafe events resulting from HIT. Software issues, human factors, and implementation challenges could be better analyzed with requirements to share knowledge.

The medical personnel in the primary care office are overwhelmed with the volume of patient care and the transition to electronic medical record keeping. The physician in the primary care practice who spearheaded the implementation of electronic documentation indicated that even with the changes they have made, there are still many hours spent with patients on the telephone, during and after office hours. Another member of the medical staff reports requesting patient records from other providers and institutions. While they wait to receive this documentation, they must rely on the information provided by the patients. Re-evaluation of workflow design and documentation tasks would be appropriate to support effective utilization of EHR.

The impact of EHR utilization in the case of Mr. S affects the transfer of knowledge about his previous care. Thorough utilization of the features in the EHR would allow his new provider a view of the care he previously was provided and the stability or fragility of the conditions which the patient was being cared for. User centered features which support the use of this technology would prevent misuse or non-use of complex data interfaces, reducing the opportunities for medical errors.

Computerized Provider Order Entry

Computerized Provider Order Entry (CPOE) has the benefit of legibility of patient orders. In the outpatient setting, medication orders can be directed to the patient's pharmacy. Although not widely studied, HIT has the capacity to track patients who meet their treatment goals. The lack of data on harmful events prevents improvements to the HIT system. CPOE systems have a more effective impact when designed for specific clinical environments and providers, with significant attention to workflow. In the case of Mr. S., patient compliance issues which may have prevented him from meeting treatment goals received little attention according to the medical documentation. Although medications for his diabetes and cardiac condition were ordered, there was no way to identify the level of patient compliance, other than the treatment goals, which he did or did not achieve. Additionally, patient phone calls to the office did not specify the detail of conversation with the nurse and whether he called for a question about his medication, symptoms, or follow up visit. This information would be helpful to the clinician in the primary care setting to help the patient meet healthcare goals.

Alerts in an EHR are effective depending on how they affect workflow (Bates, 2003). In one study, elderly patients received fewer undesired medications after the implementation of computer decision support. Alerts appear in the form of bells, flags, and pop up windows that appear while clinicians are accessing electronic medical records or entering orders in to a computer system.

Many alert systems require the clinicians to acknowledge the alert by clicking or entering an acknowledgement in the system. Alert systems must be clinically relevant in order to be effective and not cause the clinicians to ignore the alert because they appear too frequently.

Decision Support

Clinicians have the ability to use decision support systems, which are commonly integrated in to EHR systems. This feature provides evidence based information which can be accessed through the electronic medical record to support the delivery of safe care options for patients.

Utilization of HIT by consumers is growing and includes a variety of tools that patients can use to engage in their care. Patient engagement tools such as patient portals have the potential to increase patient knowledge of treatment and illnesses (Zhou, 2011). Patients who are supported in the utilization of these tools may be able to better manage their chronic illnesses and more effectively communicate with health care providers. Health literacy can be improved with access to these technologies. Opportunities for geriatric patients such as Mr. S. to utilize patient portals and telemedicine would enable him to interact with and acquire medical information relevant to his health. Although his primary method of contact with his primary care provider was by phone, his primary care office did not have a patient portal or other patient engagement tool with which he would have access to information or receive guidance using these technologies. Patient portals would allow Mr. S. to enter his own health history electronically, receive notifications for his immunizations and other lab work.

Solutions and Recommendations

Increased communication opportunities between users and developers of HIT would positively contribute to future development. Mandatory reporting of adverse events will enable analysis of root causes of medical errors including software and human error. A system with opportunity for shared learning around adverse events will support a culture of patient safety (Bates, 2003).

FUTURE RESEARCH DIRECTIONS

Informatics may be an essential tool for helping to improve patient care quality, safety, and efficiency. However, questions remain about how best to use existing technologies and evaluate the effects on the healthcare system. A great deal of research has been done on clinician behavior, but most work to date has shown implementation can be successful. Benefits in regard to clinical outcomes are not as clearly defined. Use of data for disease registries has potential, to influence health and public policy. Although additional studies are warranted, it is becoming clear that information technology is a key tool for improving patient safety.

CONCLUSION

Health information technology can provide a valuable source of data, which can be used to monitor clinical activities including detection, documentation, analysis, tracking, and identifying medical errors. Future research and policy should be guided by the efforts of multidisciplinary teams working cooperatively to improve patient safety (Bodenheimer, 2010).

REFERENCES

Ash, J. S., Sittig, D. F., Dykstra, R., Campbell, E., & Guappone, K. (2009). The unintended consequences of computerized provider order entry: Findings from a mixed methods exploration. *International Journal of Medical Informatics*, *78*(S1), S69–S76. doi:10.1016/j.ijmedinf.2008.07.015

Bates, D. W., & Gawande, A. A. (2003). Improving safety with information technology. *The New England Journal of Medicine*, *348*(25), 2526–2534. doi:10.1056/NEJMsa020847

Bodenheimer, T., & Pham, H. H. (2010). Primary care: Current problems and proposed solutions. *Health Affairs*, *29*(5), 799–805. doi:10.1377/hlthaff.2010.0026

Einbinder, J. S., & Bates, D. W. (2007). Leveraging information technology to improve quality and safety. *Yearbook of Medical Informatics*, *2007*, 22–29.

Feldstein, A. C., Vollmer, W. M., Smith, D. H., Petrik, A., Schneider, J., Glauber, H., & Herson, M. (2007). An outreach program improved osteoporosis management after a fracture. *Journal of the American Geriatrics Society*, *55*(9), 1464–1469. doi:10.1111/j.1532-5415.2007.01310.x

Nanji, K. C., Rothschild, J. M., Salzberg, C., Keohane, C. A., Zigmont, K., & Devita, J. (2011). Errors associated with outpatient computerized prescribing systems. *Journal of the American Medical Informatics Association*, *18*(6), 767–773. doi:10.1136/amiajnl-2011-000205

Niazkhani, Z., Pirnejad, H., Berg, M., & Aarts, J. (2009). The impact of computerized provider order entry systems on inpatient clinical workflow: A literature review. *Journal of the American Medical Informatics Association, 16*(4), 539–549. doi:10.1197/jamia.M2419

Poon, E. G., Gandhi, T. K., Sequist, T. D., Murff, H. J., Karson, A. S., & Bates, D. W. (2004). I wish I had seen this test result earlier! Dissatisfaction with test result management systems in primary care. *Archives of Internal Medicine, 164*(20), 2223–2228. doi:10.1001/archinte.164.20.2223

Ryan, J. (2007). Will patients agree to have their literacy skills assessed in clinical practice? *Advance Access, 23*(4), 603–611.

Schillinger, D. (2002). Association of health literacy with diabetes outcomes. *Journal of the American Medical Association, 288*(4). doi:10.1001/jama.288.4.475

Shah, N. R., Seger, A. C., Seger, D. L., Fiskio, J. M., Kuperman, G. L., & Blumenfeld, B. (2006). Improving acceptance of computerized prescribing alerts in ambulatory care. *Journal of the American Medical Informatics Association, 13*(1), 5–11. doi:10.1197/jamia.M1868

Smith, D. H., Perrin, N., Feldstein, A., Yang, X. H., Kuang, D., & Simon, S. R. (2006). The impact of prescribing safety alerts for elderly persons in an electronic medical record—An interrupted time series evaluation. *Archives of Internal Medicine, 166*(10), 1098–1104. doi:10.1001/archinte.166.10.1098

Wright, A., Pang, J., Feblowitz, J. C., Maloney, F. L., Wilcox, A. R., & Ramelson, H. Z. (2011). A method and knowledge base for automated inference of patient problems from structured data in an electronic medical record. *Journal of the American Medical Informatics Association, 18*(6), 859–867. doi:10.1136/amiajnl-2011-000121

Zhou, Y. Y., Unitan, R., Wang, J. J., Garrido, T., Chin, H. L., Turley, M. C., & Radler, L. (2011). Improving population care with an integrated electronic panel support tool. *Population Health Management, 14*(1), 3–9. doi:10.1089/pop.2010.0001

Chapter 7
Good IT Requires Good Communication

Charles H Andrus
Saint Louis University, USA

Mark Gaynor
Saint Louis University, USA

EXECUTIVE SUMMARY

Electronic Medical Records (EMR) in academic medical centers often have additional complexity to them due to structural and organizational differences. Often the hospital operates independent of the medical school such as the physicians often work for the medical school, while the nurses and other ancillary departments work for the hospital. Such differences require special consideration when making changes to an EMR. The case study concerns an academic medical center where there are two ways to access the EMR. One methodology is to use a clinical computer on clinical floors within the hospital. A second methodology is the use of Citrix servers to access the EMR. Due to organizational differences, the EMR users access the system via two separate sets of Citrix servers. The hospital's support staff controls one set of Citrix servers and the academic support staff controls the other set. Physicians and mid-level providers utilize the academic Citrix servers, but nursing and other ancillary departments use the hospital's Citrix servers. With the servers controlled by separate teams, careful coordination is needed to ensure uniformity across the servers for a consistent user experience.

DOI: 10.4018/978-1-4666-2671-3.ch007

CASE STUDY

Over the past few weeks, the acute care EMR team worked with their in-house developers, John and Jason, to design and create a new module to improve clinical workflow in the electronic medical record. The hospital of the academic medical center owned the acute care EMR; therefore the EMR IT staff were hospital employees. The clinicians who tested and reviewed the module believed it offered increased efficiency to the workflow for the organization. Further, the new module also excited the Clinical Analytics Team because the module provided additional data for rich data analysis to improve patient care and generate regulatory reports with greater ease.

The EMR team, excited by the acceptance and overall enthusiasm around the new module contacted the hospital's Information Systems Support team (IS Support) to inquire the necessary steps required to place the module into production. The manager of IS Support, Mike, said it required an installation into the SQL database and an installation to all the hospital clinical PCs and Citrix servers. He further explained the physician group had a separate set of Citrix servers managed by a different team that would also need to install the module. Mike estimated it would take a week for each of these tasks to be done, though he believed each respective team could do them simultaneously. Therefore, Mike told the EMR team in two weeks the module would be in place and could be used in the EMR. In addition, Mike volunteered to create work requisitions for the install and coordinate between the various support teams for both the hospital and academic Citrix servers. The EMR team communicated a three-week timeline to the clinicians in the hospital, which included the academic physicians, just as an additional precaution.

Three days prior to the installation of the module by the support teams, Mike e-mailed John to explain the EMR was having production problems that needed to be fixed prior to introducing a new module. Therefore, Mike recommended the install be pushed back two days; however, this still allowed the EMR team to meet their go-live deadline for the clinicians. John verbally communicated this information to several key members in the EMR team. Everyone agreed they could still meet the intended deadline.

On Sunday, three days later, Jason tested the module on the hospital's clinical PCs and Citrix servers. He also noticed the support team still had not made the appropriate changes to the database and that the Citrix servers did not yet have the module. Thus, he sent an e-mail to John and Mike explaining he noticed the discrepancy in the Citrix servers. Mike responded he would look into it tomorrow. Mike included other IS Support members were on the response e-mail, however, the e-mail did not include any EMR IT staff.

At 8:30 AM on Tuesday, John just sat down to an off campus meeting. He was excited since he knew the module would go-live soon, support just needed to make sure it was installed on all the correct PCs and servers prior. He decided to check his e-mail before the meeting began. He saw three new e-mails with the subject simply "Call me!" from Betsy, an EMR team member. John immediately excused himself from the room and called her. Betsy explained she had placed the link to the new module into the EMR this morning and clinicians excitedly began using it. However, the clinicians reported they were unable to use the module from the Citrix servers and were very upset. Julie, the manager of the EMR team, was very upset because the team was losing user credibility, especially since the EMR had production problems last week.

John could not believe it. What had gone wrong? He immediately called Julie to discuss the current status. Julie explained they had taken the link out of production so it would not negatively impact the clinicians until they could resolve the problem. She then explained that she had just spoken with Mike and who claimed he never realized there was a specific go-live date. He also claimed he did not realize he should have installed the module on the Citrix servers at the same time as the clinical PCs. Mike further stated he had not yet contacted the academic Citrix server support group.

After tremendous pressure from Julie, Mike's team was able to install the module on every PC and Citrix server. However, it took 24 hours from the initial mistake to resolve the issue. Some clinicians had noticed the mistake and it hurt the EMR team's credibility. Luckily, the clinicians considered the module a complete success, which improved the overall credibility of the EMR team. Yet John and Mike thought to the future and realized there were several new modules required in the coming months with similar installations. They had to make sure everything went smoothly so their programs were not blamed for interfering with patient care. They thought about what they could have done better to mitigate such a disaster.

LESSONS LEARNED

This case occurred not because of poor development or configuration, but rather repeated miscommunications. Many people conversed verbally and via e-mail about mission critical information, yet not all information was sent to each stakeholder. Part of the disaster could have been avoided if the EMR team knew the Citrix servers were not ready, which would have occurred if all communication were more robust. The EMR team could have delayed the link install, thereby preventing the clinicians from experiencing unnecessary errors. Though some credibility might have been lost with the inability to meet the go-live date, much less credibility would have been lost in comparison.

The EMR team also should have taken a more active role in making sure the module was installed by IS Support. Though trust of other teams is an important aspect of the workplace, status reports are necessary to ensure an IT project proceeds as planned. The EMR IT team should establish a well-defined roadmap in the so each stakeholder is aware of the expectations. If more status reports had occurred, the communication and overall installation would likely have improved. Most importantly, one should not assume a change was made successfully. Instead, status reports and inquiries are vital to ensure the project completes each milestone on the roadmap.

Chapter 8
Telehealth Implementation:
The Voice of Experience

Mary DeVany
University of Minnesota, USA

Marilyn Penticoff
University of Minnesota, USA

Karla Knobloch-Ludwig
Infectious Disease Specialists, USA

Aris Assimacopoulos
Infectious Disease Specialists, USA

Stuart Speedie
University of Minnesota, USA

EXECUTIVE SUMMARY

Improving the opportunity to access care by infectious disease specialists and improve the overall quality of care received is the core mission demonstrated by this clinic through the on-going and continued development of their telehealth services program. This focus does not remove the need for the clinic to adhere to sound business practices. Instead, this case demonstrates that both focuses can be appropriately accomplished. Current regulatory issues will continue to pose challenges, but these barriers are not significant enough to shut down the enthusiasm for continuing this service or for future expansion plans. This study will discuss the benefits of telehealth not only to patients, but also to the clinic practice as a whole.

DOI: 10.4018/978-1-4666-2671-3.ch008

ORGANIZATION BACKGROUND

Infectious Disease Specialists, PC (IDS) is a small independently owned and operated clinic providing clinical services for patients requiring an Infectious Disease (ID) specialist. This clinic has been in active practice since 2001. There are currently three providers (all MDs) with a fourth coming in 2012. At this time there are no Physicians Assistant's (PA) on staff. A Nurse Practitioner (NP) focusing on wound care has recently joined the practice. A previous office manager, working during the time of initial implementation, was generally supportive of advancing this effort. However, their current office manager has extensive knowledge of telehealth, having first worked in their clinic when they initiated telemedicine services, then also working in a hospital-based telehealth services program, before returning to the clinic as manager. This knowledge base has been very beneficial as they plan and develop the expansion of their current clinic services.

The number of physicians who specialize in infectious diseases practicing in this extended service area is very limited and highly regionalized. There are currently 8-10 physicians that serve the entire state of South Dakota (and into neighboring states). These physicians are located in Sioux Falls (the eastern-most border) and Rapid City (the western-most border), approximately 350 miles apart. The service area of this Sioux Falls-based healthcare practice is highly rural and it reaches into southwestern Minnesota, northwestern Iowa, and northeastern Nebraska, and southeastern North Dakota. They actively serve approximately 50 clinical locations and receive referrals from 70+ providers throughout the region (see Figure 1).

While remaining an independent clinic, the IDS clinic office space has been located on the main campus of one of the two major health systems in the region, both systems headquartering out of Sioux Falls. Because of the presence of an active telehealth program being operated within this hospital, this particular location allowed for their initial exposure to the idea of telehealth, in general, and specifically patient-focused telemedicine services.

SETTING THE STAGE

Infectious Disease Specialists (IDS) is based out of Sioux Falls, the largest city in South Dakota, which also is home to the region's two largest healthcare systems. Unfortunately, the availability of infectious disease specialists remains extremely limited. The highly rural and frontier nature of the region also makes accessing specialized care services very challenging for patients and their families.

Prior to the implementation of telehealth, the services of an ID specialist were accessed through one of the following ways: 1) the patient would come to the physi-

Figure 1. Primary service region of IDS

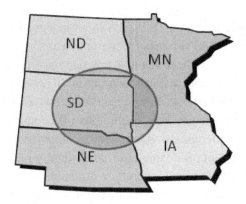

cal location of the clinic for an in-person appointment, often from hours away; 2) if the patient's illness was at a critical level, the patient would likely be transferred to a Sioux Falls-based hospital for care and the ID specialist would see them as an in-patient; 3) the physician would schedule time to come to a community for a periodic (maybe monthly or quarterly) outreach clinic, requiring the physician to leave Sioux Falls and putting in extensive "wind-shield" time; or 4) the patient's primary care provider would pick up the telephone and discuss the case with the ID specialist, hoping for additional insight regarding his patient's illness. The final option was a frequent occurrence and one for which the specialist's time and expertise was not compensated. An unfortunate outcome was that often providers would simply "wing it," sometimes leading to further complications. In many cases, patients simply did not or could not gain access to these specialized services, which many times meant that their overall care was compromised, sometimes significantly.

In an effort to enhance the quality of care patients receive, increase access to their services, reduce the amount of time spent out of their office on outreach clinics, and reduce the number of un-paid "curb-side consults," IDS began investigating the potential utilization of telehealth technologies as part of their clinic offerings.

Their initial steps into telemedicine services were encouraged by the lead physician in the practice. Quickly he became their champion for the development, and then expansion, of telemedicine services within their clinic. The understanding of the benefits telemedicine services had for patients, as well as the clinic practice itself, developed into a vision for long-term service availability and over-all expansion. As the clinical champion, he has worked to encourage and educate those within his own clinic as well as those in the greater healthcare community, both locally and nationally, about the value telemedicine services had for a highly rural region with limited (often highly limited) specialized clinical resources.

Their introduction, and their on-going service development, was initially encouraged through a partnership developed with the hospital's telehealth staff. The telehealth program's clinical coordinator (a registered nurse) worked closely with the rural locations from where the patients were seen, educating them on proper patient presentation skills and the collection of important patient information needed prior to and during a patient interaction. She also worked with the IDS clinic providers and staff, training them on equipment operation and learning their clinical needs, in order to support and encourage a smooth and successful patient event.

Early on in their program, this clinic conducted an informal chart review to evaluate the impact of their initial services and to raise awareness regarding the need to improve the care patients were receiving regarding their various diseases. This review indicated that, prior to IDS becoming involved in their care, approximately one quarter of the patients reviewed were on an inappropriate dose of antibiotics, or they were on an antibiotic that was not even necessary. In an age when the use of antibiotics appears to be increasing and where "super-bugs" are becoming resistant to the antibiotics we rely on, this is an issue of major concern.

The providers in this clinic understood that their ability to positively impact a patient's care was being hampered by their inability to provide their level of specialty care when a patient most needed it. This often resulted in several things: a delay in the delivery of appropriate care (or the provision of inappropriate care); an increased cost of that care, some of which may have been covered by insurance (increased hospital stay), and some which were often shouldered by the patient and family (increased travel expenses); a decrease in that patient's quality of life (increased stress, decreased overall health); and an increase in the length of time required to successfully manage the care of that patient.

CASE DESCRIPTION

Clinical telemedicine services were initiated in fiscal year 2002 purely as a test and any real level of growth did not occur until about three years following that first trial consult. As indicated in Figure 2, the number of patients seen annually by telemedicine has seen significant growth every year since the service was implemented.

Technology Concerns

The primary concern regarding the use of this technology was, as is usually the case for telemedicine services, will the technology allow for an adequate transfer of patient information to provide a beneficial and accurate clinical service to the patient. The secondary concern was whether the interaction could be performed in a manner

Figure 2. Number of telemedicine patients seen annually since service began

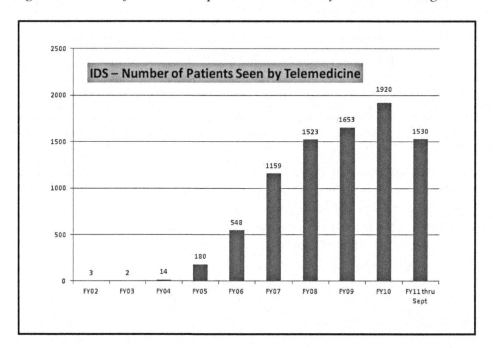

that would be similar enough to an in-person patient visit, in both experience and in time used, to make it a functional component of a clinic practice. In general, the question was whether the technology would get in the way of quality patient care.

In order to answer the question of technology getting in the way of quality patient care, this clinic conducted a research study, published in 2008, that compared the outcomes of patients seen utilizing telemedicine technologies to patients seen through standard in-person visits. This study indicated that, for the illnesses studied, the care received through the use of telemedicine technologies was very similar in quality to the care received in-person. (Assimacopoulos, 2008) This study focused on in-patient (hospital-based) services and lends support to the premise that telehealth services are an effective form of healthcare delivery, especially for rural patients.

Technology Components

The primary technology utilized in this practice is interactive videoconferencing. For the first couple of years, the physicians used a room-based video unit located in the hospital's telehealth department. This option, while cost-effective from an equipment perspective, was challenging from a practice management perspective. Whenever a patient was to be seen for a telemedicine visit, the physician was required to leave their practice space, take time away from their clinic practice (and patients) to walk over to the telemedicine room in the middle of the hospital. This also meant that the tools and processes they knew in their own work environment were not easily accessible and could not be easily and smoothly followed.

Later, the clinic obtained equipment to be located within their clinic space. This allowed for a smoother practice management process. A nurse and/or physician could easily go from seeing a patient in-person in one clinic room, then move over to the clinic room next door where they would see their next patient for a telemedicine visit. This allowed them to follow their standard clinic processes for scheduling, patient records, and on-going patient communications.

In addition to the standard videoconferencing unit, this practice also utilizes an electronic stethoscope and a hand-held auxiliary examination camera. These tools allow the provider access to more of the information they would normally collect during a traditional patient visit: heart sounds, lung sounds, a closer view of the skin or body part, a look inside a patient's mouth, and more. While the provider does rely on the nurse presenting the patient at the remote location to serve as their hands in many situations, these additional tools increase the providers ability to obtain much of the same information as they would have in an in-person visit. During the visit, they are also able to provide direction and encouragement to remote personnel to assist them in obtaining additional patient images and information.

Management and Organizational Concerns

The primary goal was to allow patients the opportunity to have their care supported by an ID physician while not being forced to leave their home community for every appointment. This goal proved obtainable, but it took time to identify the appropriate steps to implementation.

Organizational preparation was an important component to this successful program. Training for both sides of the patient event was significant and required several focuses. One obvious piece was becoming familiar with the actual equipment being used for the interaction. In order for the patient information to be transmitted successfully and completely, knowledge of how to operate all components of the equipment and the necessary peripheral equipment (electronic stethoscope, auxiliary camera, etc.) is required. This responsibility falls more heavily on the location where the patient is located since the images originate there.

Ensuring that the connection and interaction is successful is often facilitated through the implementation of formal processes. The development of these processes is something that has occurred over years but now they occur simultaneously with the equipment component to facilitate a smooth service initiation. Developing these processes has required an understanding of clinic operations from both the specialists' perspective and the remote facility's perspective. Expectations must be realistic when establishing the processes for scheduling, equipment testing, patient presentation, and other aspects of a successful telemedicine patient event. This goal was accomplishable because there was a sincere focus on improving patient care. Unfortunately, this is not a one-time event when a new site comes on line. Because of the turnover of staff at all locations, training on both equipment and process is an on-going need and focus.

Another component of training revolves around being able to build and manage a relationship through the technology. This applies not only to the relationship with the patient but also to the relationship with the local healthcare provider assisting the patient. It is likely that the remote provider is not highly versed in the care of infectious disease patients and may require direction during the patient visit. The specialist needed to develop a method for communicating through the equipment that could provide adequate and professional, yet kindly, direction to the healthcare provider assisting the patient. It is important to provide any direction in a manner that builds skills without diminishing the worth of these professionals. Appropriate communication through the technology is important in order to build and enhance the relationship with patients as well. A patient may not be able to identify specifically what made them feel uncomfortable about the telehealth visit, just simply that they did not like it. The physicians at IDS have learned the importance of eye contact through the equipment. This works to build and enhance the relationships with their patients, and ultimately positively impacts their care as well.

As with many things, if people do not know about something, they will not know to use it. Making patients and remote healthcare locations aware that these telemedicine services are available is important. IDS has approached this in three ways. The first is to work with personnel at regional hospitals and clinics where telemedicine technologies are available to make them aware of their services and to confirm technological connectivity. The second is to communicate with healthcare providers in the region to make them aware that services are available to assist their patients, often from within their own community. The third is to inform their patients directly. This is done either at the time of their in-person visit, where they share various options for follow-up, or in supplemental information like their website, where their option for telemedicine is described (see Figure 3).

CURRENT CHALLENGES FACING THE ORGANIZATION

This clinic deals with various challenges in the on-going provision of telemedicine services. These challenges are not viewed as overwhelming, but they are issues that require regular attention, understanding, and planning.

Figure 3. Website snapshot

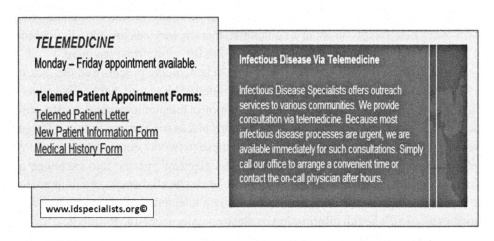

Service expansion is a challenge that really has two prongs. The first is the co-ordination, support, and management of additional locations that are interested in receiving services. The second is having enough professionals to provide the services needed by those locations. Both of these issues will need to be appropriately managed in order to maintain a strong and consistent service, not only for the newly served locations, but also for those who are long-standing as IDS service facilities.

The laws and regulations that direct both provider licensing and hospital credentialing pose a fairly daunting barrier for continued and expanded telemedicine services. Healthcare providers are required by law to be licensed in the state(s) where they provide services. This includes the state where their primary clinic is located, the states where they go, in-person, to provide outreach clinics, and the states where their telemedicine patients are located. Obtaining these licenses is often complicated, time consuming and expensive. Additionally, these licenses must also be renewed, which requires replicating this expensive process at every renewal.

Credentialing is a process required by hospitals to adequately identify providers, understand their skills and their ability to appropriately care for the patients receiving services within their walls. It is a process that requires physicians to provide proof of their education, their licenses, places where they practice, adverse events, and more. They are required to provide this information for each hospital where they provide services, both in-person and by telemedicine technologies. This process is also highly time consuming (requiring updates when additional facilities are added) and very costly since often original documents are required.

While current reimbursement policies cover most patient services provided by this clinic, it still requires knowledge and understanding of the special requirements to ensure telemedicine services are reimbursed to their fullest level. To add to the complication, internal organizational reimbursement (billing) processes, often connected to the HIT requirements and processes, need to be consulted and addressed with every new facility in order to guarantee that the services are actually making it through the financial maze of the organization for appropriate payment.

An electronic medical record supports the telemedicine process and the lack of a fully operational and fully integrated electronic health record can be viewed as a significant challenge to the successful continuation of telemedicine services. Because patient information is often "housed" in various electronic formats within different health systems' HIT networks, and because these networks currently are not fully interconnected to allow for easy and seamless electronic access and exchange of that information when needed for patient care, it can be challenging gaining access to a patient's complete medical file. Following a telemedicine event, the provider updates a patient's health information by electronically accessing the medical record through a password process, unique to each facility, and then dictating directly into that patient's medical record. A different method is often necessary for each facility where services are provided making it a cumbersome, time-consuming process.

Keeping equipment up-to-date can be expensive and complicated. This includes not only the maintenance of current equipment, but also planning for the next generation of technology. Making sure that the equipment which is relied upon to provide patient care is always available is challenging. The cost of service contracts and the time involved with trouble-shooting are on-going issues, both budgetarily and functionally. In addition, equipment changes regularly and it is important to plan for the next generation, even while still fully utilizing current technology. Because of the current need to reach their patients in an appropriate healthcare facility (for reimbursement purposes), the need for compatibility with regional health systems' telehealth networks is a vital component surrounding the success of this clinic service. While the flexibility of the technology is shifting to allow connection into patients' homes, workplaces, and other locations, the regulatory environment has not made this option currently available. However, planning and preparing for this change is a piece of equal importance to maintaining current operations.

Bringing a new site on line requires time and patience. Because not everyone is equal in their acceptance and understanding of telehealth technologies and telemedicine services, this can be a challenging task. As indicated above, understanding and teaching appropriate process and skills for telemedicine events can be challenging and time consuming. Having an interested and willing provider at the patient location is often the key to success. Even if primary care providers and clinic administration are supportive, a nurse that is a begrudging patient presenter can quickly sabotage the service.

SOLUTIONS AND RECOMMENDATIONS

Recently, the clinic has rehired as clinic manager, a nurse that initially served as their primary telehealth nurse coordinator. This has helped to ensure the continuation of strong support for on-going telemedicine services. There are plans being considered for the addition of new services and providers. However, in order to continue with current plans for service continuation and expansion, the challenges indicated above will need to be addressed as part of their overall strategic plan since it is not likely that they will be fully resolved in the near future.

In November of 2011, the clinic moved into a new location, several miles away from their previous place of business. This new location is detached from the campuses of both major health systems, removing the perception of allegiance to one system over the other, simply based upon clinic location. It is anticipated that this will encourage service expansion to facilities from all regional health systems. Additional efforts will likely be needed in order to equalize relations with the various regional health systems and the communities and patients they serve. This new location will also better support the additional providers that are scheduled to join the practice, both physicians and nurse practitioners. It is anticipated that the addition of these providers will help to support the current requests for services, as well as the anticipated increase over the next few years.

Unfortunately, the provider licensing challenges are not expected to be resolved in the near future. While it is an issue that is currently receiving a level of attention at the federal level, it is also an issue that could be highly contentious as it is of importance to states' and their right to protect their citizens. It is also a financial issue for the state licensure boards. There is certainly value to the establishment of a license structure and process that allows providers to cross state borders in a simpler manner than is currently in place. However, with the special interests surrounding this issue, a quick resolution is not anticipated. Knowing this, it is anticipated that the clinic must continue to approach their licensure requirements in a manner similar to their current process. This established process, while costly and time-consuming, is a known challenge that currently cannot be addressed without changes at both state and federal levels. Work should also begin at a state level to educate regulatory leaders regarding this issue.

The credentialing process is another challenge that is outside of the control of the clinic. This process (specific to hospitals) is established and directed by those facilities. It will be helpful to the clinic to educate the client facilities regarding the recent change/relaxation of the credentialing requirements by the Centers for Medicare and Medicaid Services. This change allows a hospital, which is receiving the specialty services to accept, by agreement, the credentials from the hospital of the provider's primary services. This applies when a patient is seen by telemedicine either as an inpatient at the remote hospital, or when the patient enters the hospital as an outpatient visit. Fortunately, this process does not apply to services provided to locations outside of the hospital structure. When possible, opportunities should be considered for providing services in other appropriate locations.

Reimbursement is yet another area of challenge where the clinic does not have a great deal of control. While additional patient services are submitted every year to be added to the "allowed" list, the overall process is arduous and slow. It is important to evaluate all new services to determine if they are covered under the already approved codes and if they fall within the current rules. This is another area where building awareness among regulatory and legislative leaders, at both state and federal levels, regarding the importance of expanding telehealth reimbursement coverage could prove helpful.

Regarding the internal, electronic process of getting paid for the service(s) provided, it will often fall to the clinic staff to educate each new service location regarding the processes that will be necessary in order to get the covered service through the organization's financial billing process and appropriately paid by the payer (Medicare, Medicaid, insurance, etc.). This includes establishing a location code for telehealth (if necessary) and other processes unique to each organization's electronic billing system.

Even though a fully interoperable health information exchange is not currently in place, the current ability to access patient records electronically is critical to this service. Ultimately, improving patient care is the primary focus. Even though the current process is far from seamless, it provides access to important information for the specialists as they provide their care, and then back to the primarily care provider as they manage the on-going care of their patient. Avoiding duplicated records, duplicated tests, and the risk of missing information are all reasons why this access is valuable.

Equipment and technology are ever changing. Staying on top of what is considered legacy (i.e. room-based videoconferencing equipment), current (i.e. desktop units), and future technologies (i.e. Web-based solutions and smartphone-based applications) is a never-ending task. Understanding where the current and future technologies fit in with the current regulatory requirements is very difficult and industry messages are often mixed. Unfortunately, this is not expected to change. The decision is often where do they want to lead and where would they rather follow. This determination will likely vary with each service opportunity that is identified and it often centers on two points: 1) identifying what is the level of acceptable risk, and 2) what will the budget support.

Currently, the willingness of the partner facilities and referring providers to assist with the telemedicine services is critical to the on-going success of this service. It is a piece that IS within their control. This clinic has developed an understanding of the value of being flexible, supportive, and patient with new providers and new facilities. Understanding that not everyone is comfortable using technology is one key to establishing a successful service. Working with healthcare facilities to identify those individuals interested in this expanded service will support their ability to provide a successful service. In addition, remembering the value of on-going training for active sites will help to maintain and enhance current services. This is sometimes the most difficult of the challenges because it revolves around individuals and relationships, which are ever changing.

CONCLUSION

Over these past years, the providers and leaders of this clinic have determined that the benefits for both their patients and their strategic planning out-weigh those challenges indicated above. They have determined that telemedicine is a service that makes sense in the rural area they serve. Their level of telemedicine services have expanded over the years to a point where some weeks they will see more telemedicine patients than they do in-person clinic patients.

Now that the foundation is in place and the system is polished and refined, they have found that there is no real difference in seeing patients in-person or face-to-face via telemedicine. They have also found that a patient's compliance with their care plan, for both the follow-up with inpatient discharges as well as the chronically ill patients, have risen with the ability to see them in their hometown setting and not burdening them with excessive travel. It is an option, which is automatically offered to patients, allowing them the opportunity to decide how they would like to schedule their follow-up visits. It is strongly encouraged for those who find it difficult to come on-site for appointments.

Infectious Disease Specialists, LLC is excited about what they see as their future with telemedicine, specifically from two viewpoints: 1) as a vital component to the financial success of their over-all clinic practice and 2) as a tool they can use to improve the care of their patients, especially those residing in the more rural and frontier communities of their service area. Success in both areas allows them to stay focused on their primary mission, providing quality patient care.

REFERENCES

American Telemedicine Association. (2011). *Removing medical licensure barriers: Increasing consumer choice, improving safety and cutting costs for patients across America*. Retrieved November 15, 2011, from http://www.fixlicensure.org

Assimacopoulos, A., Alam, R., Arbo, M., Nazir, J., Chen, D., Weaver, S., ... Ageton, C. (2008, October). A brief retrospective review of medical records comparing outcomes for inpatients treated via telehealth versus in-person protocols: Is tele-health equally effective as in-person visits for treating neutropenic fever, bacterial pneumonia, and infected bacterial wounds?. *Telemedicine and e-Health*, 762-768.

Department of Health and Human Services, Centers for Medicare and Medicaid Services. (2011). Medicare and medicaid programs: Changes affecting hospital and critical access hospital conditions of participation: Telemedicine credentialing and privileging. *Federal Register*, *76*(87), 25550–25565. Retrieved from http://www.gpo.gov/fdsys/pkg/FR-2011-05-05/pdf/2011-10875.pdf

Department of Health and Human Services, Centers for Medicare and Medicaid Services. (2011). *Medicare learning network: Telehealth services, rural health fact sheet series*. Retrieved from https://www.cms.gov/MLNProducts/downloads/TelehealthSrvcsfctsht.pdf

Physician Licensure. (2011). *Center for telehealth and e-health law*. Retrieved November 15, 2011, from http://www.ctel.org/expertise/physican-licensure/

KEY TERMS AND DEFINITIONS

Center for Medicare and Medicaid Services: This federal agency, housed within the U.S. Department of Health and Human Services, regulates much of the healthcare provided in the United States and provides for a significant amount of the payment (reimbursement) of those services.

Credentialing: The process used by healthcare organizations to establish the qualifications of licensed professional and assess their clinical background and legitimacy. The process is generally an evaluation of a healthcare professional's current licensure, training or experience, and competency to provide a particular service or procedure.

Electronic Stethoscope: A device that allows for auscultated sounds such as heart and lung sounds to be transmitted from one location to another via electronic communications.

Frontier: Describes an area with scarce population (6 people or less per square mile) and highly limited healthcare services (primary care, or otherwise). Again, depending on the program, the applicable definition will vary.

Healthcare Provider: This can include a physician, a Physician's Assistant (PA), an advanced practice nurse, a clinical social worker, a dentist, a nurse, a physical/occupational therapist, or others.

Infectious Diseases: Diseases caused by the entrance into the body of organisms (as bacteria, protozoans, fungi, or viruses) which grow and multiply there (Webster's Medical, 2012).

Interactive Videoconferencing: Two-way, interactive video and audio signals which allows both ends of the connection to see and hear each other in "live time" throughout the course of the event.

Rural: When used for healthcare purposes, this indicates communities and areas outside of large urban centers, which have limited access to healthcare services, especially specialized care. This designation varies depending upon which federal program is being considered. There are three primary definitions utilized (US Census Bureau, Federal Office of Management and Budget, and USDA Economic Research Service), the main factors considered are population and distance from an urban area.

Telehealth: An "umbrella-term" used to describe the exchanging of health-related information from one location to another utilizing some form of electronic communications to improve a patient's health and/or wellness.

Telemedicine: The utilization of telehealth technologies for the purposes of actual patient care, often utilizing interactive audio/video technologies (but not exclusively).

Chapter 9
Avera Medical Group Pierre's Implementation of an eConsult Program:
Bringing Specialty Practices to Patients in Rural South Dakota

Ann Pommer
Avera Medical Group Pierre, USA

EXECUTIVE SUMMARY

The manner in which health care is delivered to patients has evolved significantly through the years. Technology has played an important role in that evolution. This case study explores one way health care organizations are investing in advanced health care technologies to deliver services to patients when the patients are not in the same room as the providers. This study explores the implementation of an eConsult program, also known as telemedicine, at Avera Medical Group Pierre. This study will discuss the process of implementing an eConsult program, the equipment needed to provide eConsults, privacy, and billing concerns, and the facility's future plans for expanding the telemedicine services they offer. Overall, this case study strives to show that implementing telemedicine can be a relatively easy process of embracing technology, which can greatly benefit patients.

DOI: 10.4018/978-1-4666-2671-3.ch009

ORGANIZATIONAL BACKGROUND

Avera Medical Group Pierre is located in Pierre, South Dakota. It is a multi-specialty clinic and ambulatory surgical center that provides services to the more than 17,000 residents in Pierre and Fort Pierre areas. More than 30 providers work at Avera Medical Group Pierre. This includes family practice and internal medicine physicians, general surgeons, and specialists in obstetrics and gynecology, orthopedics, urology, podiatry, neurology, and physical medicine and rehabilitation. On an average day, between 200 to 400 patients come through the doors of Avera Medical Group Pierre to use the clinic's services or to undergo a procedure in the ambulatory surgical center.

Avera Medical Group Pierre was once known as Medical Associates Clinic and was provider-owned and operated. On January 1, 2009, it became part of Avera, which has headquarters in Sioux Falls, South Dakota. Avera McKennan Hospital and several clinics are located in Sioux Falls. Other regional hospitals in the organization, along with additional healthcare facilities, are in 300 locations in South Dakota and the surrounding states. Avera Medical Group Pierre has been in growth mode ever since becoming part of Avera by actively recruiting new physicians and expanding health services the clinic and surgical center offer. Part of that expansion included implementing an eConsult program.

SETTING THE STAGE

Avera Medical Group Pierre has always embraced technology to improve operations. In 2005, the clinic converted its paper medical record process to an Electronic Health Record (EHR) system. As of 2011, approximately 90% of the clinic's documentation processes take place electronically. The EHR system the clinic integrated has components including computerized physician order entry, a laboratory information system, and a clinical decision support system. The conversion to an EHR has sped up coding and billing, record retrieval, transcription documentation management, and other processes. Technology can also be found in the Radiology Department where staff use a picture archiving and communication system, which has improved operations associated with medical images. The clinic also encourages its patients to use technology. On the clinic's website are forms for patient information, notice of privacy practices, and HIPAA acknowledgement. Patients can print these forms at their convenience and fill out prior to their appointment at the clinic. This process speeds up registration time, which can be a great benefit for patients who are not feeling well.

Key Players

- **Marnie Burke, MPA, RN:** Director of Patient Care at Avera Medical Group Pierre.
- **Cathy Niklason:** eConsult Coordinator for Avera.
- **Laurie Gill:** Clinic Administrator at Avera Medical Group Pierre during the time the eConsult program was implemented.

CASE DESCRIPTION

Beginning Steps

Telemedicine is defined as the use of interactive audio and visual technologies to exchange medical information for diagnostic, monitoring, and therapeutic purposes when clinicians and patients are separated by distance. The distance that some of Avera Medical Group Pierre's patients live from some specialists was a fundamental factor in deciding to bring telemedicine to the clinic. The cities of Pierre and Fort Pierre, connected by a bridge spanning the Missouri River, are in a very distinct rural area. The cities are centrally located in South Dakota. The nearest large cities are Rapid City, which is almost 170 miles to the west, and Sioux Falls, which is more than 220 miles to the east. Several of Avera Medical Group Pierre's patients live in the small towns that surround Pierre and Fort Pierre, such as Blunt, Onida, and Highmore. A number of patients live farther away in towns such as Faulkton and Chamberlain. Some of Avera Medical Group Pierre's doctors perform outreach services and travel to nearby towns to see patients. However, even with the outreach services, Avera Medical Group Pierre did not feel it was meeting the demand it wanted in services offered to patients. Prior to the implementation of the eConsult program at the clinic, referring patients to a specialist usually meant sending them on a long drive to Sioux Falls or Rapid City. An important reason for bringing an eConsult program to the clinic was so patients did not have to leave the Pierre and Fort Pierre areas in order to receive specialty care that was not physically offered at the clinic.

When the clinic and ambulatory surgical center became part of Avera at the beginning of 2009, it was during a rough economic time for the United States. That tough economy did not overlook Avera. However, a grant was available that made the idea of bringing an eConsult program to the clinic a possibility. Discussions began in January 2011, and Laurie Gill, administrator of Avera Medical Group Pierre at the time, immediately agreed to the idea. In March 2011, Cathy Niklason, eConsult Coordinator for Avera, traveled to Pierre with other staff members to install the equipment. They also trained Avera Medical Group Pierre staff members on how to operate the equipment, schedule eConsult appointments, and bill eConsult services. The first patient to use telemedicine at Avera Medical Group Pierre was seen on April 27, 2011, less than four months after initial discussions about implementing an eConsult program.

An eConsult Encounter

An eConsult encounter begins the same way as a face-to-face patient encounter: the primary care physician refers the patient to a specialist. The specialist will send the patient a patient information packet to complete and bring with to the visit. From this point on, elements involved with an eConsult start to differ from a regular consultation. On the day of the appointment, the patient returns to the primary care physician's office (referred to as the originating site) and checks in at the reception desk. The nurse takes the patient to the eConsult exam room, takes the patient's vitals, completes a nursing assessment, and reviews the eConsult process with the patient. The nurse faxes the assessment and vitals, along with the patient information packet if necessary, to the specialty clinic (referred to as the distant or specialty site). After the documentation is faxed, the nurse advises the specialty site that the patient is ready for the eConsult to begin. The specialty site initiates the call to the originating site and the eConsult begins telephonically with the patient viewing the doctor on a television monitor and vice versa. The specialty site provider completes documentation in the patient's medical record at the specialty site and sends a copy to the referring provider. Both the originating and specialty sites bill for their parts in the eConsult.

Environment and Technology Components

The entire process of implementing the eConsult program at Avera Medical Group Pierre took only four months. A reason for this quick process could be attributed to the fact that Avera already had 58 facilities offering eConsults before implementing the program at the Pierre clinic. Avera has six staff members dedicated to eConsults. When an eConsult program is implemented at one of the Avera facilities, the eConsult staff provides that facility with an information and training manual. The manual is a brief 25 pages, but it has critical information that is helpful during the training process and can also serve as a reference down the line. It includes information on eConsult basics, the referral and scheduling process, eConsult certification requirements, and equipment specifications. There can be unique challenges associated with a patient encounter that involves cameras, monitors, electronic stethoscopes, and other equipment that is not used during a face-to-face patient encounter. The manual was created to aide facilities with some of those challenges.

The manual also covers the requirements Avera established regarding the exam room and equipment for eConsults. These requirements ensure good quality transmission, safety, and the best possible experience for patients. After the initial implementation, and every two years thereafter, eConsult staff members come to the facility to complete an assessment. If everything meets the Avera eConsult requirements, the facility receives internal certification. The certification process is a good way for eConsult staff members to check for outdated equipment that needs to be replaced, any processes that may need updating, and other issues that need to be addressed.

One requirement for the exam room is that it must be within close proximity to the normal patient flow without disruption. It must also mirror a normal exam room setting and size. The walls must be a neutral color such as tan, beige, or light blue, and free from patterns so the background is not distracting during the eConsult. The exam room should not have windows as they might create a glare on the monitors. The room should have all internal walls as an external wall might allow disruption in the transmission feed. Avera Medical Group Pierre converted an existing exam room that had no windows and had four internal walls into its telemedicine exam room. This room is used only for eConsults and not for other patient encounters. This allows the equipment to remain set up at all times thus eliminating the need to move the equipment into the exam room before each eConsult. Avera Medical Group Pierre's eConsult exam room has two rows of seating so the patient can have family members present and/or the referring physician. This provides a unique aspect with telemedicine because it is rare in face-to-face ambulatory encounters for the referring provider to sit in on a consultation.

Avera Medical Group Pierre links to physicians in Sioux Falls using a point-to-point connection across Avera's secure network. This is a direct connection that allows for authentication and transmission encryption, which provides greater security in the transmission. Point-to-point also allows for data compression, which provides better visual and audio feeds. Some Avera facilities that provide eConsults are not able to establish a point-to-point connection, so they use out-of-network bridged calls that require a modem. While this still works, the quality might not be as good as connections achieved through point-to-point.

The most essential equipment for an eConsult is a camera, speaker, and monitor. Avera Medical Group Pierre uses a video camera and speaker made by Polycom. A beneficial feature of the Polycom system is its ability for parties on both ends of the video feed to be able to zoom in and out. The Polycom system provides a High-Definition (HD) image so clear you can see pores on a person's skin. For the monitor, Avera Medical Group Pierre uses a standard HD one. The Avera eConsult team recommends that the monitor be wall-mounted or on an approved cart. Both the monitor and the camera should be at a comfortable eye level for patients. At Avera Medical Group Pierre, the monitor is mounted on the wall facing the patient seating area (see Figure 1).

There are options other than using a Polycom system for video conferencing. Most computers today come with an HD cam already installed. This would work for telemedicine purposes, and some Avera facilities use it for their eConsult nutrition program, but it may not have the capability of zooming in and out. Another issue with a computer HD cam is that the computer would need to be configured to enable it to connect with other equipment that may be used during the eConsult.

Another option comes from the growing field of mHealth, which is the practice of medicine and public health supported by mobile devices. One product is FaceTime, a mobile application from Apple that allows a person to make video calls from their Mac to an iPad 2, iPhone 4, iPod Touch, or another Mac. There is discussion about FaceTime possibly being used in telemedicine. The first thought that might come to mind is whether transmitting data via an Apple product would allow for secure transmission. According to Apple, it would be secure. FaceTime users have their own unique identifications which would allow for audit trails, and calls are fully encrypted which create secure transmission. However, as is the issue with HD cams, there may be the problem of not being able to zoom in and out or connect to other telemedicine equipment.

Figure 1. Avera medical group pierre's econsult exam room

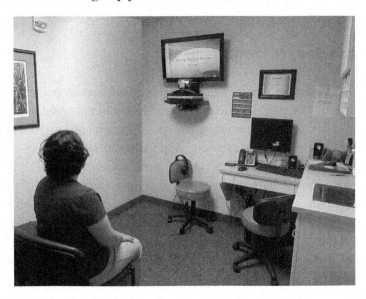

Two other pieces of equipment used in telemedicine are a stethoscope and an otoscope. When most people visualize a doctor in their head, they probably imagine a person in a white coat with a stethoscope around his or her neck. A stethoscope is still used during an eConsult, although it is an amped up version of the average stethoscope. The one Avera Medical Group Pierre uses is a TR-1/EF Telephonic Telescope manufactured by Telehealth Technologies. The stethoscope is connected to a box that is connected by a cable to the Polycom video unit. The provider at the specialty site can listen to the stethoscope using a headset. Avera facilities not on Avera's network that use bridged calls need to connect the stethoscope to the modem in order to transmit the audio. The quality is not as good as stethoscopes connected using point-to-point. Even though the tone and rhythm sound the same using either connection, the stethoscope connected to a modem may pick up background noise.

There are otoscopes facilities can purchase that are compatible with telemedicine video conferencing systems. The otoscope would connect to the video conferencing system essentially the same way as a stethoscope would, but instead of outputting sound to the provider at the specialty site, it would output images of the outer-ear canal, eardrum, middle ear, lower sinuses, or upper throat.

Another piece of equipment used during an eConsult is one found in most offices, and that is a fax machine, which transmits patient documents between the two sites. Avera recommends that the fax machine not be in the actual exam room but near it. At Avera Medical Group Pierre, there is a fax machine in the nurses' area just outside the eConsult exam room.

Care requirements for the equipment are that it must pass Avera quality of service and biomedical certification. To ensure the equipment is in proper working order, each unit must be rebooted one time per week, and a monthly call-in for equipment check is required if the eConsult equipment is not used frequently.

Privacy and Record Ownership

Information management and the electronic transmission of patient information are not new topics in the health information field. Health information professionals are familiar with issues of transmitting patient information through email, fax, and EHR systems. Telemedicine presents a unique transmission security concern: the transmission of audio and visual of the actual patient encounter. The line used to transmit the audio and visual from Avera Medical Group Pierre to one of the specialty sites is a secure line. One of the reasons for using an exam room with no exterior walls for eConsults is to ensure that the transmission is secure and uninterrupted.

The ownership of a medical record belongs to the facility that creates the record. With telemedicine services, two separate facilities are entering record information on the same patient for the same encounter, but each creates its own note. When a patient comes to Avera Medical Group Pierre for an eConsult, the nurses' assessment and vital signs belong to Avera Medical Group Pierre. The remainder of the documentation created by the specialty site during the eConsult belongs to the specialty site.

Billing Issues

The billing of telemedicine services is similar to the billing of radiological services when they are divided into technical and professional components. The specialty or distant site bills for the professional services and submits an appropriate CPT or HCPCS code with modifier GT, which means "via interactive audio and video telecommunications system." The originating site bills the facility services and submits HCPCS code Q3014, "telehealth originating site facility fee."

Avera Medical Group Pierre did not encounter any billing problems during the implementation of the eConsult program. As the originating site, the clinic submits only the facility charge for an eConsult, Q3014, and that code was already loaded in the billing system and EHR. The Business Office submits most of its insurance claims electronically through electronic data interchange. Sometimes claims are rejected and sent back to the business office due to issues with codes or insurance information. However, there were no issues with electronically submitting claims with Q3014 on them.

When it comes to billing and reimbursement for eConsults, the question arises: Will an insurance company pay for an eConsult or consider it not medically necessary or not a covered benefit? That depends on the insurance company and its policies. Medicare accepts telemedicine codes as long as they meet medical necessity requirements and are of a particular code range. The insurance companies to which Avera Medical Group Pierre has submitted telemedicine facility charges are Medicare, Medicaid, BlueCross BlueShield, Dakotacare, and Avera Health Plan. Some companies have reimbursed the eConsult while others have denied it as not a covered benefit and made the patient responsible for payment of the charges. Perhaps one day when insurance companies are evaluating whether or not a service is medically necessary, the geographic location of the patient will matter.

ADVANTAGES AND DISADVANTAGES

The biggest advantage in offering patients telemedicine services, according to Marnie Burke, MPA, RN, Director of Patient Care at Avera Medical Group Pierre, is that it saves patients time and money associated with driving to another town to see a specialist. It also allows Avera Medical Group Pierre to broaden its range of services.

The obvious disadvantage of telemedicine is that the provider and the patient are not physically in the same room. There is equipment, such as a stethoscope and otoscope, which can bring more elements into the eConsult. However, nothing can replace some of the benefits of a face-to-face encounter. Another disadvantage is the possibility of technical difficulties. No patient wants to be in the middle of a discussion with his or her doctor when all of sudden the image of the doctor freezes. The information and training manual Avera provides its facilities includes a section on a variety of possible technical problems that could arise during an eConsult. Some are having sound but no picture, hearing yourself repeated back, the exam camera does not work, or the connection drops during the session. The manual lists a few techniques to troubleshoot each problem. If troubleshooting does not work or if the problem is not listed in the manual, Avera provides the pager and phone number of eConsult staff members to contact for assistance.

CHALLENGES

The implementation process of the eConsult program at Avera Medical Group Pierre was quick and simple. The only challenge they experienced was a setback to the initial planned specialty, which was endocrinology. The partnership with that specialty physician did not develop, but the clinic was able to partner with other specialties without a long delay in providing the first eConsult at the clinic.

Once telemedicine is established at a facility, some challenges could still develop. Small facilities may not be able to dedicate an exam room solely for telemedicine encounters. The equipment would then have to be moved into an exam room and the connection re-established before each eConsult. Other challenges may be due to the type of facility that is providing telemedicine. For example, hospitals that offer telemedicine services have a requirement that clinics do not need. Any physician who connects to a hospital at the specialty site needs to be credentialed with that particular hospital. In the clinic setting, the physician need only be licensed.

RECOMMENDATIONS

To make an eConsult a good experience for both the patient and the provider, there are some aspects to remember regarding audio and visual transmission. Ensure the camera captures all the people in the exam room. When communicating back and forth, there could be a short delay in the audio transmission so it would be a good idea to pause before responding. If the patient requests to discuss something privately during the eConsult, mute the microphone to respect that request. When using the stethoscope, mute the other microphones to reduce background noise so the stethoscope microphone is clearly heard. A very important tip is to remember that the microphone is very sensitive and can pick up even the slightest noise.

For facilities interested in implementing telemedicine, Cathy Niklason says that a key component in the success of an eConsult program is having support from the facility administrator and the referring physicians. Having the administrators on board with telemedicine creates a very positive atmosphere and will contribute to the success down the line. If physicians support the eConsult idea, they are more likely to refer their patients to the specialist via the eConsult rather than sending them to another town to see a physician face-to-face. A recommendation Marnie Burke, MPA, RN, offers to other clinics is to obtain good equipment because the picture quality will be better. To facilities still deciding whether or not they should implement telemedicine, Burke says, "Go for it. Absolutely do it because it enhances what we can do for patient services."

FUTURE PLANS

Once initial telemedicine services are established in a facility, there are updates and improvements that can be done to enhance those services. Telemedicine is still fairly new to Avera Medical Group Pierre. However, six months after the first eConsult was performed, the clinic already expanded the telemedicine services offered. What started out as a working connection with one specialty has grown to a working connection with several additional specialties, including pulmonology, liver disease, hematology and oncology, hematology and transplant, midlife care for women, dermatology, radiation oncology, and nutrition services.

Avera Medical Group Pierre has plans for further expanding its telemedicine specialties. For example, they have received training with North Central Heart Institute for cardiology eConsults. Coordinating with some specialties will require purchasing new equipment. The clinic recently acquired an AMD-2500 General Exam Camera manufactured by AMD Global Telemedicine. It will be able to be positioned over patients' bodies for clear, close-up visuals of the skin. This will allow Avera Medical Group Pierre to work with dermatology and infectious disease specialties.

Since the implementation of the eConsult program at Avera Medical Group Pierre, the clinic has performed approximately 60 eConsults as of November 2011, with additional appointments scheduled. One day, Avera Medical Group Pierre would like to be the specialty site that connects with distant patients. For now, the clinic is the one helping patients connect with distant doctors. For those patients who no longer have to drive 200 miles to see a specialist, coming to Avera Medical Group Pierre for an eConsult is a benefit worth staying in town.

ADDITIONAL READING

American Telemedicine Association. (2012). *American telemedicine association.* Retrieved from http://www.americantelemed.org/i4a/pages/index.cfm?pageid=1

Apple Inc. (2012). *Apple - FaceTime.* Retrieved from http://www.apple.com/mac/facetime/

Avera. (2012). *Avera medical group pierre - Pierre, SD - Avera.* Retrieved from http://www.avera.org/clinics/pierre/index.aspx

Global Medicine, A. M. D. Inc. (2012). *Telemedicine equipment and telehealth technologies.* Retrieved from http://www.amdtelemedicine.com

Polycom, Inc. (2011). *Polycom.* Retrieved from http://www.polycom.com/

Products, R. N. K. Inc. (2011). *Telehealth technologies.* Retrieved from http://www.telehealthtechnologies.com/

KEY TERMS AND DEFINITIONS

Clinical Decision Support System: A knowledge system that analyzes patient data to help health care providers make clinical decisions.

Computerized Physician Order Entry: A process of electronic entry of physician instructions for the treatment of patients communicated over a computer network to the medical staff or other departments, such as pharmacy, laboratory, or radiology.

Current Procedural Terminology (CPT): A code set maintained by the American Medical Association that consists of five-digit numeric codes that describe physician services and procedures.

Distant or Specialty Site: Refers to the location of the physician or other medical professional.

Electronic Data Interchange: The transfer of data between different companies using networks or the Internet.

Electronic Health Record (EHR): A longitudinal electronic record of patient health information generated by one or more encounters in any care delivery setting. Included in this information are patient demographics, progress notes, problems, medications, vital signs, past medical history, immunizations, laboratory data, and radiology reports.

Health Insurance Portability and Accountability Act (HIPAA): A law enacted in 1996 that is composed of the Privacy Rule and the Security Rule. The Privacy Rule provides federal protections for personal health information held by covered entities and gives patients rights regarding that information. It permits the disclosure of personal health information needed for treatment, payment, and health care operations. The Security Rule specifies a series of administrative, physical, and technical safeguards for covered entities to assure the confidentiality, integrity, and availability of electronic protected health information.

Healthcare Common Procedure Coding System (HCPCS): A standardized code set that identifies medical services, supplies, and equipment. It consists of two levels. Level I codes are CPT codes, and Level II codes are five-digit alpha-numeric codes that describe medical equipment, drugs, orthotics, prosthetics and supplies.

mHealth: The practice of medicine and public health that is supported by mobile devices.

Originating Site: Refers to the location of the patient.

Picture Archiving and Communication System: A system of hardware and software that is dedicated to the storage, retrieval, management, distribution, and presentation of images. It replaces hard file copies with digital images that can be used and seen by several different medical professionals and different medical automation systems simultaneously.

Point-to-Point Connection: A direct connection between two points on the same network.

Telemedicine (eConsult): The use of interactive audio and visual technologies to exchange medical information for diagnostic, monitoring, and therapeutic purposes when clinicians and patients are separated by distance.

Chapter 10

Florida Health Information Exchange:
A Journey to Improving Care through the Exchange of Patient Health Information

Alice Noblin
University of Central Florida, USA

Kelly McLendon
Health Information Xperts, USA

Steven Shim
Harris IT Services, USA

EXECUTIVE SUMMARY

Florida began the journey to health information connectivity in 2004 under Governor Jeb Bush. Initially these efforts were funded by grants, but due to the downturn in the economy, the state was unable to support growth in 2008. The American Recovery and Reinvestment Act of 2009 provided funding to further expand health information exchange efforts across the country. As a result, Florida is now able to move forward and make progress in information sharing. Harris Corporation was contracted to provide some basic services to the health care industry in 2011. However, challenges remain as privacy and security regulations are put in place to protect patients' information. With two seemingly opposing mandates, sharing the information versus protecting the information, challenges continue to impede progress.

DOI: 10.4018/978-1-4666-2671-3.ch010

ORGANIZATION BACKGROUND

Efforts toward building a Health Information Exchange (HIE) in Florida began in 2004. The Agency for Health Care Administration (AHCA) laid the foundation for a statewide HIE by organizing health care stakeholders and providing initial funding to local Regional Health Information Organization (RHIO) projects through its grants program. Florida is working to achieve a secure and sustainable approach to health information technology adoption and exchange resulting in better health care outcomes with lowered total costs. The development of a HIE that protects privacy and aligns with national exchange standards is the goal of AHCA. Leveraging existing networks to best achieve widespread adoption is one way to achieve the goal. In 2010, the Office of the National Coordinator for Health Information Technology (ONC) provided grant funds to significantly advance Florida's plans to build a statewide health information infrastructure. The provision of sustainable services to meet the meaningful use criteria established by ONC is an important focus of the HIE.

Key services to be implemented include:

- A patient look-up service
- A provider directory
- Secure messaging
- Public health reporting

This case study aims to describe the historical journey of the HIE in the State of Florida from 2004 to the present. Significant financial resources from the stimulus package in 2010 have allowed the HIE to move forward by providing the key services above to allow sharing of patient data. As has occurred throughout the nation, privacy concerns have been at the forefront of all networking efforts in Florida. In addition to describing the current structure and services available, we will chronicle the ongoing efforts to create and maintain the processes of privacy and security compliance which will ultimately improve user confidence in the HIE.

SETTING THE STAGE

Health Information Exchange within the State of Florida began as an Executive Order from Governor Jeb Bush in May, 2004. Governor Bush established an advisory board (Governor's Health Information Infrastructure Advisory Board [GHIIAB]) to advise AHCA in the creation and implementation of a Florida Health Information Technology (HIT) infrastructure (Greaves, et al., 2007). In addition to supporting local data exchanges (RHIOs), the state was working on development of an overarching network to bring the local exchanges together, which has become the current HIE.

Florida Health Information Network

The Florida Health Information Network, Inc. (FHIN) was created in 2005 to implement a statewide infrastructure, connecting the RHIOs and other networks in the state. The vision of the FHIN was to provide a secure network for exchange of necessary medical information to improve continuity of care (Rosenfeld, Koss, Caruth, & Fuller, 2006). The FHIN Grants Program provided initial support of $2 million to advance electronic health information exchange in local communities (Takach & Kaye, 2008). Assistance was provided to the new RHIOs through the following: planning grants to develop strategic plans; implementing grants to demonstrate exchange of information between at least two (nonaffiliated) provider organizations; and, training grants to support provider use of EHR systems. The FHIN grants program required a dollar for dollar match from the RHIOs. It was felt that the matching program requirements improved the RHIOs chances of long-term success and sustainability.

The initial goal of the FHIN was to provide a data set consisting of hospital inpatient and outpatient encounters including laboratory results and diagnoses, as well as medications and demographic information (Rosenfeld, et al., 2006). Claims data for Medicaid patients would also be included, as well as Department of Health (DOH) public health information.

In 2007, the FHIN released a White Paper, Architectural Considerations for State Infrastructure (Greaves, et al., 2007). This paper proposed that the FHIN would enable health care providers to access a patient's medical records from any provider database connected to the network, regardless of location. Collaboration among the public and private sectors, state and local governments, providers, employers, consumers, health plans and payers would enable connectivity among RHIOs and other health information networks in Florida via a central server.

Recommendations from this document provide more detail as to how the FHIN planned to address technical concerns which were initially raised by the GHIIAB (Greaves, et al., 2007):

- **Central Authority for Technical Standards:** Setting standards and certification requirements including state-level security specifications.
- **Network Security:** Secure and encrypted communications along with detailed logs would be kept by both the requesting and responding entities.
- **Authentication of Users:** The state server would manage the transactions between the RHIOs, state agency databases, and other health information

sources. The FHIN would credential physicians in RHIOs as well as those directly connected to the FHIN with the use of digital signatures and role-based authentication.

- **Patient Consent:** Use of a statewide patient authorization system with the use of a Personal Identification Number (PIN) to allow the patient to control who accesses the information.
- **Master Patient Index:** Use of a common set of fields for identification including name (first and last), phone number, date and location of birth, or a personal identification number.
- **Minimal Clinical Dataset:** Specific data fields identified by each RHIO that would be available to the requesting physician upon request.

This undertaking met with obstacles that seriously impacted its activities. One of the major obstacles encountered in implementing a statewide network was legal and regulatory issues surrounding existing privacy laws (Rosenfeld, et al., 2006). To provide consent for access to information, patients would have a PIN to provide to the caregiver at the time of the encounter. Unlike other state exchanges and RHIOs nation-wide, the FHIN specifically recommended against an opt-in or opt-out consent model initially due to the additional costs of implementing such a system. For emergency purposes, physicians were to be allowed to "break the glass" and view a patient's record (Greaves, et al., 2007, p. 40). This would have required an audit trail and a letter to the patient notifying him/her of this access. Significant issues were found with each of these process steps and designs.

In March 2010, the Office of the National Coordinator (ONC) announced the State Health Information Exchange Cooperative Agreement Program awardees as part of the Health Information Technology for Economic and Clinical Health (HI-TECH) Act. Florida received $20,738,582 (HHS, 2012). Following an Invitation to Negotiate, this federal funding resulted in Florida awarding a contract to Harris Healthcare Solutions to create the Florida HIE infrastructure.

Through the designated state entity (AHCA), Florida looked to Harris to create a Florida Health Information Exchange Infrastructure under the ONC funding. The infrastructure was to include open source technologies where appropriate and give the highest priority to privacy, security, and interoperability with existing and future electronic patient medical records. The patient lookup service will enable participating users to locate and retrieve patient records. The structure of the HIE will be a network of networks without a centralized master patient index. An authoritative provider directory will be established for all providers to facilitate communication between physicians. Secure messaging to facilitate sharing of clinical summaries (a meaningful use criterion) will be provided. This resource for providers will use national standards to ensure security. Public health reporting will be provided in conjunction with the Florida Department of Health.

See Table 1 for the categories of key stakeholders who will need to become engaged early on to ensure success of the Florida HIE.

CASE DESCRIPTION

The American Recovery and Reinvestment Act (ARRA) provides for incentive payments to hospitals and physicians who engage in the meaningful use of electronic health records. Meaningful use is a set of standards meant to ensure that EHRs are not only purchased, but utilized for certain key functions. The HIE meaningful use standards aim to provide health records for the treating physician (from a prior episode of care) to improve quality of care and coordination of care, as well as patient access to health information. HIE services must take into account the scope of data exchange and location of the records.

Table 1. Adoption stakeholders

Stakeholder	Description
Patients	Make informed decisions working with provider
Active Physicians and other Providers	Licensed Practicing Healthcare Providers in Florida. Includes physicians, nurses, physician assistants, nurse practitioners.
RECs	Regional Extension Centers will recruit solo and small general medical physician groups to adopt EHRs and participate in the HIE.
RHIOs	Regional Health Information Organizations will provide local data exchanges
Hospital and Other Private HIEs	Private hospitals, hospital systems, Integrated Health Networks or other groups who have formed private HIEs
Long-Term Care Facilities	Long term and transitional care facilities
Mental Health Facilities	Mental Health and Behavioral Health Facilities
Labs (LabCorp, Quest, and state labs)	Labs that might use the HIE to provide patient information via lookup
FQHCs	Federally Qualified Health Centers
DOH	Florida Department of Health maintains a physician licensing database that provides the basis for the provider directory. County health departments provide primary care including referrals to specialists.
Hospitals and Clinics	Public and private hospitals operating within the state
Surescripts	E-Prescription network
State Immunization Records	Children's Immunization Records, Florida SHOTS

In Florida, the HIE is federated, meaning data is housed locally, not in a centralized format (AHCA, 2011). However, data can be linked together across the multiple RHIOs (Rosenfeld, et al., 2006) The HIE will serve as the location for patient information exchange but the provider will maintain the data. This will allow providers to query for patient records across various participating networks.

See Figure 1 which shows the nodes on a network that are connected through the HIE.

Patient Lookup Services

Patient Lookup enables the search and retrieval of a patient's health information, such as labs, medication history, and discharge summaries from different sources ("pull" function). AHCA recognizes that the majority of patient care is local, and that the goal of local HIE efforts will be connecting providers with local sources of patient data. In order to add value to the local HIE and help them achieve critical mass and provider adoption, the Florida HIE will provide access to and by the Florida Department of Health (DOH). This includes the county health departments who provide primary care treatment to many Floridians (AHCA, 2011). The coordination of care for these patients, including referrals for specialty care and laboratory tests, will be accomplished through the local HIE.

In addition, because many patients who use the county health departments for primary care are on Medicaid, the HIE will also be connected to the Medicaid Health Information Network. The patient lookup services will be important for verification of benefits, history of visits and medications, and laboratory test results. The health

Figure 1. Multiple options for health information exchange

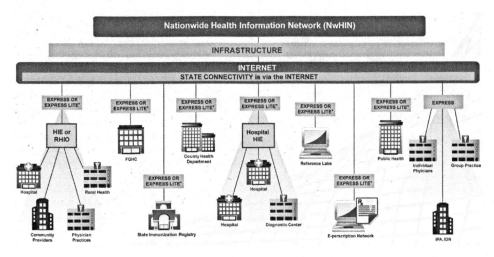

departments can also take advantage of the Medicaid Health Information Network for e-prescribing services at no charge.

The typical workflow for Patient Lookup Services is illustrated in Figure 2.

If the provider has a Master Patient Index (MPI) in place, the Florida HIE will provide an Express Lite option which will allow the provider to connect directly to the FHIN. If the provider does not have an MPI in place, then a different option is available, called Express, which the provider can use to connect to the FHIN or potentially create its own HIE (Shim, 2011). With either Express Lite or Express, a Connect Gateway is utilized for exchange of data over the Internet.

Both Express and Express Lite will need to connect to appropriate provider systems to create and package information conforming to the required standard profiles. These profiles are typically unique variations of the base standards such as the Clinical Document Architecture (CDA), Continuity of Care Document (CCD), Continuity of Care Record (CCR), and HITSP C32 which builds upon the HL7 CCD component.

Provider Directory

A provider directory is required by the State HIE Cooperative Agreement. It must allow providers who are authorized (network authentication) the ability to route various documents within the HIE. The DOH maintains a physician-licensing database that is updated daily (AHCA, 2011). This is the basis for the provider directory that will also include healthcare organizations participating in the HIE. The ability to facilitate physician to physician messaging is the ultimate goal.

Figure 2. Patient lookup service

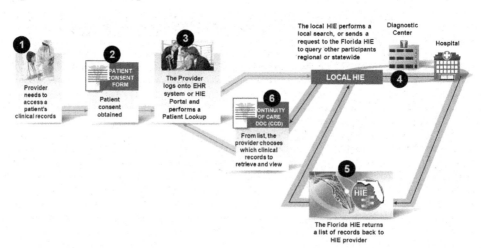

Direct Messaging Services

The Florida HIE supports a Direct Secure Messaging (DSM) service to all subscribers to support communication between physicians or organizations for transition of care or referral purposes. DSM can also support the provision of clinical documents or information in response to medical information requests. The service integrates with the provider directory to easily locate and communicate with the other Florida HIE subscribers. Supported national and best practice security standards enable the transmission of encrypted information directly to trusted recipients via the Internet. The service is hosted at the Florida HIE data center and can be accessed securely by subscribers using a Web enabled client. In this manner, providers are able to meet the requirements of meaningful use incentives. Harris has developed P2P Direct to meet the ONC Direct specifications for secure messaging in Florida (Shim, 2011). The Direct specifications represent a national standard model meant to streamline transmission of encrypted health information directly to known trusted recipients over the Internet.

Figure 3 provides an overview of the Florida HIE services.

Public Health Reporting

Public health reporting is done in coordination with the Florida Department of Health and Florida stakeholders. Secure messaging enables alert reporting to targeted

Figure 3. Platform provides flexibility for participants

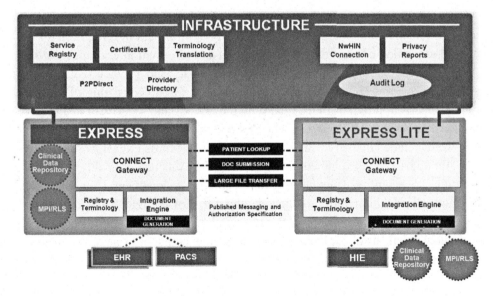

providers, and also enables the providers to easily submit required data to public health authorities (AHCA, 2010). This allows for efficient and timely notification of communicable disease and other disease outbreaks, which can in turn allow for increased public awareness.

CURRENT CHALLENGES FACING THE ORGANIZATIONS

Privacy and Security rank among the most difficult challenges HIE organizations are required to manage. HIEs are new concepts without any real precedence, and despite several years of thought modeling and tentative trials, the core principles have not been well defined and established; case law has not been created nor have regulatory enforcement precedents been set. In this atmosphere of formative establishment of what will eventually become 'best practices,' regulatory requirements are driving HIEs to make decisions on the fly and probably adjust them as time moves forward creating better, deeper levels of experience.

The exchange of health information in Florida will be based on what are called 'Trust Agreements' (Participation) that establish the obligations and assurances between the FHIN, Harris Corporation and other health care organizations in the network (AHCA, 2011). Consumers will have the ability to explicitly grant permission for disclosure and use of sensitive data as required by state and federal law through the use of consents and authorizations.

Legal Policy

AHCA and Florida stakeholders do realize that the privacy and security of health information, including integrity and availability of information, is required for successful utilization of electronic health records and information exchange services. As part of the national Health Information Security and Privacy Collaboration (HISPC) project, AHCA established a Legal Work Group consisting of legal and policy experts to provide advice regarding the privacy and security of health information exchange (AHCA, 2011). The Legal Work Group made recommendations that were included in the Florida Electronic Health Records Exchange Act of 2009. The Act updated and explained laws related to the exchange of health information including accessibility of medical records for emergency treatment. To encourage use of standardized authorizations statewide, the Act allowed AHCA to adopt uniform patient authorization forms. AHCA's participation in the national HISPC produced an in-depth analysis of applicable legal requirements that has served as a resource in policy development (AHCA, 2011).

Trust Agreements

AHCA and Florida stakeholders, upon the advice of the Legal Work Group, have developed recommended standardized documents and processes to facilitate HIE in Florida. These agreements are in general referred to as 'Trust Agreements.' Draft agreements and policies for the Florida HIE from June 2011, provide some details in the following statements (Turner, 2011).

- Direct Secure Messaging Service will be provided as a Web-mail client via Web browser for a participant to utilize. A separate account is required for each user with a username and password to login.
- Availability of central infrastructure and help desk response times will be specified in the vendor's contract with AHCA.
- Audit trail data of transactions for a terminated participant will be retained for seven years.
- Established file size and mailbox limits, which will be posted on the vendor's website.
- Verification of the accuracy of any messages as well as verification of what information a participant is authorized to send, receive, use or disclose is not the role of the vendor.
- Participant agrees to accurately complete and maintain registration information in the Provider Directory.

Disclaimers

The following disclaimers are found in the Trust Agreements, which serve to limit expectations and liabilities (Turner, 2011).

- Accuracy of Patient Record Matching. Each participant acknowledges that there could be errors or mismatches when matching patient identities between disparate data sources.
- Accuracy of Health Data. Participants are not liable for the clinical accuracy or completeness of data provided. Data may not include a full and complete medical history.
- Reliance on a System. Participant users may not rely upon the availability of a particular Participant's Health Data.
- Use of Network in an Emergency. Participant and Participant Users are responsible for determining the appropriate use of the Network for communications or transactions concerning or supporting treatment in an emergency or other urgent situation.

- Patient Care. Health Data obtained through the Network is not a substitute for information deemed necessary for the proper treatment of a patient.

Privacy Compliance

There are numerous elements in the Trust Agreements and the HIE statute to protect privacy of Protected Health Information (PHI). None of them are designed to supersede HIPAA or federal behavioral, alcohol and similar regulations.

In the event of a medical emergency when the patient or his/her legal representative is unable or unavailable to authorize access, the participant user may access the information. Written documentation in the patient's record immediately following the disclosure shall be made by the requesting participant user. The patient or the patient's legal representative must be notified of the emergency access within seventy-two (72) hours of such emergency access (Turner, 2011).

Another set of statements inside Trust Agreements that guide privacy include creation of a Minimum Data Set for Patient Lookup and Delivery Services (Turner, 2011).

- Encounter information for each emergency department visit, primary care or hospital visit (depending on participant type) shall include: patient demographic information, reason for visit, treating health care provider(s), date and place of visit, diagnoses, and procedures.
- Vital signs, discharge summaries, medications, alerts (i.e., allergies), immunizations, patient functional status, laboratory test results, and other diagnostic test results available electronically.

In summation, the privacy implications for the FHIN vendor, participant organization and the State of Florida are based upon HIPAA and similar protective regulations, however, the nuances are different enough that privacy compliance will need to be carefully considered and evolved as more infra-structure and regulations are implemented.

HIPAA Security Compliance

In executing upon the HIE statute, AHCA has required the Harris Corporation to develop a security and disaster back-up plan designed to counteract disturbances to business activities and protect critical business from the effects of major failures. The disaster back-up plan aligns with HIPAA requirements for developing a disaster recovery plan and procedures for testing the network and remediating any faults. The FHIN will be required to evaluate the need for periodic security risk assessments and maintain compliance with the HIPAA Security Rule and National Institute of Standard and Technology (NIST) guidelines. The evaluation should include the entire list of standards and implementation specifications required by 45 CFR Parts 160 and 164, including security policies, access controls, asset management, business continuity management and other forms of compliance. The evaluation will also address human resources, the physical environment, and information systems maintenance.

SOLUTIONS AND RECOMMENDATIONS

Patient Consent and Authorization

Florida law requires patient authorization for disclosure of some sensitive health data, except in medical emergencies. Two universal authorization forms (Universal Patient Authorization Form for Full Disclosure of Health Information for Treatment and Quality of Care and Universal Patient Authorization Form for Limited Disclosure of Health Information for Treatment and Quality of Care) were recently issued to enable compliance with Florida law for disclosures of such sensitive and non-sensitive health data (Turner, 2011). The forms can be used by a patient (or his/her authorized legal representative) to authorize a healthcare provider to obtain the patient's records from another provider or through an HIE. These authorizations may be used to authorize access only if permitted by both federal and state law (i.e. additional specific authorization is required for behavioral health, substance abuse, HIV and STD information, which is considered "super confidential").

Network Monitoring, Audit Trail, and Disaster Recovery

The Florida Health Information Network will include system capabilities to enable network-monitoring procedures that will create an audit trail for every transaction involving protected health information (AHCA, 2011). Audit controls included in the network will be capable of logging and tracking changes to data. In addition, queries and transactions will be recorded. The ability to track exceptions and activity in the HIE databases and in transmitting data will be developed. The state HIE network will require authentication through the use of digital certificates by the participating systems.

Harris Corporation has developed and maintains a tested and actionable plan for back-up of software and data, and a disaster recovery plan for restoring the system in the event the production systems are destroyed or damaged. Utilities capture the Harris based HIE audit log from different software solutions, i.e. Fair Warning for application systems and Security Information and Event Management (SIEM) requirements beyond privacy. Event management is built into the SIEM layer to manage issues arising from audit and security log monitors.

The technical architecture of FHIN will ensure that strong access control, secure data transfer based on established transmission standards and the use of encryption techniques are essential elements in its implementation (AHCA, 2011). Access control is the first line of defense in securing medical records and is maintained by limiting access to a select few (authorized) systems from participants who have signed agreements and worked closely with FHIN to manage secure connections limited to specific data sets. Unauthorized access to protected health information will be prevented by strong authentication processes (e.g., digital certificates) as well as access controls.

Harris executes the network layer of access controls and only accepts connections from a list of locations and systems. Application level access control is the responsibility of the provider sites. In keeping with the nature of health information access requirements the access controls utilized are relatively weak, but are considered adequate for the Florida HIE as it is within each participant's own site.

The Florida Health Information Network architecture also has security measures in place to prevent the unauthorized access to protected health information while it is being transmitted over the telecommunication network. The HIE has implemented integrity controls to ensure the detection of unauthorized users attempting to access or modify personal health information in transmission (AHCA, 2011). Policies and procedures provide the detailed requirements for securely transmitting protected health information at both the hardware and software levels, as well as requirements for reporting breaches to the security of the data. In addition, the Florida Health Information Network encrypts the data exchanged through a secure communication channel to meet HIPAA Security Rule standards (AHCA, 2011).

Data transfer standards are employed for data exchange among different health care participants and the Florida Health Information Network to enable health information exchange among all partners. For the exchange of clinical data among health care facilities, the Florida Health Information Network supports the HL7 2.x Clinical Document Architecture (CDA) standards, the ASTM Continuity of Care Record (CCR) standard using extensible markup language and HL7 3.x Continuity of Care Document (CCD) (AHCA, 2011). By supporting these standards, the exchange of clinical data among hospitals, clinics, and physician practices can be more widely enabled and supported, for EHR systems providing CCD or CCR.

Security for the FHIN has been well designed. The security models and architecture are congruent with HIPAA security and include proactive monitoring which is highly important.

FUTURE RESEARCH

Interstate Policy Development

AHCA and Florida stakeholders wish to engage in privacy-protected health information exchange with neighboring states and other states consistent with federal and state law. As an initial step, the AHCA has reached out to appropriate parties in Alabama and Georgia. Objectives of this outreach include comparison of state laws, status of health information exchange and plans, comparison of trust agreements, user agreements, and patient authorization policies and forms, and identification of appropriate legal vehicles for interstate health information exchange.

CONCLUSION

The main challenge to implementing a statewide network is the management of many, varied issues, including patient identity, privacy and security. HITECH brought additional funding which enabled the HIE project to launch, but HIPAA privacy regulations were also strengthened with steeper penalties. Therefore, it is of primary importance that HIEs have privacy and security policies and procedures in place, including appropriate privacy and security administrative, physical, and technical safeguards.

Having adequate consents and authorizations has proven to be a challenging issue, especially in light of laws governing substance abuse, mental health and other super confidential patient health information. These issues must be resolved by participant stakeholders, especially compliance, privacy, security officers, and health information management staff. Harris Corporation (the vendor) also needs to be involved with continued efforts to solve privacy and security questions and issues that will arise at a faster rate as more participants are added.

It is also very important that patient identity be well managed. Issues surrounding keeping master patient indexes clean and maintaining the highest levels of data integrity are still being identified and resolved. High integrity and accurate MPI data is vital to maintaining privacy and security along with wrongful disclosure / breach prevention. Both the users and Harris' systems in reality have roles to play in maintaining patient identity accuracy.

However, the HIE has made progress, and currently the services are secure messaging between providers of care and patient lookup, which reflects the first foray into patient identity management. As the Florida HIE provides additional service options, challenges for privacy safeguards and the other issues continue to evolve.

The HIE actively works with stakeholders from the State of Florida, Harris Corporation and prospective connected healthcare organizations to solve these issues and move forward into a fully operational mode.

REFERENCES

AHCA. (2010). *Legal agreements for participation in the FHIN.* Florida Legal Work Group Memorandum. Retrieved November 14, 2011 from http://ahca.myflorida.com/schs/AdvisoryCouncil/AC061710/TabD-UpdateOnLegalWorkGroup.pdf

AHCA. (2011). *State health information exchange cooperative agreement program strategic and operational plans.* State Health Information Exchange Cooperative Agreement Program. Retrieved November 14, 2011 from http://www.fhin.net/pdf/floridaHie/StrategicandOperationalPlansApproved.pdf

Bourret, C., & Salzano, G. (2006). Data for decision making in networked health. *Data Science Journal, 5,* 64–78. doi:10.2481/dsj.5.64

Department of Health and Human Services. (2011). *Website.* Retrieved November 14, 2011, from http://www.hhs.gov/ocr/privacy/hipaa/administrative/breachnotificationrule/index.html

Greaves, P., Sullivan, C., Nguyen, H., McBride, J., Rawlins, L., & Kragh, J. … David, B. (2007). *Florida health information network architectural considerations for state infrastructure draft white paper.* Prepared for Governor's Health Information Infrastructure Advisory Board. Retrieved November 14, 2011 from http://www.oregon.gov/OHA/OHPR/HIIAC/WebOnlyMaterials/FloridaWhitePaper4.19.07.pdf?ga=t

Menachemi, N., & Brooks, R. G. (2006). EHR and other IT adoption among physicians: Results of a large-scale statewide analysis. *Journal of Healthcare Information Management, 20*(3), 79–87.

Miller, R., & Sim, I. (2004). Physicians' use of electronic medical records: Barriers and solutions. *Health Affairs, 23*(2), 116–126. doi:10.1377/hlthaff.23.2.116

Rosenfeld, S. Koss, Caruth, & Fuller. (2006). Evolution of state health information exchange: A study of vision, strategy, and progress. *The Agency for Healthcare Research and Quality.* Retrieved November 14, 2011 from http://www.avalerehealth.net/research/docs/State_based_Health_Information_Exchange_Final_Report.pdf

Shim, S. (2011). *The evolution of health information exchanges.* Paper presented at the meeting of the Florida Health Information Management Association. Orlando, FL.

Sullivan, C. (2008). *Florida's RHIO initiative: Recycling lessons learned into new strategies for health information exchange.* Paper presented at the HIMSS 2008 RHIO/HIE Symposium. Orlando, FL.

Takach, M., & Neva, K. (2008). *Using HIT to transform health care: Summary of a discussion among state policy makers.* State Health Policy Briefing. Retrieved November 14, 2011 from http://nashp.org/sites/default/files/shpbriefing_usinghit.pdf?q=Files/shpbriefing_usinghit.pdf

Turner, C. (2011). *Florida HIE subscription agreements and policies.* State Consumer Health Information and Policy Advisory Council Interoffice Memorandum. Retrieved November 14, 2011 from http://b.ahca.myflorida.com/schs/Advisory-Council/AC062211/TABDLegalWorkgroupReport.pdf

U.S. Department of Health & Human Services. (2011). *The office of the national coordinator for health information technology.* Retrieved November 14, 2011 from http://healthit.hhs.gov/portal/server.pt?open=512&objID=1488&mode=2

ADDITIONAL READING

Adler-Milstein, J., Bates, D., & Jha, A. (2009). U.S. regional health information organizations: Progress and challenges. *Health Affairs, 28*(2), 483–492. doi:10.1377/hlthaff.28.2.483

Adler-Milstein, J., Bates, D., & Jha, A. (2011). A survey of health information exchange organizations in the United States: Implications for meaningful use. *Annals of Internal Medicine, 154*(10), 666–671.

Adler-Milstein, J., Landefeld, J., & Jha, A. (2010). Characteristics associated with regional health information organization viability. *Journal of the American Medical Informatics Association, 17*, 61–65. doi:10.1197/jamia.M3284

Adler-Milstein, J., McAfee, A., Bates, D., & Jha, A. (2008). The state of regional health information organizations: current activities and financing. *Health Affairs, 27*(1), w60–w69. doi:10.1377/hlthaff.27.1.w60

Brailer, D. (2005). Interoperability: The key to the future of health care system. *Health Affairs,* 519–w521.

Dixon, B., Zafar, A., & Overhage, J. (2010). A framework for evaluating the costs, effort, and value of nationwide health information exchange. *Journal of the American Medical Association, 17*(3), 295–301.

Halamka, J., Overage, J., Ricciardi, L., Rishel, W., Shirky, C., & Diamond, C. (2005). Exchanging health information: Local distribution, national coordination. *Health Affairs, 24*(5), 1170–1179. doi:10.1377/hlthaff.24.5.1170

Hincapie, A., Warholak, T., Murcko, A., Slack, M., & Malone, D. (2011). Physicians' opinions of a health information exchange. *Journal of the American Medical Informatics Association, 18*, 60–65. doi:10.1136/jamia.2010.006502

Johnson, K., Unertl, K., Chen, Q., Lorenzi, N., Nian, H., Bailey, J., & Frisse, M. (2011). Health information exchange usage in emergency departments and clinics: The who, what, and why. *Journal of the American Medical Informatics Association, 18*(5), 5690–5697. doi:10.1136/amiajnl-2011-000308

Kaelber, D., & Bates, D. (2007). Health information exchange and patient safety. *Journal of Biomedical Informatics, 40*(6), S40–S45. doi:10.1016/j.jbi.2007.08.011

Shapiro, J., Kannry, J., Lipton, M., Goldberg, E., Conocenti, P., & Stuard, S. (2006). Approaches to patient health information exchange and their impact on emergency medicine. *Annals of Emergency Medicine, 48*(4), 426–432. doi:10.1016/j.annemergmed.2006.03.032

Tzeel, A., Lawnicki, V., & Pemble, K. (2011). The business case for payer support of a community-based health information exchange: A Humana pilot evaluating its effectiveness in cost control for plan members seeking emergency department care. *American Health & Drug Benefits, 4*(4), 207–216.

Vest, J., & Gamm, L. (2010). Health information exchange: Persistent challenges and new strategies. *Journal of the American Medical Informatics Association, 17*(3), 3288–3294.

Vest, J., & Jasperson, J. (2010). What should we measure? Conceptualizing usage in health information exchange. *Journal of the American Medical Informatics Association, 17*, 302–307.

Voigt, C., & Torzewski, S. (2011). Direct results: An HIE tests simple information exchange using the direct project. *American Health Information Management Association, 82*(5), 38–41.

KEY TERMS AND DEFINITIONS

HIE Models, Federated: Providers of care operate within Internet connected networks. HIE participants exchange data within a structure where the providers themselves maintain the patient identification and storage of patient data. The HIE maintains provider of care directories, look-up services, messaging, data secure data transport and a wrapper of basic privacy and security functionalities, i.e. audit logs, privacy and security. As time goes forward these Federated HIE's will connect to other HIE's and RHIO's building out the National Health Information Network (NHIN).

Master Patient Index: Commonly adopted set of data fields for patient identification, typically name, date of birth and similar demographics, plus the provider name and location of treatment.

Office of the National Coordinator for Health Information Technology (ONC): United States government agency, a part of HHS (Health and Human Services) responsible for HITECH provisions including HIE's, and Medicare and Medicaid incentive programs commonly referred to as Meaningful Use.

Patient Consent: A patient authorization system with the allowing the patient to control who accesses their Protected Health Information (PHI). There are several consent models: No consent where a patient's health information is automatically included and patients cannot opt out; Opt-out with the default for health information of patients to be included automatically or the patient can opt out completely; Opt-out with exceptions where the default is for health information of patients to be included, but the patient can opt out completely or allow only select data to be included; Opt-in with a default that no patient health information is included and patients must actively express consent to be included, but if they do so then their information must be all in or all out; and, Opt-in with restrictions with a default of no patient health information made available, but the patient may allow a subset of select data to be included. In Florida part of the 'trust agreements' are two universal authorization forms (Universal Patient Authorization Form for Full Disclosure of Health Information For Treatment and Quality of Care and Universal Patient Authorization Form for Limited Disclosure of Health Information For Treatment and Health Information Exchange).

Protected Health Information (PHI): Defined under HIPAA Privacy rules as "any information, whether oral or recorded in any form or medium" that is created or received by a health care provider, health plan, public health authority, employer, life insurer, school or university, or health care clearinghouse"; and relates to the past, present, or future physical or mental health or condition of an individual; the provision of health care to an individual; or the past, present, or future payment for the provision of health care to an individual." In addition, data transmitted or maintained in any other form or medium, that includes paper records, fax documents, and oral communications. The information also must be personally identifiable by one of the 18 identifiers described within HIPAA.

Regional Health Information Organization (RHIO): There is no standardized definition of a RHIO; but common parlance is that a RHIO is synonymous with a local or regional Health Information Exchange.

Trust Agreements: Based on Federal NHIN language AHCA (the Florida Agency for Health Care Administration) and Florida stakeholders recommended standardized documents and processes to facilitate HIE in Florida. These agreements are in general referred to as 'Trust Agreements.' There are several areas covered by the 'Trust Agreements' such as patient authorization forms, direct, secure Messaging Service, availability of central infrastructure and help desk, and an audit trail of data transactions.

Chapter 11

Health Information Technology Collaboration in Community Health Centers:
The Community Partners HealthNet, Inc.

Elizabeth J. Forrestal
East Carolina University, USA

Xiaoming Zeng
East Carolina University, USA

Leigh W. Cellucci
East Carolina University, USA

Michael H. Kennedy
East Carolina University, USA

Doug Smith
The Community Partners HealthNet, Inc., USA

EXECUTIVE SUMMARY

Health-Center-Controlled Networks (HCCNs) are collaborative ventures that provide health information technologies to Community Health Centers (CHCs). Community Partners HealthNet (CPH), Inc. is a HCCN. CPH's member organizations are non-profit health care organizations that provide primary health care to individuals in medically underserved areas. As non-profits, they must regularly seek grant funding from foundations and state and federal agencies to provide quality, accessible health care. Consequently, initiatives to adopt and implement Health Information Technologies (HIT) require individual CHCs to carefully consider

DOI: 10.4018/978-1-4666-2671-3.ch011

how best to incorporate HIT for improved patient care. This case study describes CPH, discusses the collaboration of six individual CHCs to create CPH, and then explains CPH's on-going operations.

ORGANIZATION BACKGROUND

Community Partners HealthNet, Inc. (CPH) is a non-profit, federally-funded, Health-Center-Controlled Network (HCCN). The federal Health Resources and Services Administration (HRSA) defines an HCCN as: "A group of safety-net providers (a minimum of three collaborators/members) collaborating horizontally or vertically to improve access to care, enhance quality of care, and achieve cost efficiencies through the redesign of practices to integrate services, optimize patient outcomes, or negotiate managed care contracts on behalf of the participating members....HCCNs … exchange information and establish collaborative mechanisms to meet administrative, IT [information technology], and clinical quality objectives" (HRSA, 2012). Benefits of being an HCCN include federal financial incentives and favorable status in the awarding of federal grants (HRSA, 2012). CPH's member organizations began with six Community Health Centers (CHCs) in North Carolina. By 2011, it had expanded to include six multi-site CHCs (including three of the original members) and eight Rural Health Clinics (RHCs) in North Carolina and Texas (Community Partners HealthNet, 2012).

Health Care Environment

CPH's member organizations are ambulatory safety-net health care providers (also known as "essential community providers" and "providers of last resort" [Lewin & Altman, 2000, p. 54]). The Institute of Medicine (IOM) has defined "core safety net provider" as a set of:

providers that organize and deliver a significant level of health care and other health-related services.... These providers have two distinguishing characteristics: (1) by legal mandate or explicitly adopted mission they maintain an "open door," offering services to patients regardless of their ability to pay; and (2) a substantial share of their patient mix is uninsured, Medicaid, and other vulnerable patients (Lewin & Altman, 2000, p. 21).

Examples of core ambulatory safety-net providers are CHCs, RHCs, migrant clinics, free clinics, public health department clinics, and emergency rooms of public and teaching hospitals.

CHCs and RHCs have a 50-year history in the U.S health care system. Early roots of CHCs were in the Migrant Health Act of 1962 and the Economic Opportunity Act of 1964 (Bureau of Primary Health Care, 2008; Lefkowitz, 2005). These acts provided federal support for medical care delivered in migrant health centers and neighborhood health centers. In the mid-1970s neighborhood health centers became known as CHCs (Bureau of Primary Health Care). RHCs were established under the Rural Health Services Act of 1977 (Office of Rural Health Policy, 2006). In the 1980s and 1990s, Congress expanded the concept of CHCs to cover care provided to homeless people and residents of public housing under the McKinney Homeless Assistance Act of 1987 and the Disadvantaged Minority Health Improvement Act of 1990, respectively (Bureau of Primary Health Care). The Federally Qualified Health Center (FQHC) program is an extension of the migrant and CHC programs. The FQHC program was established under the Omnibus Budget Reconciliation Act (OBRA) of 1989 and expanded under the OBRA of 1990. Under these acts, FQHCs receive specially enhanced Medicare and Medicaid reimbursements (Office of Rural Health Policy). The Health Centers Consolidation Act of 1996 consolidated four federal primary care programs (community, migrant, homeless, and public housing) under section 330 of the Public Health Service Act (Bureau of Primary Health Care).

CHCs are non-profit, patient-governed, and community-directed organizations (North Carolina Community Health Center Association [NCCHCA], 2011). Strategic direction and community oversight are provided by boards of directors in which the majority of the board members receive medical care at the CHC (HRSA, 2011). The purpose of CHCs is to increase access to comprehensive basic health care. Fulfilling that purpose, in 2010, CHCs provide care to 20 million people at more than 7,900 sites. They are the largest network of primary care providers in the United States (National Association of Community Health Centers [NACHC], 2010). Primary care is defined as the:

provision of integrated, accessible health care services by clinicians who are accountable for addressing a large majority of personal health care needs, developing a sustained partnership with patients, and practicing in the context of family and community (Donaldson, Yordy, Lohr, & Vanselow, 1996, p. 1).

Primary care services are general medical services provided to ambulatory patients. These services include family practice, pediatrics, obstetrics and gynecology, and preventive services. Primary care services include well-baby checks, immunizations, and prenatal and post-natal care. Also included are treatments for childhood diseases and common chronic conditions, such as hypertension, angina, back pain, arthritis, depression, and diabetes mellitus. Primary care providers include physicians, nurse practitioners, and physician assistants.

The majority of the patients of CHCs have limited access to health care services. Factors limiting access include financial, geographic, language, cultural, and other barriers (NCCHCA, 2011). Therefore, most of the patients have low incomes, are uninsured or have Medicaid, and are members of racial or ethnic minorities (NACHC, 2010). They may live in urban or rural areas. Patients facing these types of barriers are known as medically underserved or vulnerable patients. HRSA designates Medically Underserved Areas/Populations (MUA/Ps) as areas or populations with one or some combination of the following statuses:

- Health Professional Shortage Areas (HPSAs) defined by HRSA as having shortages of primary medical care, dental, or mental health providers,
- Residents with shortages of personal health services,
- High infant mortality,
- High poverty, or
- High elderly population.

MUAs may be whole counties, groups of contiguous counties or other civil divisions, or groups of urban census tracts. MUPs may include groups of persons who face economic, cultural, or linguistic barriers to health care. They are sometimes called vulnerable patients or populations. Included in medically underserved populations are migratory and seasonal agricultural workers, the homeless, and residents of public housing.

FQHCs receive federal grant funding under section 330. FQHCs provide services using a sliding fee scale (fee adjusted to ability to pay). Benefits of the FQHC designation include:

- Start-up grant funding up to $650,000.
- Capped, cost-based Medicare and Medicaid reimbursement.
- Medical malpractice coverage through the Federal Tort Claims Act.
- Eligibility to purchase prescription and non-prescription medications for outpatients at reduced cost through the 340B Drug Pricing Program.
- Access to Vaccine for Children Program.
- Eligibility for various other federal grants and programs.

Two additional types of FQHCs exist (although not among CPH's member organizations). Look-Alikes are health care organizations that are similar to FQHCs in terms of eligibility requirements and benefits, except that they do not receive the section 330 grant funding (Office of Rural Health Policy, 2006). Outpatient health programs/facilities operated by tribal organizations or urban Indian organizations under the Indian Self-Determination Act and Indian Health Care Improvement Act, respectively (Office of Rural Health Policy).

RHCs increase access to primary and preventive health care in rural areas. RHCs must be located in non-urbanized areas with health professional shortages (HPSA or Governor-designated; Office of Rural Health Policy, 2006). Generally, similarities exist between FQHCs and RHCs in terms of eligibility requirements and benefits. Key differences are that RHCs:

- Must be in non-urbanized areas (unlike FQHCs which may be in urban areas).
- Are ineligible for 340B Drug Pricing Program.
- Have narrower scopes of services.
- Must have mid-level practitioners (nurse practitioner, physician assistant, or nurse midwife) on site and available to see patients 50% of the time.

Community Partners HealthNet (CPH), Inc. Environment

The organization's mission statement is "Community Partners HealthNet, through shared resources, serves the participating community health centers in their commitment to provide quality, accessible health care to the populations in underserved areas" (Community Partners HealthNet, 2012).

Plans and actions taken follow the organization's values of service and the providing of quality, accessible care for the specific constituency. As the Chief Executive Officer/Chief Information Officer of CPH Doug Smith explained, "CPH was needed. I knew it was the right thing to do." CPH allows for small health centers to centralize information that can, in turn, be used not only to improve patient quality, but also allows for the health centers to have access to such information at a more affordable cost. Instead of each facility having its own staff to train staff, implement information technology, write reports, and manage data activities, CPH provides the services. Smith noted, "It was obvious that this [CPH] would serve all of us to work together."

CPH is an Application Service Provider (ASP). For its member organizations in North Carolina and Texas, CPH's services include:

- Delivering and supporting information technology and administrative services,
- Managing a data warehouse, and
- Tracking clinical outcomes.

The information technology and administrative services include Electronic Health Records (EHRs), Electronic Dental Records (EDRs), and Practice Management Software (PMS; Community Partners HealthNet, 2012).

CPH has 7.0 full-Time Equivalents (FTEs) exclusive of Smith. Smith also serves as the director/CEO of Greene County Health Care, Inc. (GCHC), a CHC-member of CPH. His position at CPH is donated by GCHC. Moreover, in addition to the 7.0 FTE assigned exclusively to CPH, GCHC provides personnel support whose contribution to CPH is co-mingled with the clinic's mission. The positions at CPH include a report writer whose primary responsibility is to generate the reports requested by CPH members. Smith explained, "We can track clinical outcomes and process measures and offer feedback to the Medical Director" (See Table 1 for a sample report).

Also working at CPH are hardware technical support staff that back-up data and work with other sites if there are connectivity issues. For CPH's electronically-stored patient data, support staff members also ensure compliance with the Health Insurance Portability and Accountability Act (HIPAA) of 1996. Moreover, they work with the other CPH members to assure the data's safety during inclement weather (e.g., checking on the site during a recent hurricane). In addition, there are two training and support staffers for the member sites. Key to CPH's success in EHR implementation, data warehousing, and data reporting is the member centers' follow through in staff training. CPH staff train the staff members at each member site so they can use the health information technology (e.g., properly add a provider or specialist to EHR or a pharmacy to EHR's contract manager) and stay updated regarding meaningful use requirements and ICD-10 readiness as well as EHR user preferences on CPH's purchased certified ambulatory practice management and EHR system.

The staff number is small, but each staff member was hired with the understanding and desire for continued learning. Smith stated, "We 'grew our own.'" Smith originally hired local personnel who (a) had extensive IT experience, (b) endorsed the mission of CPH, and (c) possessed the desire to learn more about health infor-

Table 1. Sample report from Community Partners HealthNet, Inc.

Measures and Goals			
Category	CVD		
Group	Patients with hypertension		
Total Number of Patients in Group	1431		
Event Name	Patient Events	Achieved %	Target %
BP<140/90 mm HG	756	52.83	50

mation technology and the administrative responsibilities that accompany it. More recently hired staff members have already had some training and experience in the field. For example, two recent hires included a director of a health center's Management Information Systems (MIS) and an individual with 20-years' experience in second-level support at a large, multinational technology and consulting corporation. Nonetheless, all staff members endorse the service mission of community and rural health centers—to provide quality, accessible health care to the populations in underserved areas.

SETTING THE STAGE

CPH evolved from discussions among directors of North Carolina CHCs in the late 1990s. These leaders were discussing the mutual creation of a health maintenance organization. As part of this discussion, leaders established functional task forces, such as MIS and finance. Doug Smith, one of the CHC directors, was a member of the MIS task force.

Political forces terminated the discussion of the mutual health maintenance organization. However, Doug and other directors continued to consider a shared information network. Concomitantly, HRSA, through grant funding, was supporting the establishment of Health-Center-Controlled Networks (HCCNs). Deciding to go forward on the shared information network, Doug and five other directors applied for the federal funding.

Smith served as the driver, identifying the need for health information technology for the CHCs. He gained support among his colleagues for the notion that economies of scale could be realized if the health centers used CPH as an HIT and data warehousing service provider. Cost savings could accrue to the health centers because, in economies of scale, cost per unit decreases as the scale increases. Along with the CEOs' support, Smith also had physician champions from CHCs. Patient care could be improved via physicians making decisions informed by data. Finally, Smith took the lead role in gaining support from North Carolina Senators and Congressmen. Smith served as the lead champion and entrepreneur for CPH.

An interview with Dr. Thomas Maynor, Chief Operating Officer of Robeson Health Care Corporation (one of the original member centers), provided insight into the impetus for forming this shared information network. Original members of CPH shared a vision for improving the quality of health care delivered, establishing best practices, reducing costs, and making decisions informed by the aggregation of information in a data warehouse. The data warehouse would be made possible by the adoption and implementation of an integrated HIT system that included a PMS, an EHR, and an electronic dental record across the shared information network. Members of CPH participate in shared governance. The CEOs of each of the participating CHCs serve on the governing board which routinely meets quarterly, but which has met as often as monthly. Active participation by the CEOs enhances buy-in into the network; further strengthening this support is the CEOs' practice of bringing staff members to the board meetings to discuss initiatives and concerns within their functional areas of expertise. Work groups are also hosted by CPH (T. Maynor, personal communication, October 27, 2011).

Three of the six original members remain with CPH. New recruits are drawn by the mission of CPH, its track record as an established HCCN, and the dedication and reputation of its leadership. Ms. Lucy Ramirez, CEO of Nuestra Clinica del Valle, acknowledged these as factors in her clinic's decision to join CPH approximately three years ago. Her clinic had been participating in a network seeking to implement an EHR. Delays in implementation and her discovery that the new EHR would not interface with a legacy practice management system, despite previous assurances from the vendor that it would both contributed to the termination of the contract with the vendor and search for a new shared information network. As a positive deciding factor to transition to CPH, Ms. Ramirez cited her familiarity, through working together at national CHC meetings, with Mr. Doug Smith, CEO of CPH, and the successes achieved at CPH. In the brave new digital world, geographic boundaries pose few problems. Although her clinic is located in Texas, Ms. Ramirez participates in board meetings via telephone conference, and her staff members are active participants in working groups addressing clinical operations, billing and revenue cycle management, compliance, and performance improvement (L. Ramirez, personal communication, October 27, 2011).

Dr. Maynor and Ms. Ramirez shared a common perspective about the advantages of being a member of CPH—access to an EHR and a PMS, on-site training, help desk and technical support requested via electronic ticket, access to the data stored in the data warehouse for reports required by the state and federal government, technical upgrades to software, support for vendor negotiations, and shared challenges to meet the emerging federal requirements related to meaningful use and patient-centered medical home certification.

CASE DESCRIPTION

Technology Concerns

The planning of CPH's EHR and data warehouse projects started in the 1990s when its initial six member CHCs faced the challenges of legacy systems that were not Y2K (year 2000) compliant and of new encounter and performance reporting from

HRSA's Bureau of Primary Health Care. The initial members also had a vision of outcome and quality-related data being used for quality improvement activities. Quality assurance organizations such as the National Committee for Quality Assurance (NCQA) now demand reporting of quality data. In the late 1990s, little reporting function existed in any of nearly 60 EHR systems reviewed. Most vendors were charging for custom reports any time a new report was needed. The decision then was to merge the data from the backend databases of the EHRs into one large data warehouse so reporting could be centralized and become a service to the member health centers. Both EHRs and data warehouse went online at the same time and CPH is the sole service provider for both systems. CPH also provides services to generate reports from the data in the data warehouse for individual member centers. The reports are used to submit data to organizations like HRSA or NCQA as well as for quality assurance at the individual member centers. The number of member centers has grown from the initial 6 to the current 14 while both the EHRs and the data warehouse are scaled up for the growth of the consortium. The initial cost of building the data warehouse, including hardware, reporting software, upload scripts, and a catalog for the reporting software was about $100,000. Having received many awards, CPH is widely regarded and recognized as a pioneering model for HIT projects because of its centralized and integrated EHR hosting, data warehousing, just-in-time reporting, and the operation and quality of its member centers.

Challenges exist for the implementation of an integrated HIT project. One challenge involves consistency. "Providers need to be consistent on what they do," Doug Smith said during the interview for this case report. Providers capture initial data during the encounters with the patients. The consistency, comprehensiveness, and accuracy of their data capture will subsequently influence the quality of their data in the EHR and the data warehouse. Providers at health centers are under tremendous pressure to provide services to large numbers of patients. Consequently, the quality of captured data is not always consistent. New providers need to be trained thoroughly in order to record all needed data for quality reporting.

The second challenge that the data warehouse project often faces is the system changes required by major EHR software updates. Because CPH does not develop the EHR software in-house, it relies on the vendor to provide periodic updates. When an update involves changes of the data model in the EHR, the data model of the data warehouse must be modified accordingly. Occasionally, but not usually, an update will require that the scripts in the reporting software be correspondingly modified. Happening once or twice a year, system updates have been and always will be a challenge because of the nature of the entire system. CPH has been working closely with the EHR vendor; the process of the system update has been made much smoother since these meetings.

As previously mentioned, CPH generates routine reports to send to federal agencies, such as HRSA, and to quality assurance entities, such as NCQA. Additionally, though, other reports on clinical quality are sent back to medical directors for quality assurance and improvement at the individual health centers. The EHR templates could then be modified based on the quality reporting in order to enhance a Quality Improvement (QI) process. Some of the CHCs (e.g., the Greene County Health Care) have shown improvements in delivering quality health care and in reducing disparities after implementing the data warehouse project. For example, the results of one study showed that "in comparison with national data...Greene County Health Care [GCHC] is doing a comparable job meeting diabetes goals for HbA1c, blood pressure, and lipid levels and in some instances is achieving better outcomes despite predominately low-income clients" (Kirk, Bertoni, Grzywacz, Smith, & Arcury, 2008, p. 281). Moreover, in one of its latest reports to HRSA, GCHC reported that disparities in terms of diabetic care do not exist within its patient population. The complete process of quality assurance with the integration of EHR and data warehouse is shown in Figure 1.

Technology Components

Data Warehouse

In computer technology, a data warehouse is a "collection of integrated subject-oriented data bases designed to support the DSS [Decision Support System] function, where each unit of data is relevant to some moment in time. The data warehouse contains atomic data and lightly summarized data. A data warehouse is a subject oriented, integrated, non-volatile, time variant collection of data designed to support management DSS needs" (Inmon, 2012). As a specialized database, its primary purpose is to store, report and analyze data. The data stored in the data warehouse are uploaded from multiple operational database systems. Often these operational database systems are heterogeneous; therefore, certain types of data transformation and calculation (e.g., summation) are performed before the data are merged into the data warehouse under a common data structure. The term for the steps involved in uploading data from operational databases to a data warehouse is called ETL (extraction, transformation and loading). Many major database vendors (Oracle, Microsoft SQL server) have integrated into their products the functionalities for implementing a data warehouse. Because the data in a data warehouse are cleaned, transformed, pre-calculated, and cataloged; they are readily used for analytic operations such as data mining, Online Analytic Processing (OLAP), statistical analysis, or other business intelligence techniques.

Figure 1. Role of CPH data warehouse project for quality assurance and improvement

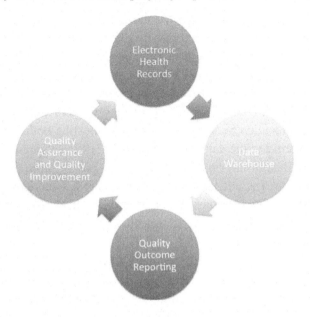

The benefits of a data warehouse are multifold:

- Supports data storage from multiple data sources. Consequentially, a centralized view can be applied to the data warehouse that allows decision makers to compare data from multiple data sources.
- Has the capability of cleaning, transforming, and cataloging data for subsequent operations. It enhances the efficiency and quality of the analysis.
- Contains, often, operational data with time stamps and location information. Thus, it will facilitate temporal and geological data analysis.
- Uses a common data structure so consistency of data is enforced, even though data may come from different sources.

A data warehouse is a specialized database different from a relational database that is often used for transactions. Most relational databases conform to relational model theory and are designed based on a data modeling technique called Entity Relationship Diagram. Tables and attributes of tables are normalized for efficient capture of transactional data. However, it is often too time consuming to run queries involving multiple relational databases along several dimensions. The schema for a data warehouse follows a dimensional template (time, location, outcome, etc.). On the other hand, the relational database follows the entity relationship diagram. The purpose of the data warehouse is for storage, reporting, and analysis. Usually, the data warehouse is not a real time system; it should not be used for ad hoc query because it will not reflect the real data distribution at the moment. Commonly, hierarchical and redundant data are stored in a data warehouse in order to improve the performance for data access and analysis. Students may consult standard texts on data warehouses, such as *Building the Data Warehouse* (Inmon, 2005), *The DataWarehouse ETL Toolkit* (Kimball & Caserta, 2004), and *Data Warehouse Fundamentals for IT Professionals* (Ponniah, 2010), for details on their implementation (see Figure 2).

CPH is an Application Service Provider (ASP) hosting both EHRs for individual member centers and the data warehouse. An EHR is a "longitudinal electronic record of patient health information generated by one or more encounters in any care delivery setting. Included in this information are patient demographics, progress notes, problems, medications, vital signs, past medical history, immunizations, laboratory data and radiology reports" (Healthcare Information and Management Systems Society, 2011).

CPH uses a vendor's certified ambulatory system to store both clinical and practice management data. The current system was selected 10 years ago by a committee of several EHR experts including one of the authors following a standard EHR selection process. In standard EHR selection processes, common criteria for vendor comparisons are: (a) technology and scalability, (b) standards and compliance, (c) user interface, (d) integration, (e) reporting and data, (f) implementation, (g) training, (h) support, (i) references, (j) leadership and response, and (k) CHC experience (Smith & Rachman, 2008). On these criteria, a vendor is rated as above average (meets most or all the criteria), average (meets some criteria), or below

Figure 2. Architecture of the data warehouse project

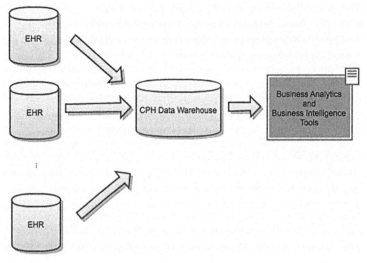

average (meets few or no criteria). After reviewing more than 50 different vendors, the committee invited four vendors of PMS/EHR systems to demonstrate their systems. The committee used scorecards for PMS and EHR to rate and rank the vendors after their demonstrations.

The system is certified, as a complete EHR supporting meaningful use, by the Office of the National Coordinator – Authorized Testing and Certification Body (ONC-ATCB). All the backend databases are running on an enterprise database management server. Using an ASP model, CPH provides services to individual member centers with charged fees. Each CHC has a dedicated database running on the server to support the transactions at the center. Each day, providers and staff at the member centers work through transparent log-ins to metaframe servers at CPH. Nothing is uploaded from the centers to CPH. The metaframe servers are connected to the main database server which houses the clinical and the PMS. Once each evening, data are extracted, transformed, and loaded into the data warehouse using the capabilities of the reporting software and the associated scripts. Selected tables from the EHR and PMS databases are used in this process; and then, time and date-stamped, as well as stamped to the originating database and server (i.e., for each CHC or RHC). The data warehouse follows a similar data schema to the relational database for the individual EHRs for the tables selected (which include all demographic and clinical data). The benefit of such similarity is simplified data transfer. Data tables are comparable between the databases and the data warehouse.

Conventionally, a data warehouse usually uses the data model called star schema in a dimensional format. Sometimes, it could be combined with a normalized relational data model to produce a snowflake data model to support both transaction and query of the data in the warehouse. However, the design of the data warehouse also needs to take into consideration the efficiency of data transfer and scalability. The model used at CPH does meet its members' needs to have a data warehouse and, to date, has been scalable to additional member health centers. Given limited human and financial resources, a normalized design may not have been a top priority at this stage. More interesting, though, is that the original design, with 10 years of data in some databases, still meets the needs of CPH, its members, and can often run reports in seconds. It is always important to benchmark the data warehouse's performance to assess its continued ability to meet the needs for increased reporting and of quality improvement requirements.

In order to track patients with different conditions (e.g., diabetes) in a data warehouse, flag fields are available and can be implemented in the EHR database, or, more commonly, the report can be based on diagnostic codes. For example, if the data warehouse needs to be used to report diabetic patient outcomes, a flag field called "diabetic" can be set on individual patients with diabetes. That information will then be uploaded and stored in data warehouse for future access and analysis.

The flag can be checked manually or automatically if certain criteria can be written as scripts running within the database. Some outcome data are pre-calculated as needed for reporting purposes. After the member centers are closed for business, the data warehouse is updated each night to prevent the uploading from impacting the performance of the centers' EHRs.

CPH staff members use enterprise-level business analytics and business intelligence software to query and analyze data from the data warehouse and to generate reports for various purposes. Business analytics tools can continuously explore and investigate business data to gain understanding and insights of the organization's performance. In contrast, business intelligence tools focus more on using a consistent set of metrics both to measure past performance and to guide future planning. Both business analytics and business intelligence applications are based on data and statistical methods. These tools have the capabilities of fetching data cataloged in the data warehouse and of producing high quality ad hoc reports for decision makers. Figure 3 is a sample report that tabulates numbers of diabetes patients by average (hemoglobin) A1c range and race. CPH staff can routinely generate such reports to support the centers' quality improvement, evaluation of health disparities, and research.

Figure 3. Sample report generated by business analytics and business intelligence software

Community Partners	Year 2005		Date: 2/21/07
HealthNet	**Diabetes Patient Average A1c Range By Race**		GCHC

Race: BLA	Patient with A1c:		
Average A1c range: 7.0 or less	Number of patients: 128	Percentage: 46.55%
Average A1c range: 7.0-7.9	Number of patients: 56	Percentage: 20.36%
Average A1c range: 8.0-8.9	Number of patients: 38	Percentage: 13.82%
Average A1c range: 9.0-9.9	Number of patients: 20	Percentage: 7.27 %
Average A1c range: 9.9 or more	Number of patients: 33	Percentage: 12.00%

Race: HIS	Patient with A1c:		
Average A1c range: 7.0 or less	Number of patients: 38	Percentage: 29.01%
Average A1c range: 7.0-7.9	Number of patients: 24	Percentage: 18.32%
Average A1c range: 8.0-8.9	Number of patients: 14	Percentage: 10.69%
Average A1c range: 9.0-9.9	Number of patients: 17	Percentage: 12.98%
Average A1c range: 9.9 or more	Number of patients: 38	Percentage: 29.01%

Race: WHI	Patient with A1c:		
Average A1c range: 7.0 or less	Number of patients: 61	Percentage: 51.26%
Average A1c range: 7.0-7.9	Number of patients: 25	Percentage: 21.01%
Average A1c range: 8.0-8.9	Number of patients: 15	Percentage: 12.61%
Average A1c range: 9.0-9.9	Number of patients: 9	Percentage: 7.56 %
Average A1c range: 9.9 or more	Number of patients: 9	Percentage: 7.56 %

Page 1

Hardware

Two servers run concurrently to support the EHRs and data warehouse. The servers are mirrored in real time so if one server is down the other could be online immediately. Both servers use the latest data storage technologies, allowing data to be stored and retrieved quickly. Both use two 640 GB I/O adapter cards from Fusion-IO as the primary storage media. I/O adapter card is one of the latest memory storage technologies based on solid state NAND Flash Memory (same category as flash drive) technology. This storage technology improves application response time; minimizes application latency; and reduces hardware infrastructure, maintenance, and energy costs. Both servers are backed up daily to another on-site server and to a remote server in a secured data center. If both servers are down, the remote server can serve as the main server for both the EHR and the data warehouse. All users access the EHR systems through the Citrix secure remote access.

Management and Organizational Concerns

Smith symbolizes transformational leadership. CPH and Green County Health Care, Inc. (GCHC) are his vocation. With Smith serving as both CEO/CIO for CPH and CEO for GCHC, the building site for CPH is adjacent to the community health center. In minutes, Smith can walk from GCHC to CPH. Thus, his presence as the leader of both facilities is apparent. This multi-leadership position is both a benefit and a concern. In order for the creation of a site such as CPH, Smith as the champion and entrepreneur was a benefit. He rallied the support from other CEOs and physicians; he spoke to the NC Senators and Congressmen; he wrote the grants for funding opportunities. Once established, he hired, trained, and guided the staff members who worked at CPH. Throughout the process, he was aware of the goodness of fit of CPH for the health centers precisely because he served as CEO of a CHC. He understood the vision for CPH—the need for data sharing, the need to organize patient information better, and the need for efficiencies in a not-for-profit environment. He also could communicate the vision with authority; he was a CEO. Nonetheless, a concern is the succession planning required to replace such a dynamic, dedicated, and transformational leader. The time and effort expended as a CEO of the CHC and the time and effort as the transformational leader for CPH takes its toll on (but also motivates) any one person. As Smith wryly admitted, he had not had a vacation since the start of CPH; by choice, he notes, and no longer true as he began a 10-day vacation following the interview for this case.

In additional to leadership, factors pursuant to CPH success included the creation of a sustainable governance structure, good reporting and training endeavors by effective staff, growth of reputation in community and rural health center leaders, and the continued securing of funding to cover CPH costs.

The governance structure is comprised of Board members from each health center site. The Board meets quarterly, monthly if needed. The meetings provide the opportunity for oversight of CPH activities as well as serve as avenues to maintain member collaborative relationships.

Ms. Beverley Stroud, CFO at Greene County Health Care, Inc. (GCHC), provides an estimated 0.20 to 0.25 FTE in support of CPH. Monthly, members of CPH pay dues and support fees. Budgeting for CPH is supported out of the CFO's office, as is the preparation of monthly invoices, and the inclusion of CPH in GCHC's financial statements (B. Stroud, personal communication, September 14, 2011). CPH charges its members quarterly dues. Benefits of membership are (a) inclusion in grant applications and any subsequent grant awards and (b) access to computer support and the data warehouse reporting functions. Support revenue is the amount paid by members quarterly and/or monthly for the specific programs used (i.e., the EHR, PMS, etc). Grant funds are also used to cover staff costs and other expenses (travel, data conversions, etc.) related to bringing new CHCs and RHCs onto the EHR. Basically, membership dues and support revenue fund ongoing operating costs. Grants pay for bringing in new centers and investments in plant, property, and equipment, if stipulated in the grant request.

CPH generated a total of $684,125 in 2010 revenue – Support Revenue ($172,234), Grants ($408,991), and Membership Revenues ($102,900). Expenses totaled $790,716. Therefore, HealthNet incurred losses of $106,591, although $231,288 was depreciation, a noncash expense (Sitterson & Barker, P.A., 2010).

As a member of CPH, GCHC and the other members derive benefits that support both the financial and clinical operations. The interface between the EHR and the PMS reduces data entry when new patients join the centers because common fields in the records are automatically populated. Some of the support responsibilities such as system maintenance and backup are performed by CPH rather than billing and other center personnel. Updates to CPT codes are performed annually. A weekly report of procedures documented in the EHR has improved billing for laboratory and x-ray procedures on a fee-for-services basis. Normally, many of these charges would have been lost. Finally, routine and ad hoc reporting of data collected by the data warehouse facilitates state and federal reporting such as annual cost reports and the Uniform Data System (UDS) reports required of community health centers (B. Stroud, personal communication, September 14, 2011).

As previously noted in "Environment," the staff members of CPH are from the local area. They possess degrees in Information Technology from local institutes of higher learning, have at least five years of prior work experience in IT, and endorse the mission of community health centers. In Smith's words, "They had to learn the application software as it was developed and as we added new capabilities."

The commitment of staff to the CPH vision was important to the success of early endeavors. For instance, understanding that any reports that were generated may or may not be accurate, based upon how the parameters were defined. To elaborate refer to Table 1, Sample Report. In this scenario, a report was requested regarding patients with hypertension. Yet, how this variable (patients with hypertension) was elucidated affects the resulting report. For example, is the requester inquiring about the number of patients who have hypertension and who have had an encounter at the health care center? OR, is the requester inquiring about the number of patients who have hypertension and who are currently being treated in the health care center? Particulars, such as the definition of the variable in question, matter, and the staff members must always be aware of such distinctions to help bring about accurate data reporting and in clarifying the question being asked by health center staff. CPH staff work with members of the CPH Quality Improvement (QI) Committee and individual health centers to design templates that capture the data consistently to meet meaningful use, patient-centered medical home, Bureau of Primary Care, or individual center QI initiatives.

Efforts placed in training the staff members of member sites were also vital to CPH success. If staff members at member sites had not been adequately trained on how to use the EHR, any information summoned for reports would be suspect and would, therefore, negate the mission of CPH. Staff members at all sites who have access to the EHR and PMS had to know how to use the systems effectively. Training was essential; Smith knew this. To this end, he hired trainers who he thought:

- Had sufficient IT experience.
- Were prepared to learn relevant health information technology, including the application software.
- Would test out new IT teaching services.
- Possessed patience to serve as a trainer.
- Had communication skills to listen to the trainees and to accommodate their teaching style to individual needs.

Crystal Beaman, currently serving as Director of Implementation and Training, was from the local area and had studied as a nursing assistant and transcriptionist. She then worked in software product engineering as she completed her college degree. With her past work experiences and her interest in CPH, Smith determined that she would be a good fit as a trainer. Beaman reported that training for a new member site is tailored to the needs of the organization. To minimize costs, remote (Web-based) training can be accomplished from the home base of CPH. Nonetheless, she does travel to each site to see that the trainees have learned the information portrayed in the remote training sessions and [to allow them] to gain further knowledge of using the EHR. This on-site encounter also presents an opportunity for face-to-face interaction with her—a CPH representative. Beaman explained, "Sometimes, if they [the trainees] are negative and frustrated in a session, it is because they missed something. We will stop, go back to where they had success, and then identify what they missed. It is important to communicate at the level they are at" (C. Beaman, personal communication, September 2, 2011).

Beaman also explained the importance of leader support at trainings. "How involved senior leadership is in supporting IT training is critical." If the center's CEO is present and engaged in the training, the rest of the trainees know the importance given to their mastering the subject matter. The CEO as IT trainer role model is not to be understated; they are leader champions.

Informal leaders may serve as HIT training champions, as well. To elaborate, Beamer has asked for pairings at trainee sites. In such cases, the pairings are with a faster learner and a slower learner. These pairings can be made across normal [usual] occupations [jobs]. For instance, if a member site had a fast learner at the front desk and a slower learner in the lab, these two staff members could be paired up, resulting in enhanced experiences for all involved.

Beaman directs training in steps, which include:

- Initial assessment to identify what is needed, equipment to be purchased, Internet upgrades if necessary, and to begin involving the staff early in the process.
- Web-based trainings to introduce staff to the basics of the EHR (clinical) and PMS (billing, scheduling appointments) packages.
- On-site trainings prior to the "go live" date to ensure staff are prepared.
- Web-based "how-to" documents and training videos.

Her final comment regarding training was that she found the presence of the "decision makers" in the training room changes the whole process. Champions of change were key to success.

Finally, key to success of CPH was funding. Smith again serves as the leader in the procurement of grants. However, Smith notes that grant funding is subject to political and competitive events and processes. As previously stated, membership fees ($15,000 per center) and support revenues do not yet cover all of CPH's operating costs. Sustainability is a potential issue regarding funding. However, based on having the infrastructure in place and a new joint marketing arrangement with the software vendor, CPH expects that, with the addition of two or three new member health centers, it will reach a break-even point.

CURRENT CHALLENGES FACING THE ORGANIZATION

CPH faces current challenges that center on sustainability issues of maintaining relationships, high quality training, and succession planning.

The first issue is that of maintaining relationships, which includes relationships with current members and growing the membership. The Board meetings are one avenue to continue collaborative environment among members. Regarding membership recruitment, there is little direct marketing activity to encourage other CHCs and RHCs to join CPH. Rather, new members generally come from those who have heard about CPH's reputation and/or Smith's reputation, or have been chosen by the NC Office of Rural Health to participate. The reputation of CPH and Smith has allowed for the growth of CPH's membership from 6 to 14. However, for increased financial support as well as QI efforts, more members are desired. To date, the funding has been directed towards building the hardware and software infrastructure, paying its staff members, providing training and IT support to members, and generating reports. There is not enough funding to budget for in-house marketing at this time.

High quality training is also important for the organization to maintain. Beaman focuses on the training initiatives and continuously looks for efficient and effective ways to train CPH members. For the last eight years, CPH has hosted a Web community that is linked to the CPH Web page. Recently, social media (information posted, sent, received, and/or exchanged via on-line) has been employed to expand training resources and capabilities. Social media may represent a change in how people send, receive and exchange information because participants, engaging in dialog (creating two-way content exchange), become both active publishers and passive recipients (Thielst, 2010). For health care organizations, social media are a means to build relationships with stakeholders. CPH's social media strategies allow for (a) continuous up-to-date tweets (via twitter), (b) notifications and links supplied on Facebook (see http://www.cphealthnet.org/ for access to these sites), (c) Website design, and (d) e-mail accounts for communications via the centers and CPH. Members can click on a training link and start a training lesson at their chosen time.

The co-mingling of executive responsibilities between GCHC and CPH represents a continuing challenge. For the present, stakeholders at GCHC seem to accept the diversion of leadership resources in exchange for the benefits provided by CPH. Acceptance of the status quo in the short term is probably acceptable, although difficulties are anticipated if the current leader should retire or change positions.

Succession planning is an issue that may be a challenge for any organization that has a transformational leader such as Smith. Succession planning is a strategy to transition from one leader to the next with minimal disruptions to work processes and employees. Dye (2010) proposes that succession planning should be a priority as strong and dependable leadership serves the needs of employees. Transformational leaders effectively communicate the organization's vision to its stakeholders, inspire their employees to strive for excellence, and provide individual attention to help employees excel. Robbins and Judge (2011) define transformational leaders as those who inspire their employees to "transcend their own self-interests" (p. 391). Necessarily, finding a successor to Smith, a transformational leader, will challenge CPH.

At CPH, Smith is transformational leader, entrepreneur, and champion. Smith's leadership with its positive attributes *is* CPH's success. He has convincingly communicated CPH's vision, hired and trained effective and loyal staff members, and procured grants and CPH members to fund the organization. Also as with single leadership, there is little to no succession planning for CPH. Smith responded that succession planning had not been a dominant thought, but GCHC could bring in a Deputy Director at some point, but not now. Of course, this issue relates to funding and the allocation of resources. Strategically, the issue addresses the need or not for a Deputy Director when the monies available are already directed toward keeping CPH's serving as the ASP and data warehouse.

SOLUTIONS AND RECOMMENDATIONS

The design of the data warehouse at CPH did not follow the conventional architecture for data warehousing. It replicated a large portion of the data model from the relational databases of the EHR. This approach's major benefit is the efficiency of data uploading from databases to the data warehouse. However, this approach may reduce the data warehouse's performance in terms of the speed of query and analysis. The scripts also create data cubes. A data warehouse usually uses the data model called star schema in a dimensional format. Sometimes it could be combined with a normalized relational data model to produce a snowflake data model to support both transaction and query of the data in the warehouse. The data model used at CPH does meet its members' needs to have a data warehouse and has been scalable so far with additional member health centers. Given limited human and financial resources, a normalized design may not be a top priority at this stage. More interesting, though, is that the original design, with 10 years of data in some databases, still meets the needs of CPH and its members, and can often run reports in seconds. Improvements in performance could be accomplished in a much cheaper fashion, including upgrading the desktop, using an application server, or moving the data warehouse DB to a separate I/O card, etc. However, the performance of the data warehouse always needs to be benchmarked in order to meet the needs of increased reporting and quality improvement requirements.

Proposed recommendations for CPH regarding sustainability issues of maintaining relationships, and succession planning include activities that align with its current mission, vision, and values. As stated earlier, CPH's mission is to serve, through shared resources, the participating community health centers in their commitment to provide quality, accessible health care to the populations in underserved areas. To that end, CPH should consider ways to increase revenue to shore up its sustainability. In terms of marketing and growth of member centers, CPH has partnered with the software vendor integrating its marketing efforts into the vendor's efforts. This relationship has resulted in CHC "leads" coming from around the country to CPH; joint CPH-vendor demos are provided to these CHCs (i.e., two demos were done in the last few weeks). Social media in health care focuses on connecting, communicating, and collaborating with like-minded constituencies. Beaman had already invested in social media ways for training. Weblogs, podcasts, YouTube (youtube.com) are examples of ways to communicate with audiences who share similar interests. They serve as a way to integrate social media into a communication strategy for membership growth.

Other methods to grow membership rely upon past strategies of CPH. New members have joined because of Smith and CPH's reputation. More engagement in research opportunities allows for more quality improvement, more recognition among peers, and perhaps more federal funding to sponsor such research endeavors. One recent example of a research partnership is the application to the Agency for Healthcare Research and Quality (AHRQ) submitted with Wake Forest University to develop (a) content for the CPH patient portal and personal health record (ePHIM) and (b) training methods and resources for staff and patients to use the portal and ePHIM.

Last is the issue of succession planning. Because leadership assets at CPH and GCHC are co-mingled, a transition plan is needed to separate the responsibilities and/or prepare for contingency situations such as departures. Planning responsibilities should be vested in the CPH Board. This recommendation is not new. Recommendations with attendant costs were presented to the Board about two years ago; the Board did not move on the recommendations. Recommendations regarding succession planning for a site such as CPH include focusing on what is realistic and what has born success in the past. Smith partly "grew his own" staff to establish CPH. The notion of "growing one's own" for succession planning might fit as well.

REFERENCES

Adair, J. (2005). *How to grow leaders: The seven key principles of effective leadership development*. London, UK: Kogan Page.

Bureau of Primary Health Care. (2008, June). *Health centers: America's primary care safety net, reflections on success, 2002-2007*. Retrieved November 8, 2011 from http://www.hrsa.gov/ourstories/healthcenter/reflectionsonsuccess.pdf

Community Partners HealthNet, Inc. (2011). *Website*. Retrieved October 17, 2011, from http://www.cphealthnet.org/index.htm

Donaldson, M. S., Yordy, K. D., Lohr, K. N., & Vanselow, N. A. (Eds.). (1996). *Primary care: America's health in a new era*. Washington, DC: National Academy Press.

Dye, C., & Garman, A. (2006). *Exceptional leadership*. Chicago, IL: Health Administration Press.

Dye, C. F. (2010). *Leadership in healthcare: Essential values and skills* (2nd ed.). Chicago, IL: Health Administration Press.

Health Resources and Services Administration. (2011a). *What are the benefits of a health center controlled network?* Retrieved October 18, 2011, from http://www. hrsa.gov/healthit/toolbox/HealthITAdoptiontoolbox/OpportunitiesCollaboration/benefitsofhccn.html

Health Resources and Services Administration. (2011b). *What is a health center controlled network?* Retrieved October 17, 2011, from http://www.hrsa.gov/healthit/toolbox/HealthITAdoptiontoolbox/OpportunitiesCollaboration/abouthccns.html

Health Resources and Services Administration. (2011c). *Program requirements*. Retrieved October 19, 2011, from http://bphc.hrsa.gov/about/requirements/hcpreqs.pdf

Healthcare Information and Management Systems Society. (2011). *Electronic health record*. Retrieved November 9, 2011, from http://www.himss.org/ASP/topics_ehr.asp

Inmon, W. H. (2005). *Building the data warehouse* (4th ed.). Indianapolis, IN: Wiley.

Inmon, W. H. (2011). Corporate information factory. *Glossary of Data Warehousing*. Retrieved November 10, 2011, from http://www.inmoncif.com/library/glossary/#D

Kanter, R. M. (2001). *Evolve: Succeeding in the digital culture of tomorrow*. Boston, MA: Harvard Business Publisher.

Kimball, R., & Caserta, J. (2004). *The data warehouse ETL toolkit: Practical techniques for extracting, cleaning, conforming, and delivering data.* Indianapolis, IN: Wiley.

Kirk, J. K., Bertoni, A. G., Grzywacz, J. G., Smith, A., & Arcury, T. A. (2008). Evaluation of quality of diabetes care in a multiethnic, low-income population. *Journal of Clinical Outcomes Management, 15*(6), 281–286.

Lefkowitz, B. (2005). The health center story: Forty years of commitment. *The Journal of Ambulatory Care Management, 28*(4), 295–303.

Lewin, M. E., & Altman, S. (Eds.). (2000). *America's health care safety net: Intact but endangered.* Washington, DC: National Academy Press.

McGinn, C. A., Grenier, S., Duplantie, J., Shaw, N., Sicotte, C., & Mathieu, L. (2011). Comparison of user groups' perspectives of barriers and facilitators to implementing electronic health records: A systematic review. *BMC Medicine, 9*(1), 46–55. doi:10.1186/1741-7015-9-46

National Association of Community Health Centers. (2010). *Fact sheet - Community health centers: The return on investment.* Retrieved October 13, 2011, from http://www.nachc.org/client/documents/CHCs%20ROI%20final%2011%2015%20v.pdf

North Carolina Community Health Center Association. (2011). *Fact sheet - Community health centers: Part of NC's health care solution.* Retrieved October 13, 2011, from http://ncchca.affiniscape.com/associations/11930/files/CHCs%20are%20 cost-saving%20-%20UPDATED%20AUGUST%202011.pdf

Office of Rural Health Policy, Health Resources and Services Administration, Department of Health and Human Services. (2006). *Comparison of rural health clinic and federally qualified health center programs.* Retrieved October 18, 2011, from http://www.ask.hrsa.gov/downloads/fqhc-rhccomparison.pdf

Ponniah, P. (2010). *Data warehousing fundamentals for IT professionals* (2nd ed.). Hoboken, NJ: John Wiley & Sons. doi:10.1002/9780470604137

Poon, E. G., Blumenthal, D., Jaggi, T., Honour, M. M., Bates, D. W., & Kaushal, R. (2004). Overcoming barriers to adopting and implementing computerized physician order entry systems in US hospitals. *Health Affairs, 23*(4), 184–190. doi:10.1377/hlthaff.23.4.184

Rao, S. R., DesRoches, C. M., Donelan, K., Campbell, E. G., Miralles, P. D., & Jha, A. K. (2011). Electronic health records in small physician practices: Availability, use, and perceived benefits. *Journal of the American Medical Informatics Association, 18*(3), 271–275. doi:10.1136/amiajnl-2010-000010

Robbins, S. P., & Judge, T. A. (2011). *Organizational behavior* (14th ed.). Upper Saddle River, NJ: Prentice Hall.

Sitterson & Barker, P. A. (2010, June 30). *Financial statements.* Snow Hill, NC: Greene County Health Care, Inc.

Smith, D. (2009). *A practical approach: Network-based economies of scale for community health.* Paper presented at the Annual Conference and Exhibition of the Healthcare Information and Management Systems Society (HIMSS). Chicago, IL.

Smith, D., & Rachman, F. D. (2008). *Economies of scale in HCCN EHR implementations.* Paper presented at Management Track, National Association of Community Health Centers [NACHC] 2008 Community Health Institute (CHI). Retrieved March 8, 2012 from http://www.softconference.com/nachc/sessionDetail.asp?SID=118996

Thielst, C. B. (2010). *Social media in healthcare: Connect, communicate, collaborate.* Chicago, IL: Health Administration Press.

ADDITIONAL READING

Agency for Health Care Research and Quality. (2011b). *Guide to reducing unintended consequences of electronic health records.* Retrieved November 12, 2011, from http://ucguide.org/

Agency for Healthcare Research and Quality. (2011a). *Website.* Retrieved November 8, 2011, from http://www.ahrq.gov/

Boonstra, A., & Broekhuis, M. (2010). Barriers to the acceptance of electronic medical records by physicians from systematic review to taxonomy and interventions. *BMC Health Services Research, 10,* 231–247. doi:10.1186/1472-6963-10-231

Certification Commission for Health Information Technology. (2011). *Website.* Retrieved November 8, 2011, from http://www.cchit.org/products/onc-atcb

Gruber, D., Cummings, G. G., LeBlanc, L., & Smith, D. L. (2009). Factors influencing outcomes of clinical information systems implementation. *CIN: Computers, Informatics. Nursing, 27*(3), 151–163.

Healthcare Information and Management Systems Society. (2011). *Electronic health record.* Retrieved November 9, 2011, from http://www.himss.org/ASP/index.asp

Inmon, W. H. (2005). *Building the data warehouse* (4th ed.). Indianapolis, IN: Wiley Publishing.

Jamal, A., McKenzie, K., & Clark, M. (2009). The impact of health information technology on the quality of medical and health care: A systematic review. *Health Information Management Journal, 38*(3), 26–37.

Kimball, R., & Ross, M. (2002). *The data warehouse toolkit: The complete guide to dimensional modeling* (2nd ed.). New York, NY: Wiley.

Lau, F., Kuziemsky, C., Price, M., & Gardner, J. (2010). A review on systematic reviews of health information system studies. *Journal of the American Medical Informatics Association, 17*(6), 637–645. doi:10.1136/jamia.2010.004838

Lefkowitz, B. (2007). *Community health centers. A movement and the people who made it happen.* Piscataway, NJ: Rutgers University Press.

Miller, R. H., & Sim, I. (2004). Physicians' use of electronic medical records: Barriers and solutions. *Health Affairs, 23*(2), 116–126. doi:10.1377/hlthaff.23.2.116

National Association of Community Health Centers. (2011). *Website.* Retrieved November 7, 2011, from http://www.nachc.org/

National Committee for Quality Assurance. (n.d.). Retrieved November 8, 2011, from http://www.ncqa.org/

Office of the National Coordinator for Health Information Technology. (2011). *Website.* Retrieved November 8, 2011, from http://healthit.hhs.gov/portal/server.pt/community/healthit_hhs_gov__home/1204

Rural Assistance Center. (2011). *Website.* Retrieved November 7, 2011, from http://www.raconline.org/

U.S. Department of Health and Human Services, Centers for Medicare and Medicaid Services. (2011). *Website.* Retrieved November 7, 2011, from https://www.cms.gov/center/fqhc.asp

U.S. Department of Health and Human Services, Health Resources and Services Administration. (2011a). *HRSA health IT adoption toolkit.* Retrieved November 7, 2011, from http://www.hrsa.gov/healthit/toolbox/HealthITAdoptiontoolbox/index.html

U.S. Department of Health and Human Services, Health Resources and Services Administration. (2011b). *State primary care offices*. Retrieved November 7, 2011, from http://bhpr.hrsa.gov/shortage/hpsas/primarycareoffices.html

U.S. Department of Health and Human Services, Office of the National Coordinator for Health Information Technology. (2011). *Website*. Retrieved November 7, 2011, from http://healthit.hhs.gov/portal/server.pt/community/healthit_hhs_gov__home/1204

KEY TERMS AND DEFINITIONS

Business Intelligence: Computer-based techniques used in identifying, extracting, and analyzing organizational (business) data, such as revenues and costs by services or by units.

Community Health Center (CHC): Non-profit health care organization that provides primary care to individuals in medically underserved areas.

Data Warehouse: Collection of integrated subject-oriented databases designed to support the Decision Support System (DSS) function, where each unit of data is relevant to some moment in time. A data warehouse is a subject oriented, integrated, non-volatile, time variant collection of data (atomic and lightly summarized) designed to support managerial decision-making.

Economy of Scale: Cost savings that accrue from operating on a larger scale; cost per unit decreases as scale of output increases.

Electronic Health Record (EHR): Longitudinal electronic record of patient health information generated by one or more encounters in any care delivery setting. Included in this information are patient demographics, progress notes, problems, medications, vital signs, past medical history, immunizations, laboratory data, and radiology reports.

Health-Center-Controlled Network (HCCN): Collaborative venture that provides health information technologies to community health centers.

Scalable: Capable of being expanded in terms of volume, site or provider, population, and geographic location.

Social Media: Information posted, sent, received, and/or exchanged via on-line.

Succession Planning: Strategy, blueprint, or outline that addresses how transitions from one leader to the next with minimal disruptions to work processes and employees.

Transformational Leadership: Type of leadership in which leaders effectively communicate their organizations' visions to stakeholders, inspire employees to excel, and help employees excel.

Chapter 12
CoRDS Registry:
An HIT Case Study Concerning Setup and Maintenance of a Disease Registry

Seth Trudeau
Sanford Health, USA

EXECUTIVE SUMMARY

The Coordination of Rare Diseases at Sanford (CoRDS) registry has been started to provide a central repository of data for participants suffering from a number of rare diseases and to provide those participants with a resource to learn more about their disease and, in a future enhancement, connect with others that are afflicted. The second purpose of the registry is to provide a resource for researchers to identify and recruit potential participants for their research studies. This case study will focus on the technical aspects of setting up a registry and providing access to participants and their medical team, who will enter data about their disease, and researchers, who will access de-identified data to include in their research. Security of the external website and access to Protected Health Information (PHI) are the main areas of concern with this registry.

ORGANIZATIONAL BACKGROUND

The CoRDS registry was started by David Pearce, PhD, who is employed by Sanford Research. Sanford Research is a partnership between Sanford Health and the University of South Dakota. Sanford Health is one of the largest rural healthcare systems in the United States with headquarters located in Sioux Falls, SD and

DOI: 10.4018/978-1-4666-2671-3.ch012

Fargo, ND. The 33 hospitals and 100+ clinics included in the health system spread across 6 states in the Midwest with a population of more than 2 million people in the covered region.

In February of 2007, Sanford Health was presented with a very generous gift of $400 million from philanthropist T. Denny Sanford with the goal of improving the human condition. An additional commitment was received from Mr. Sanford of $100 million in 2010 to focus on the way we treat breast cancer and search for new treatments and protocols. Many initiatives were started from these gifts including: a focus on pediatric care both in the Sanford Health region and around the world, an effort was started to make Sanford Research one of the top research facilities in the nation, the Sanford Project was started to bring in some of the top diabetes researchers to focus on finding a cure.

Sanford Health is using some of the most regarded software in the industry to handle all aspects of patient care, including EPIC (www.epic.com) for their Electronic Medical Record, Lawson (www.lawson.com) for Purchasing and Payroll and Velos eResearch (www.velos.com) for Clinical Trial Management Software. The Velos software will be utilized in the delivery and collection of the CoRDS registry data and information.

PROJECT BACKGROUND

In an article from Drolet and Johnson (2008), the authors reviewed a number of existing literature to formulate a more precise definition of a medical disease registry. They put forth the definition of "a medical data registry as a system functioning in patient management or research, in which a standardized and complete dataset including associated follow-up is prospectively and systematically collected for a group of patients with a common disease or therapeutic intervention" (pp. 1012-1013). They define 6 characteristics of a medical disease registry: merge-able data, standardized datasets, a set of rules for data collection, observations that are gathered over time, knowledge of outcomes through the use of follow-up, and characterizing the domain of the registry as chronic disease or acute/interventional therapy.

The CoRDS registry was initiated in June of 2010. As of October 2011, there were 98 registered patients covering 35 different rare diseases. The registry is being hosted at Sanford Research/USD in Sioux Falls, South Dakota and is supervised by Investigator David Pearce, PhD, Co-Investigator Chun-Hung Chan, PhD and coordinated by the CoRDS Administrator Liz Donohue. At this point in the registry's existence contact between the registry and its participants is done primarily through telephone and postal mail. The administrator is also working with national and local organizations to promote awareness of the registry. The business needs for this project are to automate and expand the reach of this registry through a technology solution consisting of a Web-delivered portal for participants to enter information and for researchers to pull information back out. The registry does have a Web presence (www.sanfordresearch.org/cords) with some general information and contact details, but not much else.

As was mentioned before, Sanford Health uses software developed by Velos for the management of their clinical trials. This same software has a module for the creation and delivery of a participant portal via the Internet. The experiences of Sanford Health with the existing modules of the Velos application have been positive. The software and vendor support meets our needs for clinical trial management, the participant portal, and reporting on the data collected.

The Information Technology team that supports the Velos application, and the Research department as a whole, is comprised of a Project Manager, an Interface Analyst, and three Application Support Specialists. In addition to the investigators and administrator of the registry, the CoRDS registry team has also added an assistant for the Administrator and a Web Developer to handle the presentation of the participant portal to the participants.

The information in Table 1 lists the stakeholders and their requirements that affect how the participant portal will be designed and maintained.

Table 1. Stakeholder requirements

Stakeholder	Requirements
Participants	• Ease of Use • Ability to populate as much or as little information as needed • Privacy of their data
Researchers	• Ease of querying participant data that has been de-identified • Process to gain access to the data they need
CoRDS personnel	• Ability to capture the data needed for research from the participants • Ease of participant and researcher account setup • Availability of the application and website • Ease of maintenance • Reporting needs to monitor data submissions and data use
Info Technology support	• Tracking customizations to the software • Ease of maintenance • Participant and Researcher security • Auditing capabilities
Sanford Health organization	• Branding of the external website • Policies and Procedures created and documented • Institutional Review Board approval • Security of the website, the users, and auditing of access • Privacy of participant data

CASE DESCRIPTION

Initially the participant portal and its data have been housed within the same application instance and database as the Sanford Health clinical trial data. The original plans for this registry included an installation of the Velos software and the database on a separate set of servers. Due to constraints on the implementation timeline and budget, this was moved to a future task. The implementation tasks for the computerized registry are discussed below.

Portal Security

The first step that needed to be done to get ready for the participant portal to be activated on the current platform was to secure the existing Web server by adding SSL authentication and to move the server out of the internal Sanford Health network so that it could be accessed through the Internet. An SSL certificate was purchased by Sanford Health from a Trusted Certificate Authority and the appropriate setting changes were made to the Web server and software to allow the login page to be seen externally. The SSL layer, along with the multiple levels of firewalls protecting the Sanford Health servers, adds the necessary security to the external website to prevent unsolicited intrusion into the system. The network path between the externally facing Web server and the database server, still housed within Sanford Health's network, was locked down to specific ports and certificates were created to authenticate the traffic from sender to receiver.

The next step was to setup the underlying security for users to enter the system and navigate to the data they need to access. The first piece of security is the participant account. Currently, the CoRDS administrator contacts potential participants through e-mail or over the telephone to get their mailing address. A short questionnaire and an Informed Consent form are sent to the requestor through the postal mail service. The Informed Consent form gives the potential participant all of the information that they need to know about the research study, how their data will be used, and who will have access to it. The participant is enrolled in the study as of the date on the Informed Consent form. The first piece of the project discussed here is to automate the request for enrollment and the form acquisition. The potential participants will be directed to the Sanford Health CoRDS website where they will be able to fill out a short contact questionnaire electronically. The request for access form will be sent to the CoRDS administrator for review and an account for the participant portal will be setup as quickly as possible. A personalized e-mail will be sent with the participant's login information and instructions.

Researchers that wish to use the data gathered through the CoRDS registry will need to submit the proper forms to the Sanford Health Institutional Review Board.

They will need to explain what data they would like to access and what they will use it for. Additionally, they can request contact information for participants if they are recruiting for a clinical trial. These requests also need to go through the Sanford Health Institutional Review Board. The researchers will be setup as users in the Velos system with rights limited to the de-identified data specified in their request.

The Velos software is Part 11 compliant, which means that on top of your standard username and password to enter the system, there is a second level of authentication that is done whenever someone attempts to submit a change to the data. An e-signature is assigned to each user and is requested every time a Submit button is clicked. No data entered or edited in the system will be saved to the database until the user submits the valid e-signature assigned to his/her account. This is an additional layer of security that most systems do not provide currently. Both the login password and the e-signature have been set to expire on a regular basis. Password strength for this system will follow Sanford Health's standards. At least four characters are required for the e-signature.

Title 21 CFR Part 11 of the Code of Federal Regulations deals with the Food and Drug Administration (FDA) guidelines on electronic records and electronic signatures in the United States. Part 11, as it is commonly called, defines the criteria under which electronic records and electronic signatures are considered to be trustworthy, reliable and equivalent to paper records (FDA Title 21 CFR Part 11 Section 11.1 (a)).

To ensure that researchers are viewing only the data and forms assigned to them the Velos system includes a multi-layered security tree involving study level access, organization level access, and group/individual level access (see Figure 1). Each rare disease will receive its own organization. Participants will be enrolled into the CoRDS study as a member of their respective organization (rare disease). The participant portal will display forms that will be built to gather information from the participant. These forms will be locked down by organization so that participants from each organization will only see those forms associated to their rare disease. Forms can also be assigned at the individual participant level or a group level if there are specific items that need to be cared for within each disease. All data entered into these forms will stay with the participant and will not be displayed in any other participant's access.

Portal Design

The forms for the participant portal will be designed by the CoRDS registry team and built by the Research IT team. Each form will need to go through the Sanford Health Institutional Review Board to make sure that the data being collected follows the initial intent of the CoRDS registry. They will also review whether the Informed

Figure 1. CoRDS registry design

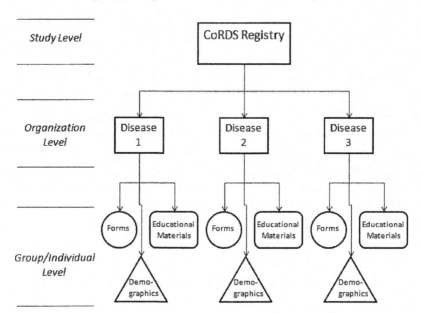

Consent form that the participants signed before being enrolled in the study needs to be reworded and signatures recollected from each participant.

Researchers that would like to view the data contained in this registry will need to submit a request form that will be reviewed by the Sanford Health Institutional Review Board. Once a researcher has been screened and approved, an account will be setup with access to the Velos system. The researcher's account will be locked down by organization (rare disease) so that they will only be able to view data from participants and forms assigned to that organization. Within the Velos application is an Ad-Hoc querying tool that will be made available to the researcher with access to pull data from custom-built database views of the data in the forms that each participant fills out. These views will be created by the Research IT team and will not contain any information deemed as Protected Health Information (PHI). These include, but not limited to, the participant's name, date of birth, social security number, medical record number, address, phone number, age, e-mail addresses. For a complete list of these items see the National Institutes of Health's website http://privacyruleandresearch.nih.gov/pr_08.asp.

Policies and Procedures

Policies will need to be developed to handle the request, approval, and setup of accounts for both researchers and participants. We will also need to develop policies to govern what access levels will be used for each type of user as well as communication plans between the CoRDS team and the participants. Sanford Health needs to be sure that it divulges all policies and practices involving the use of the registry data for audit purposes. The policies will need to be submitted to and approved by the Sanford Health Institutional Review Board.

Participants will be asked at enrollment if they would like to be contacted about research opportunities associated with their rare disease. A researcher can request that contact be made with an individual or set of participants to inform them of a new research opportunity or to gather some detailed information about their disease. If they were approved for that access the CoRDS administrator will be able to contact the participants on the researcher's behalf. All communication between researcher and participant will be done through the CoRDS registry team until the participant has declined further communication from that researcher or they have been successfully enrolled in the research trial owned by the researcher.

Future Development

A future enhancement to the registry will include an option for participants to have the ability to contact other participants suffering from the same disease. The initial goals for the registry included providing the participants with a central place to learn about their disease, see any and all research opportunities related, and be able to contact those other participants in the registry that are living with the same disorder. This information would be made available on a landing page for the participant portal after a participant logs into the system and would be disease-specific. The participants are not obligated to agree to contact from other participants, but the option will be presented to them.

CURRENT CHALLENGES

We did run into several issues during the initial phases of the project and have a couple of issues that are still in the process of being resolved at this point. The higher impact issues are listed in Table 2 and are discussed in detail in the next sections.

Timeline Skew

As happens in most organizations, timelines for projects are subject to delays and re-prioritization as other higher priority work comes in. A merger involving Sanford Health and the MeritCare Health System in Fargo, ND caused significant delays as projects came in to consolidate or merge applications and data between the two

Table 2. Issues and solutions

Issue	Solution
Research IT team's schedule affected by a merger of the organization causing delays in the project timeline.	The project was broken down into smaller steps. This allowed some work to be done for the CoRDS registry as time allowed from the other projects.
House the registry data on a separate instance of Velos or add it into the existing Velos instance.	Due to the time required from the IT team to create and maintain a new instance of Velos the decision was made to use the existing instance.
Auditing capabilities of the Velos system was identified as not being complete.	Ongoing issue working with the vendor to identify the affected audit information and resolve.
Branding the participant portal with the Sanford Health name, color and logos.	Many of the features were customizable through setting changes in the database and HTML code.

organizations. One of the larger projects that involved the Research IT team was migrating data from another Clinical Trial Management system used at MeritCare to the Velos application. The CoRDS portal project timeline, as well as a number of other projects, were delayed for more than 6 months. In order to keep the CoRDS registry project moving forward the project was broken down into easily identified pieces. This gave the Research IT team the ability to complete smaller milestones in the project as work from the merger was completed.

The original plan of creating a separate instance of Velos to house the registry data required was also revisited and was deemed to involve too much work on the part of the resource-constrained Research IT team, so the implementation plan was changed to use the existing Velos instance. This decision will be revisited post-implementation to schedule when we will move the registry to its own instance of Velos.

Auditing

During Sanford Health's use of the Velos software, issues with the usability and completeness of the auditing data had surfaced. Sanford Health and the CoRDS registry require all selects, inserts, updates, and deletes of the data to be logged. In conversations with Velos and other Velos customers it was determined that there was not necessarily any missing audit data, but that some of the audit records captured were showing that the database user used by the application was the one making a majority of the changes in the database. This was due to database triggers that were being run after an insert or update was performed by the actual Velos user. The initial change to the data was audited as the Velos user, but subsequent changes from triggers were audited as the database user. Velos is working on a process to identify the originating user in their audit tables for triggered changes. We also enabled Oracle database auditing to capture more information about each change to the data.

We are continuing to work with Velos to identify any other missing or incomplete auditing data produced by the system. This is an ongoing item of concern because of the amount of PHI involved in the system and the trust of the participants towards the registry for keeping their data secure.

Portal Branding

Given that the CoRDS participant portal will be accessed by external users, patients not necessarily seen at Sanford Health, the website must be configured to have a similar look and feel as other Sanford Health websites. The Marketing team at Sanford Health was given access to the portal in a Test instance where they compiled a list of recommended alterations. These included adding colors, fonts, and logos specific to Sanford Health and the CoRDS registry. Many of the alterations were configurable in the Velos software through the portal setup utility. Some alterations required a change to the HTML and JSP code of the application. These changes were tracked in a separate spreadsheet to be validated after each application upgrade. Once the portal has been implemented and we review the project for lessons learned we will submit these changes to Velos to see if they can become customizable through the portal setup utility.

CONCLUSION

The purpose of the CoRDS registry is two-fold. The participant portal will continue to evolve to be a beneficial resource and communication tool for people affected by rare diseases across the globe. The participants will have access to up-to-date information regarding research opportunities, treatment options, and potential cures for their diseases. A future enhancement to the registry will give the participants access to communicate with others afflicted by their disease across the globe.

Healthcare research will also benefit from having these potential research subjects identified and categorized in one place. The registry participants will be educated and informed which will improve study screening and participation. The data gathered by the forms in the participant portal will save the researchers time and money. Future research will also be able to look for similarities in diseases that may help to find common causes and cures.

With the help of technology, medical disease registries can evolve into more than just a static list of people suffering from the same chronic conditions. They can be used to connect people to educational tools, emotional support, and research into life-extending therapies and cures.

REFERENCES

Drolet, B. C., & Johnson, K. B. (2008). Categorizing the world of registries. *Journal of Biomedical Informatics*, *41*(6), 1009–1020. doi:10.1016/j.jbi.2008.01.009

Privacy Rule and Research. (2011). *How can covered entities use and disclose protected health information for research and comply with the privacy rule?* Retrieved November 5, 2011, from http://privacyruleandresearch.nih.gov/pr_08.zip

KEY TERMS AND DEFINITIONS

Auditing: Is an evaluation of a person, organization, system, process, enterprise, project or product. The term most commonly refers to audits in accounting, but similar concepts also exist in project management, quality management, and energy conservation.

Clinical Trail Management System: Is a customizable software system used by the biotechnology and pharmaceutical industries to manage the large amounts of data involved with the operation of a clinical trial. It maintains and manages the planning, preparation, performance, and reporting of clinical trials, with emphasis on keeping up-to-date contact information for participants and tracking deadlines and milestones such as those for regulatory approval or the issue of progress reports.

Informed Consent: Has been given based upon a clear appreciation and understanding of the facts, implications, and future consequences of an action. In order to give informed consent, the individual concerned must have adequate reasoning faculties and be in possession of all relevant facts at the time consent is given.

Institutional Review Board: Is a committee that has been formally designated to approve, monitor, and review biomedical and behavioral research involving humans with the aim to protect the rights and welfare of the research subjects. An IRB performs critical oversight functions for research conducted on human subjects that are *scientific*, *ethical*, and *regulatory*.

Participant Portals: Are healthcare-related online applications that allow patients to interact and communicate with their healthcare providers, such as physicians and hospitals. Typically, portal services are available on the Internet at all hours of the day. Some participant portal applications exist as stand-alone websites and sell their services to healthcare providers. Other portal applications are integrated into the existing website of the healthcare provider. Still others are modules added onto an existing electronic medical record system. The common theme for all of these portal types is the ability of the patient to interact with their medical information via the Internet.

Patient Registries: Are collections of secondary data related to patients with a specific diagnosis, condition, or procedure. They play an important role in post-marketing surveillance of pharmaceuticals.

Protected Health Information (PHI): Under the US Health Insurance Portability and Accountability Act (HIPAA), is considered to be any information about health status, provision of health care, or payment for health care that can be linked to a specific individual. This is interpreted rather broadly and includes any part of a patient's medical record or payment history.

Rare Disease: Is considered as any disease that affects a small percentage of the population. Most rare diseases are genetic, and thus are present throughout the person's life, even if symptoms do not appear immediately.

Chapter 13
Healthcare Systems using Clinical Data:
Addressing Data Interoperability Challenges

Biswadip Ghosh
Metropolitan State College of Denver, USA

EXECUTIVE SUMMARY

The use of Information Systems (IS) in healthcare organizations is increasing. A variety of information systems have been implemented to support administrative activities such as scheduling systems, insurance and billing, electronic prescriptions, pharmaceutical dispensaries, and patient health records and portals. To make a fundamental difference in the delivery of patient care, systems that support important clinical healthcare decision processes are needed that leverage the clinical knowledge embedded in patient medical records. The aggregation of clinical data from multiple sources is difficult due to data interoperability issues. The VHA case study of the CISCP system illustrates a program that effectively leveraged clinical data from multiple surgical programs to build a system to support decision-making at many organizational levels. The technical and organizational practices from the VHA case provide important lessons to address interoperability issues when building other healthcare information systems.

DOI: 10.4018/978-1-4666-2671-3.ch013

BACKGROUND

The use of Information Systems (IS) in healthcare organizations is on the increase. Among the reasons for this trend are pressures to reduce costs, which have been growing at an unsustainable rate and to improve the quality of healthcare (Warner, 2004). A variety of Information systems have been implemented in healthcare organizations such as scheduling systems, electronic medical records, computerized physician order entry, insurance and billing, electronic prescriptions, pharmaceutical dispensaries and patient health portals (LeRouge, Mantzana, & Wilson, 2007). Such applications range from automating administrative tasks such as billing, facilities management, laboratory management, and patient visit scheduling to clinical decision support and clinical program management.

The nature of organizations that participate in the United States (US) healthcare industry can vary greatly. They range from advanced practice critical care hospitals to outpatient clinics that provide primary care. Unlike in nationalized healthcare systems such as in UK or regionally organized systems such as in Canada, the US system is pluralistic where information system adoption decisions are left to each individual provider. However, the need to operate inside the US healthcare system requires each provider organization to adopt a variety of information systems to manage administrative activities, such as billing, scheduling, prescribing and storing patient medical records. Current research reports that larger the size of the healthcare organization, such as a hospital, health maintenance practice or health network (HMO), the greater the adoption of technology (Ozdemir, Barron, & Bandyopadhyay, 2011). Information systems, such as the just-in-time KM at Partners HealthCare (Davenport & Glaser, 2002) and the computerized physician order-entry system at CareGroup (Grimson, Grimson, & Hasselbring, 2000) have reduced medical errors, which cause an estimated million injuries and 98,000 deaths each year in the USA alone. Such systems have been found to be effective to facilitate coordination and mutual communication among clinicians across the many silos of specialization in the organization and have reduced medical practice errors (Aron, et al., 2011). In addition, these systems can reduce costs and help healthcare professionals to cope with information overload and to learn about and utilize current research developments into their practice. While a majority of these information systems support administrative tasks and are built using administrative or resource utilization data sets, yet to make a fundamental difference in the healthcare organization and its effectiveness in the delivery of patient care, systems that support important clinical healthcare processes are needed (Raghupathi & Tan, 2008). With the growth in the adoption of Electronic Medical Records (EMR) by healthcare providers, more patient data is now available to utilize in the practice of Evidence-Based Medicine (EBM). The Health Information Technology for Economic and Clinical Health (HITECH)

Act was passed in 2009 with goals to incent healthcare providers to establish EMR in individual medical and leverage the electronic patient data to provide better and more effective patient care (Agarwal, Gao, DesRoches, & Jha, 2010).

A classification of information systems that facilitate the processes of decision-making are referred to as Decision Support Systems (DSS). These systems support organizational decision making at different levels and for different types of decisions—from routine (operational) problems with structured solutions to very abstract wide ranging problems (strategic) that have unstructured solutions (Simon, 1977; Clark, Jones, & Armstrong, 2007). DSS can leverage the clinical data in EMR systems to improve patient outcomes by improving the delivery of care in healthcare organizations. In an healthcare organization, DSS technologies can support: (1) the general goals of reducing the uncertainty in the decision making process, such as providing a variety of tabulated data variables to assist the decision maker, (2) building a model to evaluate choices and estimating the impact of the choices on one or more objective (e.g. assessing the riskiness of possible treatment outcomes for a presenting patient using clinical data from prior cases), and (3) the capability to evaluate changes in assumptions, model inputs and parameter values on a chosen decision.

The effective utilization of these systems in a clinical context require the organizations to carefully assess their decision making needs, the preparation and training of the personnel involved in those decisions and investment into the system quality and the functionality of the DSS. Factors such as the integration of the DSS into the work tasks and workflow and the level and consistency of the data collected and input into the system and the way the output information is used and shared by the DSS can influence the success of the DSS (Clark, Jones, & Armstrong, 2007). However, medical departments work largely in silos that can limit the "holistic" view of patient data and creating data aggregation and interoperability issues. Current attempts at building large infrastructure to utilize medical records from multiple practices have met with limited success (McGrath, Hendy, Klecun, & Young, 2008). As a result, decision support systems built with clinical data to support clinical processes can be difficult to implement. Technical and organizational practices must be instituted to better utilize "holistic" clinical data on patients, so that it can be used in an organization-wide DSS.

SETTING THE STAGE: DATA INTEROPERABILITY

Healthcare organizations are relatively flat organizations that operate as professional adhocracies that have only minimal formalized coordination mechanisms (usually by mutual adjustment) between medical specializations (Mintzberg, 1983). Healthcare organizations have silos of specialized practices with minimal data/process standardization and integration. Minimal standardization and integration of clinical activities produces clinical data that cannot be easily aggregated on an organization wide basis leading to interoperability problems (Hammond, et al., 2010). Aggregating EMR data in such an environment is difficult not only due to technological issues but also from an organizational standpoint. Typically, facilities in which patient care is delivered vary widely, ranging from "basic" centers with limited scope of medical practice to highly "advanced" urban hospitals with state of the art medical technology for patient care. The patient data captured in each care setting varies. In a typical, scenario when patients receive care in multiple facilities and from several clinicians, there can be differences in their care protocols and workflows resulting in large variations in the EMR generated for patients. For example, the realization of a fully connected large UK healthcare network has been problematic (McGrath, et al., 2008). The problems include systems and semantic interoperability issues. Specifically, the meaning of the data varies by medical practice and specializations, so aggregation of data across multiple EMR systems is extremely complex. Standards are critical for interfaced medical records from multiple medical practices and systems (Adams, et al., 2010). There are over 300 EMR or EHR vendors with systems that differ in their data fields, workflows, and medical protocols. Standard for exchanging information between medical applications and the transmission of health related information is elusive (Raghupathi & Tan, 2008). Consequently, exchanging medical data in the current environment is difficult.

Semantic interoperability is defined as the preservation of meaning in information and data as it moves between systems and users or is repurposed (Goodenough, 2009). Preservation of meaning is critical for safe clinical care and for administrative decisions based on statistical analysis of healthcare data. Standards help to ensure data is semantically unambiguous (Goodenough, 2009; Hammond, et al., 2010). However, ensuring data standards are followed when building an overall health record for the patient by combining medical records is often problematic. Typically, facilities in which patient care is delivered vary widely, ranging from—basic centers with limited scope of medical practice to highly—advanced urban hospitals with state of the art medical technology for patient care. In a typical scenario, when patients receive care in multiple facilities and from several clinicians, there can be differences in their care protocols and workflows resulting in large variations in the medical records generated for patients. Additionally, the diversity in medical group practices is well documented as medicine is practiced in specialties. Each specialty has its own set of laboratory datum, medical protocols, and treatment regimens. Hence, medical records created by one specialty can be difficult to use in other practices (Gupta, et al., 2007). To aggregate data for processing, a holistic assessment of a patient is needed, yet is missing in medical records that have been generated from silo based islands of specialized care (Raghupathi & Tan, 2008). Even after establishing standards for data definitions (semantic interoperability) and standards for integration and aggregation of data from multiple systems (systems interoperability), the dynamic and piecemeal nature of medical data creates issues with building this holistic view of the patient case (Bloomrosen & Detmer, 2010).

CASE DESCRIPTION

The VHA (Veterans Health Administration) is a distributed national healthcare organization of hospitals, patient consultation offices, nursing homes, and labs established to serve veterans of military duty. The VHA medical system is the largest integrated healthcare system in the US (Kizer & Dudley, 2009). With over 150 acute care hospitals in the VHA healthcare organization and 14,000 staff physicians, it serves over ten million patients. Additionally the system has over 350 outpatient clinics, which provide treatment on 24 million annual patient visits. Approximately, forty cardiac surgical programs perform approximately 6500 open-heart surgeries annually. Given the high costs and risks of cardiac surgery, an information system using clinical data was critical for facilitating efficient management of the resources and quality of these surgical programs. Veterans are a high-risk mix of patients having pre-existing conditions and often with permanent multiple injuries that are rarely seen in other healthcare systems (Kizer & Dudley, 2009). The VHA underwent a transformation that was supported by major information technology changes after several patient care quality issues were reported in the national media (Kizer & Dudley, 2009). The goal of the IT systems was to standardize the technology platform to support a set of rationalized processes and applications that could support the entire span of the VHA network and eliminate variation in care (Venkatesh, Bala, Venkatraman, & Bates, 2007). By eliminating large un-standardized data sources and applications that could not coordinate among each other, this large scale standardization of IT and the maturation of a VHA-wide enterprise architecture played a large part in improving the nature and quality of services rendered and in enhancing the efficiency and effectiveness of internal operations (Venkatesh, Bala, Venkatraman, & Bates, 2007). The coordination among applications in the VHA allows patient data to be reused among multiple applications such as pharmacy, physician order entry, laboratory, and electronic claim processing.

Elective Cardiac surgery in any healthcare network is particularly resource intensive and cardiac surgery is the most expensive. Hospitals typically have severe budget constraints, which necessitate effective allocation of scarce resources and judicious adoption of expensive advances in medical procedures and treatment regiments. In the Veterans Health Affairs (VHA) hospital system's cardiac surgical programs, care was difficult to access and patients had long wait times for surgery, which often had adverse outcomes. VHA care had become fragmented, with significant inefficiencies in allocating resources across facilities, due to the sheer size, physical distribution, and scope of the VHA medical network. In addition, there were issues with adoption of the most effective medical treatments and procedures for a patient mix that is more acutely sick than typical patients. A VHA wide information system based on clinical data from cardiac surgical programs was highly needed to address many of these issues. The Continuous Improvement in Cardiac Surgery Program (CICSP) was established to plan, collect, and analyze clinical data using medical records from a wide variety of VHA facilities and practices. Some were internal to the VHA network and some were external affiliate facilities, such as University hospitals or contracted facilities. CICSP began collecting VHA-wide cardiac surgery data in 1987 (Shroyer, et al., 2008). It implemented an innovative analytic capability initiative that used historical outcomes of surgeries and procedures to develop statistical risk models.

This innovative system became part of VHA's ongoing transformation that began in 1995. The system has evolved since its inception to include automation and procedures that increase data completeness, and tracking of additional data variables for processes of care, resources of care and medication compliance. As new surgical procedures were adopted, the CICSP data collection was expanded to include additional variables. The Web-based dashboards, implemented in 2006 and 2008, provide views of the data in multiple categories—surgical outcomes, resources and processes of care and medications compliance. A system implementation timeline is shown in Figure 1.

VHA embraced metrics and performance management and since 2000 has scored better than private healthcare organizations on multiple outcome measures (Arnst, 2006; Longman, 2005). Measurable improvements were seen in clinical outcomes of the surgical programs over time. These improvements included decreased mortality and morbidity from surgery, shorter wait times and length of stays, greater compliance with medications, and more standardized treatments, such as the use of cardiac catheterization and combinations of medications. The success of the analytic capability also translated to better and more efficient care processes (Grover, et al., 2001). Overall costs decreased. Consequently, the cost of insuring a VHA patient was $4100/year compared to more than $6,300/year on average outside the VHA (Arnst, 2006; Kizer & Dudley, 2009).

Figure 1. System implementation time line (Shroyer, et al., 2008)

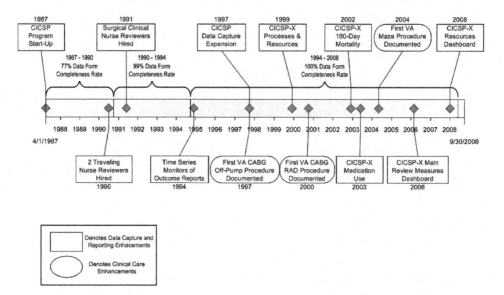

CURRENT CHALLENGES FACING THE ORGANIZATION

The CICSP system draws on clinical data in electronic medical records of patients. The systems using a multitude of variables—preoperative and postoperative data that serves as input into building the system outputs—decision models and reports. This clinical data must be aggregated from a large number of facilities and surgical programs across the country and is difficult because of semantic ("meaning of specific values") issues in the data. The collection and aggregation of input data is a challenging activity. Although VHA's advanced enterprise architecture and systems integration automated some data input such as pharmacy data and laboratory and imaging results, a majority of the patient data for the CISCP system is entered manually. The data is entered by a multitude of clinicians, such as residents, attending surgeons, department chiefs, and operating room circulating and medical nurses (Khuri, et al., 1998). Semantic interoperability becomes challenging, as agreement on meaning of specialized medical data is difficult to achieve among the variety of personnel (e.g., How is acute renal failure judged across the system?).

Using a set of interviews with key personnel associated with the CICSP system—including recording nurses and clinicians and administrators, the following challenges were identified.

A nurse reported the importance of team members from across facilities to build shared understanding:

It is better to have the team leader do site visits. The only time some of them look at charts is when they do a site visit. Her understanding is from what we tell her. If they are not reading charts on a regular basis then they lose skills.

Healthcare data is dynamic and changes rapidly with each reassessment of the patient. As clinicians visit patients and new information is collected and shared with the medical teams, the patient medical record needs to be updated. This calls for the nurses to abstract some variables after consulting multiple physician notes and other fields in the patient record. Moreover, the data input team faces multiple challenges associated with geographic dispersion of facilities and from reconciling data that originate in multiple incompatible systems, as well as in charts and scanned paper forms. A nurse interviewed explained data entry problems:

Residents think [data entry] is "not their job." Residents change twice a month, so there is perpetual training.

Staff turnover, varying processes and diversity in their work systems result in data entry that is non-uniform and that cannot be aggregated or compared. Typical data problems for the CICSP system range from misunderstanding data definitions, errors in data entry, incomplete data sets, conflicts between multiple data sources, and inaccessibility of data from remote facilities (see Table 1).

Using multiple information systems sometimes means coping with discrepancies. Data definitions may vary across systems or facilities.

Death is defined as within 30 days by us, 60 days by them.

Table 1. Data interoperability problems and resolution

Data Interoperability problem	Example
Misunderstanding data definitions	"Death is defined as within 30 days by us, 60 days by them."
Inconsistency in scales for data entry	"Acute renal failure is determined by consulting a number of data variables and is subjective."
Errors in data entry	"because voices echo in the Operating Room the nurse may not hear information from the doctors correctly"
Incomplete data sets	"We lose information if no one looks at charts."
Conflicts between multiple data sources	"There are often conflicts with drug dosage in the system."
Inaccessibility of data from remote facilities	"We cannot get data from remote sites. Their charts are not automated."

The nurses have a "bible" of definitions, which they consult constantly to check for updates.

Definitions change over time. We pull out the 'bible.'

Despite the importance of patient record systems such as VISTA Web, interviews revealed that paper forms are widely used instead. For example, anestheologists use a paper form that has been in use since 1929 by the army. Although the forms are scanned into the system, sometimes the sheets are scanned in upside down or have missing information. In the Operating Room, during preparations the circulatory nurse tries to enter data. However, because voices echo in the Operating Room the nurse may not hear information from the doctors correctly. As a result, the data from the scanned anestheologist sheet is usually more reliable. Unfortunately, when one has to get the data off a scanned sheet a problem is that the image is not a data point. As a result, trying to verify data for preoperative variables is difficult.

According to interviews with recording nurses, who are involved in data collection and cleaning, it is important to extract data from CT scans, MRI, and patient charts.

We pull data out of CT scans and MRI.

We lose information if no one looks at charts.

Procedures vary by location. Some locations have more resources.

People come from facilities in neighboring states. Some of these places have enough dollars for lab panels – 23 tests. 'We don't do lab panels.'

Although Vista Web is used, remote sites do not automate their charts.

We cannot get data from remote sites. It is difficult to get data from these remote sites as their charts are not automated.

Interviews with nurses who are involved with data collection reveal that some of the information systems are outdated and lack a user friendly GUI interface. As a result, the nurses need to check and interpret the data and use manual procedures to ensure accuracy. For example, the input program does not allow two pointers although one is available from the serum and one is available that is calculated. The nurse uses judgment to determine what data to input.

Nurses, in some cases, use Personal Digital Assistants (PDAs) to facilitate data collection on patient conditions and outcomes. They also use a Community of

Practice (CoP) discussion forum for training on how to control variation in the data collection steps across multiple patient record systems.

The reason for the high reliability is because we discuss the data in the nurses' community. It takes time.

We discuss definitions and problems on conference calls. The human factor is very important. Networking facilitates developing connections. It is a lonely job. I got to know [X] at a conference. We developed a family of camaraderie.

Although nurses try to help each other, they are not allowed to identify the patient because of privacy laws. When they call or communicate through email, they cannot see the relevant chart, making it difficult to resolve data issues. A nurse comments:

We must not identify the patient. It is hard to field if we cannot see a chart.

Collaboration among nurses doing data collection is good. However, the practice of "farming out" creates issues with accessing information. A nurse explains:

We help as much as we can. We have conference calls and use email. We talk about spinal fusions. We farm out work and this can be problematic. If a very expensive antibiotic is used, we don't know why. Because of HIPPA we are unable to get information. We need a release from the patient.

Data mining is limited when complex, legacy, and incompatible information systems are used as the source. Nurses provide intelligence that is difficult to automate. One of the nurses relates:

The workload is high with some days work for 21 hours straight. We find what computers cannot find.

Effective data collection of historical data from several sources depends on several data quality processes. A data quality manager monitors these processes, which include data concordance tests, database validation processes, and a data certification process.

A nurse explains how during a remote charts are reviewed to validate data practices:

Chart reviews are used to audit data. You cannot view VISTA Web remotely. They pick a number of charts, assess them, then they see if they matched what I gave them.

Inter-rater reliability is measured to ensure data quality. A nurse relates the procedure:

We fax inter-rater reliability. It took an entire day to do. Every CPR is different, and GUI and reports are different. There is a lack of consistency. A few years ago the reliability was .999. They would only tell a few questions. When people question data quality, we can silence criticism if we have the inter-rater reliability, but we are not told.

SOLUTIONS AND RECOMMENDATIONS

Technology Components

The CICSP system started with extracting aggregate surgical case data from the Vista system using a secure data feed. The extracted clinical variables from the medical records are needed for model generation and supporting decision making screens. Although the VHA's organizational complexity and the diversity in their multiple facilities posed a significant challenge, their enterprise architecture provided a robust infrastructure for transmission of encrypted medical data and database servers to store, clean, and process that data (Venkatraman, et al., 2008). However, variations in recording standards caused issues, such as (1) incomplete patient electronic records, (2) lack of required data variables, and (3) inconsistent classification of preoperative and postoperative variable codes. The inherent diversity and dynamic nature of the medical data collected from multiple sources meant that a fully automated solution for clinical data aggregation was not feasible (see Figure 2).

The automated procedure involved database servers that ran a battery of validation checks. Successful validation resulted in delivery to the data warehouse. Validation failures which were listed on reports as inconsistencies needed manual procedures to update patient case data. Manual procedures involved additional medical judgment. Recording nurses reassessed patient variables and conditions during follow-up visits. They manually checked new data and resolved inconsistencies. A Community of Practice (CoP) was critical for manual procedures and will be discussed in more detail in the next section.

Management and Organizational Components

Managerial and organizational practices during data collection helped to improve data quality, which was a critical factor in the aggregation of clinical data for the CICSP system. For example, management established a data certification process

Figure 2. Framework to build data interoperability

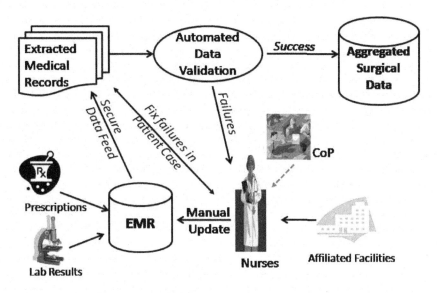

lead by a data quality manager; data concordance tests and data validation processes. Hiring two nurse reviewers in 1990 and surgical clinical nurse reviewers in 1991 were key steps in the CICSP timeline. The nurses reviewed data inputs and recorded data "hidden" in charts and scanned documents. Building a community of practice (Wenger & Snyder, 2000) for these nurses alleviated problems with the quality of data originating in multiple systems and documents. Through the participation in the community, the nurses support each other by identifying ways to use technology to more effectively collect, process, and transmit data. The interactions also build trust, identify and norms within the team, which allows the nurses to share knowledge to more effectively carry on data collection activities, which can span multiple facilities and systems. While some of the data is automatically entered into patient records—such as lab values and medication fulfillment, other patient data is manually entered by a multitude of clinical care providers. Staff turnover, varying processes and diversity in their work systems can result in data entry that is non-uniform and that cannot be aggregated or compared. Moreover, a second level of interpretation is needed by data recording nurses for variables that are coded as either the presence of a condition or not—such as heart disease. These variables need to be abstracted by the recording nurse after consulting multiple physician notes and other fields in the patient record.

OUTCOMES AND RECOMMENDATIONS

VHA strives to be an innovator for quality of care performance, accountability, and reporting using effective data collection practices and multiple output formats supporting multiple types of decision makers. The focus of the CICSP system is to support local VHA cardiac surgery programs in their self-assessment and self-improvement efforts. The onus and responsibility for using the data and outputs of the system rest on the facility personnel. The centers receive ongoing quality evaluation of their programs with the semiannual reports providing comparison and evaluations from a comprehensive review from VHA leadership. An executive board supports VHA with periodic review of cardiac surgery program performance and evaluates risk-adjusted outcomes for quality assurance. Centers identified as performing below expectations conduct a medical chart audit and may receive a site visit (Hammermeister, et al., 1994).

The success of the CICSP program rests upon the robust data collection and cleaning processes. By ensuring accuracy in the input data, the trust and reliance on the outputs of the system by the system users is enhanced. Additionally communities among the key actors enable critical knowledge sharing to support the system (see Table 2).

The VHA CICSP system applied technology and procedures in a complex organization with a distributed and diverse set of facilities, clinical care providers, and patients. This case study shows the importance of developing standard data definitions, which is important for any organization that is widely dispersed. Without standardization, data cannot be accurately compared across multiple sources. Communities of practice promote data standardization by facilitating sharing information and knowledge. This system provides an example of how a large-scale clinical data driven system can be implemented to support multiple decision makers in other healthcare organizations. The interpretation of the case study and recommendations presented in this chapter are solely those of the author. They do not in any way represent the views of the Department of VA or VHA.

Table 2. Lessons learned and practices

Lessons learned	Practices
Need to check data transmissions for errors and omissions	Leverage Automated Data transmission, checking programs on an robust Enterprise Architecture
Need to develop standard data definitions	Distribute a "bible" of standard data definitions, which are continually updated
Encourage communities of practice to facilitate information sharing and data quality	Provide face-to-face conferences, monthly conference calls, an email distribution list, a FAQ Web page and a Web-based discussion board

REFERENCES

Agarwal, R., Gao, G., DesRoches, C., & Jha, A. K. (2010). The digital transformation of healthcare: Current status and the road ahead. *Information Systems Research, 21*(4), 796–809. doi:10.1287/isre.1100.0327

Arnst, C. (2006, July 17). The best medical care in the US: How veteran affairs transformed itself and what it means for the rest of us. *Business Week*, 50–56.

Aron, R., Dutta, S., Janakiraman, R., & Pathak, P. A. (2011). The impact of automation of systems on medical errors: Evidence from field research. *Information Systems Research, 22*(3), 429–446. doi:10.1287/isre.1110.0350

Bloomrosen, M., & Detmer, D. E. (2010). Informatics, evidence-based care, and research: Implications for national policy: A report of an American medical informatics association health policy conference. *Journal of the American Medical Informatics Association, 2*(17), 115–123. doi:10.1136/jamia.2009.001370

Clark, T. D., Jones, M. C., & Armstrong, C. P. (2007). The dynamic structure of management support systems: Theory development, research focus and direction. *Management Information Systems Quarterly, 31*(3), 579–615.

Davenport, T. H., & Glaser, J. (2002). Just-in-time delivery comes to knowledge management. *Harvard Business Review, 80*(7), 107–111.

Goodenough, S. (2009). Semantic interoperability, e-health and Australian health statistics. *Health Information Management Journal, 2*(38), 41–45.

Grimson, J., Grimson, W., & Hasselbring, W. (2001). The SI challenge in healthcare. *Communications of the ACM, 43*(6), 49–55.

Grover, F. L. (2001). A decade's experience with quality improvement in cardiac surgery using the veterans affairs and society of thoracic surgeons national databases. *Annals of Surgery, 4*(234), 464–474. doi:10.1097/00000658-200110000-00006

Gupta, A. (2007). Information systems and healthcare XVII: A HL7v3-based mediating schema approach to data transfer between heterogeneous health care systems. *Communications of the Association for Information Systems, 19*, 622–636.

Hammermeister, K. E., Johnson, R., Marshall, G., & Grover, F. L. (1994). Continuous assessment and improvement in quality of care: A model from the department of veterans affairs cardiac surgery. *Annals of Surgery, 219*(3), 281–290. doi:10.1097/00000658-199403000-00008

Hammond, W. E. (2010). Connecting information to improve health. *Health Affairs, 29*(2), 285–290. doi:10.1377/hlthaff.2009.0903

Khuri, S. F. (1998). The department of veterans affairs NSQIP – The first national, validated, outcome-based, risk-adjusted and peer-controlled program for the measurement and enhancement of the quality of surgical care. *Annals of Surgery, 228*(4), 491–507. doi:10.1097/00000658-199810000-00006

Kizer, K. W., & Dudley, R. A. (2009). Extreme makeover: Transformation of the veterans health care system. *Annual Review of Public Health, 30*, 313–339. doi:10.1146/annurev.publhealth.29.020907.090940

LeRouge, C., Mantzana, V., & Wilson, E. V. (2007). Healthcare information systems research, revelations and visions. *European Journal of Information Systems, 16*, 669–671. doi:10.1057/palgrave.ejis.3000712

Longman, P. (2005). The best care anywhere. *The Washington Monthly, 37*, 1–2.

McGrath, K., Hendy, J., Klecun, E., & Young, T. (2008). The vision and reality of 'connecting for health': Tensions, opportunities and policy implications of the UK national programme. *Communications of the Association for Information Systems, 23*, 603–618.

Mintzberg, H. (1983). *Structure in fives: Designing effective organizations*. Englewood Cliffs, NJ: Prentice Hall.

Ozdemir, Z., Barron, J., & Bandyopadhyay, S. (2011). Analysis of the adoption of digital health records under switching costs. *Information Systems Research, 22*(3), 491–503. doi:10.1287/isre.1110.0349

Raghupathi, V., & Tan, J. (2008). Information systems and healthcare XXX: Charting a strategic path for health information technology. *Communications of the Association for Information Systems, 23*, 501–522.

Shroyer, A. L. (2008). Improving quality of care in cardiac surgery: Evaluating risk factors, processes of care, structures of care, and outcomes. *Seminars in Cardiothoracic and Vascular Anesthesia, 3*(12), 140–152. doi:10.1177/1089253208323060

Simon, H. A. (1977). *The new science of management decision*. Englewood Cliffs, NJ: Prentice-Hall.

Venkatesh, V., Bala, H., Venkatraman, S., & Bates, J. (2007). Enterprise architecture maturity: The story of the veterans health administration. *MIS Quarterly Executive, 2*(6), 79–90.

Venkatraman, S., Bala, H., Venkatesh, V., & Bates, J. (2008). Six strategies for electronic medical record systems. *Communications of the ACM, 51*(11), 140–144. doi:10.1145/1400214.1400243

Warner, M. (2004). Under the knife. *Business 2.0, 5*(1), 84-89.

Wenger, E. C., & Snyder, W. M. (2000, January-February). Communities of practice: The organizational frontier. *Harvard Business Review*.

Chapter 14

User and Data Classification for a Secure and Practical Approach for Patient–Doctor Profiling Using an RFID Framework in Hospital

Masoud Mohammadian
University of Canberra, Australia

Ric Jentzsch
University of Canberra, Australia

EXECUTIVE SUMMARY

Utilization and application of the latest technologies can save lives and improve patient treatments and well-being. For this it is important to have accurate, near real-time data acquisition and evaluation. The delivery of patient's medical data needs to be as fast and as secure as possible. Accurate almost real-time data acquisition and analysis of patient data and the ability to update such a data is a way to reduce cost and improve patient care. One possible solution to achieve this task is to use a wireless framework based on Radio Frequency Identification (RFID). This framework can integrate wireless networks for fast data acquisition and transmission, while maintaining the privacy issue. This chapter discusses the development of an intelligent multi-agent system in a framework in which RFID can be used

DOI: 10.4018/978-1-4666-2671-3.ch014

for patient data collection. This chapter presents a framework for the knowledge acquisition of patient and doctor profiling in a hospital. The acquisition of profile data is assisted by a profiling agent that is responsible for processing the raw data obtained through RFID and database of doctors and patients. A new method for data classification and access authorization is developed, which will assist in preserving privacy and security of data.

1. INTRODUCTION

Application of innovative architectures for secure access, retrieval, and update of data in healthcare systems continues to be needed for cost reduction and quality of service. To this end the use of Radio Frequency Identification (RFID) has been shown to be a viable and promising technology in the health care industry (Finkenzeller, 1999; Glover & Bhatt, 2006; Hedgepeth, 2007; Mohammadian & Jentzsch, 2008; Schuster, Allen, & Brock, 2007; Shepard, 2005; Angeles, 2007; Pramatari, Doukidis, & Kourouthanassis, 2005; Qiu & Sangwan, 2005; Mickey, 2004; Whiting, 2004). RFIDs has the capability to penetrate and add value to many areas of health care. RFIDs can lower the cost of some services as well as improve services to individuals and health care providers. The real value of RFID is achieved in conjunction with the use of intelligent software systems such as intelligent multi-agent systems. The integration of these two technologies can benefit and assist health care services.

Radio Frequency Identifiers (RFID) have been around for many years. Their use and projected use has only begun to be researched in hospitals (Fuhrer & Guinard, 2007). This research study considers the use of RFIDs and its potential in hospitals and similar environments. RFIDs can be more effectively used to collect data at the source thereby providing the data for monitoring patients well being in order to provide a higher level of patient health care. There are four areas where using RFIDs in their data collection role can have significant positive benefits in hospitals. These four areas are:

- **Care Tracking:** This is getting the right care to the right patient at the right time;
- **Quality of Care:** Improving the services given to the right patient at the right time in a timely manner;
- **Cost of Care:** Finding ways to be effective in the use of available resources such that the cost per patient per incident does not adversely increase to the cost of the resources; and

- **Service of Care:** More timely information to enable a more informed decision by providing more knowledge about an individual's need for care (Mohammadian & Jentzsch, 2007, 2008).

RFID tags and readers are commonly associated with inventory and tracking goods in such places as manufacturing and warehousing, but hospitals are starting to apply RFID to new purposes (Kowalke, 2006). RFID technology does not require contact or line of sight for communication, like bar codes. RFID data can be read through the human body, through clothing, read wirelessly, and through non-metallic materials and are wireless. This makes RFIDs an appropriate technology to fit into the health care environment.

Both research and practical application of the use of RFIDs in hospitals continues to be of importance. For hospitals, this has meant the potential of managing inventories in a more efficient manner. Inventories in hospitals take on a variety of differences roles than those found in manufacturing. The nature of the inventory and assets in a hospital can include various types of equipment (that is often very expensive, comes in many sizes, and uses), drugs (that come in a variety of sizes, shapes, color, and governing regulations), beds, chairs, as well as patients (the primary reason hospitals exist) and staff.

People tracking can be looked at from three perspectives:

1. **On-Going Full Time:** This is often referred to as human chipping. People are tagged such that the tagging is an integral part of the person 24/7. This type of human tracking (chipping) is not considered herein.
2. **Part Time:** People acquire some type of tag as part of their work and/or task environment. RFIDs are well suited for this type of tagging by staff in the health care industry.
3. **Casual:** These tags are used on and as need basic as part of the conditions or circumstances that people find themselves in. This type of tagging using RFIDs would be suitable for patients in the health care environment.

The percentage of worldwide radio frequency identification projects related to people or people tagging has increased from eight percent to 11 percent since 2005 (Tindal, 2008). The healthcare sector has yet to quantify or provide evidence of the benefit to people tagging. Human chipping (on-going full time tagging) is not new but does bring up a lot of ethical questions and is not considered herein (Angeles, 2007).

RFIDs are used in hospitals for tracking high-value assets and setting up automated maintenance routines to improve operational efficiencies. However, the use of RFIDs in tracking beds and tracking mobile equipment is in its infancy. RFIDs are used to monitor equipment for example how long a bed was used at a particular location to determine a sterilization schedule as well as bed location tracking. However RFID technology is already being deployed across the pharmaceutical industry to combat drug counterfeiting, drugs shelf life tracking (Kowalke, 2006). The management of patients and their condition is paramount in a hospital. RFIDs can assist in asset and personnel tracking, patient care, and billing where unnecessary expenses will be cut, the average length of stay of a patient is reduced, where more patient lives will be saved due to timely efficient services, and where patient records are actively continuously updated to provide better patient care (Kowalke, 2006).

The health sector is already taking up people-tagging where it allows nurses to radio their location if they are being assaulted, reduce mother baby mismatches and baby theft, help severe diabetics with getting correct treatment, and monitoring disoriented elderly patients without the need for a dedicated member of staff (Tindal, 2008).

The need is not to keep track of staff but be able to locate the staff with the particular skills that are needed at the right time and place. Staff wearing badges with RFIDs embedded can be found to help provide that needed and timely care that a patient may need. However, privacy concerns have been aired over patient tracking using RFIDs.

There is a need for more research into applications and innovative architectures for secure access, retrieval and update of data in healthcare systems (Finkenzeller, 1999; Glover & Bhatt, 2006; Hedgepeth, 2007; Mohammadian, 2008; Schuster, Allen, & Brock, 2007; Shepard, 2005; Angeles, 2007; Pramatari, Doukidis, & Kourouthanassis, 2005; Qiu & Sangwan, 2005; Mickey, 2004; Whiting, 2004). Although many organizations are developing and testing the possible use of RFIDs the real value of RFID is achieved in conjunction with the use of intelligent software agents for processing and monitoring data obtained via RFIDs. Thus, the issue becomes the integration of these two great technologies for the benefit of assisting health care services.

This research study considers a framework using RFID and Intelligent Software Agents for managing patients' health care data in a hospital environment. A fuzzy data classification system is also developed to improve the application of regulatory data requirements for security and privacy of data exchange.

This manuscript is divided into six sections. Next section considers issues relate to RFID patient scenario and data collection and profiling. Section three is based on the patient to doctor profiling and intelligent software agents. This section covers also RFID background and provides a good description of RFIDs and their components (Mohammadian & Jentzsch, 2007, 2008). This section discusses several practical cases of RFID technology in and around hospitals. It will list three possible applicable cases assisting in managing patients' medical data. Section four discusses the important issue of maintaining patients' data security and integrity and relates that to RFIDs. Last section provides conclusion and further directions for this research study. Part of the research study presented in this chapter is already published in journal and conferences in the past few years. The reference to these publications is provided in this manuscript when appropriate.

2. RFID PATIENT SCENARIO

A patient upon arrival to a hospital can be issued with an RFID tag embedded in their wrist band, which can contain such patient information as:

- Their patient number;
- Their surname;
- First name;
- Reason admitted to the hospital;
- Date and time of admission;
- Their doctor's name; and
- On-going monitoring data.

Monitoring could include such things as: heart rate, blood pressure, patient temperature, and some other vital signs that are particular to the patient's case. Monitoring would be settable to the need of the patient. For example, once an hour might be sufficient for most patients, but for others every 15 minutes might be sufficient. This illustration shows how a particular section of a hospital might be configured according to the needs of that section. Each patient has a patient-tag. Each patient's bed has a bed-tag. Spaced out within rooms, hallways, and hospital staff stations are receivers. Every 15 minutes the receiver interrogates the bed and the patient tags. The patient's vital signs are sent to the patient database where the patient's condition is recorded. The patient care profile is then updated with this information. If anything is out of range or an exception is identified the nearest nurse station to the patient is then contacted.

2.1. Data Collection

Large amount of health care data such as patients, doctors, nurses, institution itself, drugs and prescriptions, diagnosis is collected and stored in hospitals. It is not feasible or effective to use RFID to collect and retrieve such large amount of data. This chapter concentrates on a subset with the understanding that all areas could, directly or indirectly, benefit from the use of RFID and intelligent software agents in a health care environment.

The RFID (Bhuptani & Moradpour, 2005) provides the passive vehicle to obtain the data via its monitoring capabilities. The intelligent software agent provides the active vehicle in the interpretation profiling of the data and reporting capacity. By investigating and analyzing patient data the patient's condition can be monitored and abnormal situations can be reported on time. Using this information an evolving profile of each patient can be constructed and analysed. Analyzing the data can assist in deciding what kind of care a patient requires, the effects of ongoing care, and how to best care for this patient using available resources (doctors, nurses, beds, etc.) for the patient. The intelligent software agent builds a profile of each patient as they are admitted to the healthcare institution by analyzing the recorded and stored data about each patient. The same way a profile for each doctor is developed based on stored data about each doctor. Therefore, patients and doctors profile can be correlated to obtain the specialization and availability of the doctors to suit the patients.

3. INTELLIGENT AND MULTI-AGENT SYSTEMS

A Multi-Agent System (MAS) consists of a set of intelligent agents that are connect together to perform tasks in an environment to achieve a common goal. To achieve a common goal successfully the agents cooperate and collaborate with each other. The cooperation and collaboration is performed by such tasks as sharing knowledge or competition. Multi-agent systems are shown to be useful in diverse application applications (Balaji & Srinivasan, 2010). This is due to the benefits offered by multi-agent systems such as increased efficiency, reliability, and scalability. In a multi-agent system, each agent is required to perform its task and collaborate and/or compete with other agents by modifying the environment in which agents operate. The agents are distributed in the agent environment and agents communicate with each other by passing messages/requests. An agent's actions affect other agent's actions, environment, and decision. Multi-Agent systems provide several benefits. Some of the benefits include:

- **Parallel Computation:** Several agents can perform task simultaneously in parallel fashion. This in turn can increase the efficiency of the system in which they operate.
- **Reliability:** It is possible that one or more agents can fail to finalize their operations. In such a case, it may be possible to delegate the process of such agents to other agents.

- **Scalability:** It is possible to increase the number of agents with the increase in the size or complexity and workload of the system in which the agents operate (Balaji & Srinivasan, 2010).

3.1. Patient Profiling

Profiling is combined with personalization, and user modeling (Wooldridge & Jennings, 1995). The use of profile in hospitals and healthcare so far has been limited. Tracking of information about consumers' interests by monitoring their movements online is considered profiling or user modeling in e-commerce systems. By analyzing the content, URLs, and other information about a user's browsing path/click-stream a profile of a user behavior is constructed. However patient profiling differ from user profiling in e-commerce systems. The patient profiling is useful in a variety of situations such as providing a personalized service based on the patient and not on symptoms or illness to a particular patient as well as assisting in identifying the medical facilities in trying to prevent the need for the patient to return to the hospital any sooner than necessary. Patient profiling also assist in matching a doctor's specialization to the right patient. A patient profile can assist in providing information about the patient on continuous bases for the doctors so that a tailored and appropriate care can be provided to the patient.

3.2. Patient to Doctor Profiling

A patient or doctor profile is a collection of information that can be used in a decision analysis situation between the doctor, domain environment, and patient. A static profile is kept in pre-fixed data fields where the period between data field updates is long such as months or years. A dynamic profile is constantly updated as per evaluation of the situation in which the situation occurs. The updates may be performed manually or automated. The automated user profile building is especially important in real time decision-making systems. The profiling of patient doctor model is based on the patient/doctor information. These are:

- The categories and subcategories of doctor specialization and categorization. These categories will assist in information processing and patient/doctor matching.
- Part of the patients profile based on their symptoms (past history problems, dietary restrictions, etc.) can assist in prediction of the patients needs specifically.

- The patients profile can be matched with the available doctor profiles to provide doctors with information about the arrival of patients as well as presentation of the patients profile to a suitable, available doctor.

A value denoting the degree of association can be created form the above evaluation of the doctor to patient's profile. The intelligent agent based on the denoting degrees and appropriate, available doctors can be identified and be allocated to the patient (Mohammadian & Jentzsch, 2008).

In the patient/doctor profiling the intelligent agent software will make distinctions in attribute values of the profiles and match the profiles with highest value. It should be noted that the intelligent agents create the patient and doctor profiles based on data obtained from the doctors and patient namely:

- Explicit profiling occurs based on the data entered by hospital staff about a patient.
- Implicit profiling can fill that gap for the missing data by acquiring knowledge about the patient from its past visit or other relevant databases if any and then combining all these data to fill the missing data. Using legacy data for complementing and updating the user profile seems to be a better choice than implicit profiling. This approach capitalizes on user's personal history (previous data from previous visit to doctor or hospital).

The proposed intelligent agent architecture allows user profiling and matching in such a time intensive important application. The architecture of the agent profiling systems using RFID is given in Figure 1.

Profile matching (Doan, Lu, Lee, & Han, 2003) performed is based on a vector of weighted attributes using an intelligent agent system. To get this vector, the intelligent agent uses a rule-based system to match the patient's attributes (stored in patient's profile) against doctor's attributes (stored in doctor's profile). If there is a partial or full match between them then the doctor will be informed (based on their availability from the hospital doctor database). Such a rules based system is built based on the knowledge of domain experts. This expert system is extensible as new domain knowledge can be added to its knowledge base as rules. Large amount of research in the area of profiling in e-commerce, schema matching, information extraction, and retrieval has shown promising results (Do & Rahin, 2002; Doan, Lu, Lee, & Han, 2003). However, profiling in healthcare is new and innovative.

Staff and patient/doctor profiling and profile matching could be the missing link in providing more tailored healthcare professionals and facility to patients in a hospital environment. Profile matching may consist of:

Figure 1. Agent profiling model using RFID (Mohammadian & Jentzsch, 2008)

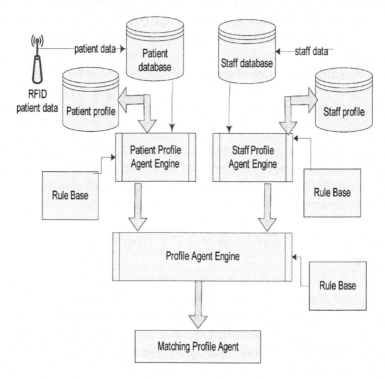

- Determining the matching algorithms required for matching patient/doctor profile,
- Determining the availability of staff and facilities required for a given patient,
- Understanding of government policies related to patient healthcare.

Another issue related to patient/doctor profiling is defining the level of matching of the patient and doctor profile. It is not always possible to provide the services of the doctor/s and facilities identified as exact match for a patient healthcare because the matching doctor may be unavailable or unreachable. Some guidelines include issues such as the critical nature of the patient illness, its level of sensitivity and regulatory rules.

As such, the rules that govern patient/doctor profile matching can be expressed in human linguistic terms, which can be vague and difficult to represent formally. Fuzzy Logic (Zadeh, 1965) has been found to be useful in its ability to handle vagueness. In this research study the profiling patient/doctor and matching is based on fuzzy logic. The profiling matching system consists of a fuzzy rule based system and an inference engine between a patient profile and doctor/s profile.

The matching between a patient profile and doctor/s is then divided into the following classes: *"total match," "medium match," "low match,"* and *"no match."* Based on these class categories a weighted match of patient/doctor profile can be identified. The doctors then can be categorized and ranked based on the matching profile value. The doctors can be classified into classes based on their matching profile as well as their availability such as *"highly available," "more and less available,"* and *"not available."* Of course, the data about availability of the doctors are obtained and updated and the profiling agent continuously checks such information from the staff database. The matched doctors then is ranked as: *"high," "medium," "low,"* and *"zero."* A fuzzy rule for the profile matching system then may look like:

IF *patient_doctor_profile* is total match and *doctor_availability* is highly available Then *doctor_ranking* = high

The integration of RFID capabilities and intelligent agent techniques provides promising development in the areas of performance improvements in RFID data collection, inference and knowledge acquisition and profiling operations (see Table 1).

Due to the important role of intelligent agents in this system, it is recognized that there is a need for a framework to coordinate intelligent agents so that they can perform their task efficiently.

Intelligent agent coordination (Wooldridge & Jennings, 1995; Odell & Bigus, 1998; Shaalana, El-Badryb, & Rafeac, 2004) has shown to be promising. The Agent Language Mediated Activity Model (ALMA) agent architecture currently under research is based on the mediated activity framework. We believe that such a framework is able to provide RFID with the necessary framework to profile a range of internal and external medical/patient profiling communication activities performed by a multi-agent system.

4. RFID DESCRIPTION

RFID or Radio Frequency Identification is a progressive technology that is easy to use and well suited for collaboration with intelligent software agents. Basically, an

Table 1. Fuzzy rule base for patient_doctor_profile_match

Patient_doctor_profile_match				
Availability	**Total match**	**Medium match**	**Low match**	**No match**
Highly available	high	high	low	Zero
More and less available	medium	medium	low	Zero
Not available	zero	zero	zero	Zero

RFID can be read-only, volatile read/write; or write once/read many times. RFID are non-contact; and non-line-of-sight operations. Being non-contact and non-line-of-sight will make RFIDs able to function under a variety of environmental conditions and while still providing a high level of data integrity (Finkenzeller, 1999; Glover & Bhatt, 2006; Hedgepeth, 2007; Mohammadian & Jentzsch, 2008; Schuster, Allen, & Brock, 2007; Shepard, 2005). A basic RFID system consists of four components namely, the RFID tag (sometimes referred to as the transponder), a coiled antenna, a radio frequency transceiver and some type of reader for the data collection.

4.1. Transponders

The reader emits radio waves in ranges of anywhere from 2.54 centimeters to 33 meters. Depending upon the reader's power output and the radio frequency used and if a booster is added that distance can be increased. When RFID tags (transponders) pass through a specifically created electromagnetic zone, they detect the reader's activation signal. Transponders can be on-line or off-line and electronically programmed with unique information for a specific application or purpose. A reader decodes the data encoded on the tag's integrated circuit and passes the data to a server for data storage or further processing.

There are four major frequency ranges that RFID systems operate at. As a rule of thumb, low-frequency systems are distinguished by short reading ranges, slow read speeds, and lower cost. Higher-frequency RFID systems are used where longer read ranges and fast reading speeds are required, such as for vehicle tracking, automated toll collection, asset management, and tracking of mobile equipment (see Table 2).

Table 2. Four major frequency ranges

Frequency	Range	Applications
Low-frequency 125 - 148 KHz	3 feet	Pet and ranch animal identification; car key locks
High-frequency 13.56 MHz	3 feet	library book identification; clothing identification; smart cards
Ultra-high frequency 915 MHz	25 feet	Supply chain tracking: Box, pallet, container, trailer tracking
Microwave 2.45GHz	100 feet	Highway toll collection; vehicle fleet identification

4.2. Coiled Antenna

The coiled antenna is used to emit radio signals to activate the tag and read or write data to it. Antennas are the conduits between the tag and the transceiver that controls the system's data acquisition and communication. RFID antennas are available in many shapes and sizes. They can be built into a doorframe, bookbinding, DVD case, mounted on a tollbooth, embedded into a manufactured item such as a shaver or software case so that the receiver tags the data from things passing through its zone (Finkenzeller, 1999; Glover & Bhatt, 2006; Hedgepeth, 2007; Schuster, Allen, & Brock, 2007; Shepard, 2005). Often the antenna is packaged with the transceiver and decoder to become a reader. The decoder device can be configured either as a handheld or a fixed-mounted device.

4.3. Types of RFID Transponders

RFID tags can be categorized as active, semi-active, or passive. Each has and is being used in a variety of inventory management and data collection applications today. The condition of the application, place, and use determines the required tag type.

Active RFID tags are powered by an internal battery and are typically read/write. Tag data can be rewritten and/or modified as the need dictates (Finkenzeller, 1999; Glover & Bhatt, 2006). The semi-active tag comes with a limited battery. The battery is used to power the tags circuitry and not to communicate with the reader (Shepard, 2005). Passive RFID tags operate without a separate external power source and obtain operating power generated from the reader. Passive tags, since they have no power source embedded in themselves, are consequently much lighter than active tags, less expensive, and offer a virtually unlimited operational lifetime. However, the trade off is that they have shorter read ranges, than active tags, and require a higher-powered reader.

4.4. Transceivers

The transceivers/interrogators can differ quite considerably in complexity, depending upon the type of tags being supported and the application. The overall function of the application is to provide the means of communicating with the tags and facilitating data transfer. Functions performed by the reader may include quite sophisticated signal conditioning, parity error checking, and correction. Once the signal from a transponder has been correctly received and decoded, algorithms may be applied to decide whether the signal is a repeat transmission, and may then instruct the transponder to cease transmitting or temporarily cease asking for data from the transponder. This is known as the "Command Response Protocol" and is used to circumvent the problem of reading multiple tags over a short time frame. Using interrogators in this way is sometimes referred to as "Hands Down Polling." An alternative, more secure, but slower tag polling technique is called "Hands Up Polling." This involves the transceiver looking for tags with specific identities, and interrogating them in turn.

4.5. Hospital Environment

In a hospital environment, in order to manage patient medical data we need both types; fixed and handheld transceivers. Transceivers can be assembled in ceilings, walls, or doorframes to collect and disseminate data. Hospitals have become large complex environments. In a hospital, nurses and physicians can retrieve the patient's medical data stored in transponders (RFID tags) before they stand beside a patient's bed or as they are entering a ward. Given the descriptions of the two types and their potential use in hospital patient data management we suggest that:

- It would be most useful to embed a passive RFID transponder into a patient's hospital wrist band;
- It would be most useful to embed a passive RFID transponder into a patient's medical file;

Doctors should have Netbook or tablets equipped with RFID or some type of personal area network device. Either would enable them to retrieve some patient's information whenever they are near the patient, instead of waiting until the medical data is pushed to them through the hospital server.

After examining both ranges for Active and Passive RFID tags, we can suggest the following:

- *Low frequency range tags* are suitable for the patients' band wrist RFID tags. Since we expect that the patients' bed will not be too far from a RFID reader. The reader might be fixed over the patient's bed, in the bed itself, or over the doorframe. The doctor using his/her Netbook, tablet, or smart phone would be aiming to read the patient's data directly and within a relatively short distance.
- *High frequency range tags* are suitable for the physician's tag implanted in their Netbook or tablets. As physicians move from one location to another in the hospital, data on their patients could be continuously being updated.

Hospital patient data management deals with sensitive and critical information (patient's medical data). *Hands Down polling* techniques in conjunction with multiple transceivers that are multiplexed with each other, form a wireless network. The reason behind this choice is that, we need high speed for transferring medical data from medical equipment to or from the RFID wristband tag to the nearest RFID reader then through a wireless network or a network of RFID transceivers or LANs to the hospital server. From there it is a short distance to be transmitted to the doctor's smart phone, Netbook, tablet, a small laptop, or even the desktop through a Wireless LAN (WLAN) or wired LAN.

The "Hand Down Polling" techniques as previously described, provides the ability to detect all detectable RFID tags at once (i.e. in parallel). Preventing any unwanted delay in transmitting medical data corresponding to each RF tagged patient. Transponder programmers are the means, by which data is delivered to Write Once, Read Many (WORM) and read/write tags. Programming can be carried out off-line or on-line. For some systems re-programming may be carried out on-line, particularly if it is being used as an interactive portable data file within a production environment, for example, data may need to be recorded during each process. Removing the transponder at the end of each process to read the previous process data, and to program the new data, would naturally increase process time and would detract substantially from the intended flexibility of the application. By combining the functions of a transceiver and a programmer, data may be appended or altered in the transponder as required, without compromising the production line.

It can be concluded from this section that RFID systems differ in type, shape, and range; depending on the type of application. Low frequency range tags are suitable for the patients' band wrist RFID tags. Since we expect that the patients' bed not to be too far from the RFID reader, which might be fixed on the room ceiling or doorframe. High frequency range tags are suitable for the physician's Netbook or other wireless capture device. As physicians move from one location to another in the hospital, long read ranges are required. On the other hand, transceivers which deal with sensitive and critical information (patient's medical data) need the Hands Down polling techniques. These multiple transceivers should be multiplexed with each other forming a wireless network.

4.6. Applications of the RFID Technology in a Hospital

The following section describes steps involved in the process of using RFID in an hospital environment for patient information management:

1. A biomedical device equipped with an embedded RFID transceiver and programmer will detect and measure the biological state of a patient. This medical data can be an ECG, EEG, BP, sugar level, temperature, or any other biomedical reading. After the acquisition of the required medical data, the biomedical

device will write this data to the RFID transceiver's EEPROM using the built in RFID programmer. Then the RFID transceiver with its antenna will be used to transmit the stored medical data in the EEPROM to the EEPROM in the patient's transponder (tag) which is around his/her wrist. The data received will be updated periodically once new fresh readings are available by the biomedical device. Hence, the newly sent data by the RFID transceiver will be updated (and may be accumulated as needed) to the old data in the tag. The purpose of the data stored in the patient's tag is to make it easy for the doctor to obtain medical information regarding the patient directly via the doctor's Netbook, tablet, smart phone, or even a small laptop.

2. Similarly, the biomedical device will also transfer the measured medical data wirelessly to the nearest WLAN access point. Since high data rate transfer rate is crucial in transferring medical data, IEEE 802.11b or g is recommended for the transmission purpose.

3. Then the wirelessly sent data will be routed to the hospitals main server; to be then sent (pushed) to:

   a. Other doctors available throughout the hospital so they can be notified of any newly received medical data.

   b. To an on-line patient monitoring unit or a nurse's workstation within the hospital.

   c. Or the acquired patients' medical data can be fed into an expert (intelligent agent) software system running on the hospital server and to be then compared with other previously stored abnormal patterns of medical data, and to raise an alarm if any abnormality is discovered.

4. Another option could be using the in-built-embedded RFID transceiver in the biomedical device to send the acquired medical data wirelessly to the nearest RFID transceiver in the room. Then the data will travel simultaneously in a network of RFID transceivers until reaching the hospital server.

5. If a specific surgeon or physician is needed in a specific hospital department, the medical staff in the monitoring unit (e.g. nurses) can query the hospital server for the nearest available doctor to the patient's location. In our framework, an intelligent agent can perform this task. The hospital server traces all doctors' locations in the hospital through detecting the presences of their wireless mobile device; e.g. Netbook, tablet, smart phone, or small laptop in the WLAN range. Physicians may also use RFID transceivers built-in the doctor's wireless mobile device.

6. Once the required physician is located, an alert message will be sent to his\her Netbook, tablet, smart phone, or laptop indicating the location to be reached immediately including a brief description of the patient's case.

7. The doctor enters into the patient's room or ward according to the alert he/ she has received. The doctor wants to check the medical status of a certain patient and interrogates the patient's RFID wrist tag with his RFID transceiver equipped in his\her Netbook, tablet, smart phone, or laptop.

4.7. Practical Cases using RFID Technology

This section explains in details three possible applications of the RFID technology in three applicable cases. Each case is discussed step-by-step.

Those cases cover issues as acquisition of Patient's Medical Data, locating the nearest available doctor to the patients location, and how doctors stimulate the patient's active RFID tag using their Netbook, tablet, smart phone, or laptop in order to acquire the medical data stored in it.

Case 1: Acquisition of Patient's Medical Data

Case one will represent the method of acquisition and transmission of medical data. This process can be described as follows:

A biomedical device equipped with an embedded RFID transceiver and programmer will detect and measure the biological state of a patient. This medical data can be an ECG, EEG, BP, sugar level, temperature, or any other biomedical reading.

After the acquisition of the required medical data, the biomedical device will write -burn this data to the RFID transceiver's EEPROM using the built in RFID programmer. Then the RFID transceiver with its antenna will be used to transmit the stored medical data in the EEPROM to the EEPROM in the patient's transponder (tag) which is around his/her wrist. The data received will be updated periodically once new fresh readings are available by the biomedical device. Hence, the newly sent data by the RFID transceiver will be accumulated to the old data in the tag. The purpose of the data stored in the patient's tag is to make it easy for the doctor to obtain medical information regarding the patient directly via the doctor's Netbook, tablet, smart phone, or laptop.

Similarly, the biomedical device will also transfer the measured medical data wirelessly to the nearest WLAN access point. Since high data rate transfer rate is crucial in transferring medical data, IEEE 802.11b, g, or n is recommended for the transmission purpose (with n being optimal) (see Figure 2).

Then the wirelessly sent data will be routed to the hospitals main server; to be then sent (pushed) to:

*   Other doctors available throughout the hospital so they can be notified of any newly received medical data.

Figure 2. Acquisition of patient data (Mohammadian & Jentzsch, 2008)

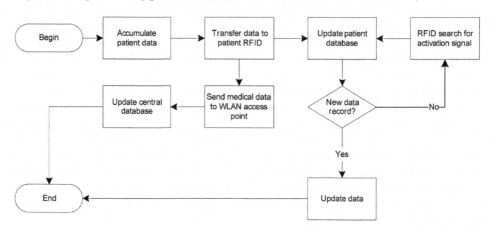

- To an on-line patient monitoring unit or a nurse's workstation within the hospital.
- Or the acquired patients' medical data can be fed into an expert (intelligent) software system running on the hospital server. To be then compared with other previously stored abnormal patterns of medical data, and to raise an alarm if any abnormality is discovered.

Another option could be using the in-built-embedded RFID transceiver in the biomedical device to send the acquired medical data wirelessly to the nearest RFID transceiver in the room. Then the data will travel simultaneously in a network of RFID transceivers until reaching the hospital server.

Case 2: Locating the Nearest Available Doctor to the Patient's Location

This case will explain how to locate the nearest doctor who is needed urgently to attend an emergency medical situation. This case can be explained as follows:

If a specific surgeon or physician is needed in a specific hospital department, the medical staff in the monitoring unit (e.g. nurses) can query the hospital server for the nearest available doctor to the patient's location. In our framework, an intelligent agent can perform this task.

The hospital server traces all doctors' locations in the hospital through detecting the presences of their wireless mobile device; e.g., Netbook, tablet, smart phone, or laptop in the WLAN range (see Figure 3).

Figure 3. Locating nearest doctor (Mohammadian & Jentzsch, 2008)

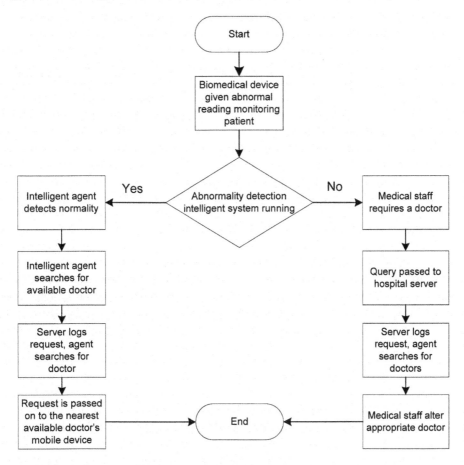

Another method that the hospital's server can use to locate the physicians is making use of the RFID transceivers built-in the doctor's wireless mobile device. Similarly, to the access points used in WLAN, RFID transceivers can assist in serving a similar role of locating doctor's location. This can be described in three steps, which are:

- The fixed RFID transceivers throughout the hospital will send a stimulation signal to detect other free RFID transceivers—which are in the doctors Netbook, tablet, smart phone, or laptop, etc.
- Then all free RFID transceivers will receive the stimulation signal and reply with an acknowledgement signal to the nearest fixed RFID transceiver.

- Finally, each free RFID transceiver cell position would be determined by locating to which fixed RFID transceiver range it belongs to or currently operating in.

After the hospital server located positions of all available doctors, it determines the nearest requested physician (pediatrics, neurologist, etc.) to the patient's location. Once the required physician is located, an alert message will be sent to his\ her Netbook, tablet, smart phone, or laptop indicating the location to be reached immediately. This alert message could show:

- The building, floor and room of the patient (e.g. 3C109);
- Patient's case (e.g. heart stroke, arrhythmia, etc.); and
- A brief description of the patient's case.

If the hospital is running an intelligent agent as described in the our proposed framework on its server, the process of locating and sending an alert message can be automated. This is done through comparing the collected medical data with previously stored abnormal patterns of medical data, then sending an automated message describing the situation. This system could be used to assist the staff in the patient monitoring unit or the nurse's workstation who observe and then sends an alert message manually.

Case 3: Doctor Stimulates the Patient's Active RFID Tag using their PDAs in Order to Acquire the Medical Data Stored in It

This method can be used in order to get rid of medical files and records placed in front of the patient's bed. Additionally, it could help in preventing medical errors— reading the wrong file for the wrong patient and could be considered as an important step towards a paperless hospital. This case can be described in the following steps:

The doctor enters into the patient's room or ward. The doctor wants to check the medical status of a certain patient. Therefore, instead of picking up the 'hard' paper medical file, the doctor interrogates the patient's RFID wrist tag with his RFID transceiver equipped in his\her Netbook, tablet, smart phone, or laptop.

The patient's RFID wrist tag detects the signal of the doctor's RFID transceiver coming from his\her wireless mobile device and replies back with the patient's information and medical data.

If there was more than one patient in the ward possessing RFID wrist tags, all tags can respond in parallel using Hands Down polling techniques back to the doctor's wireless mobile device. Another option could be, the doctor retrieving only the patient's number from the *passive* RFID wrist tag. Then through the WLAN the doctor could access the patient's medical record from the hospital's main server.

RFID technology has many potential important applications in hospitals, and the discussed three cases are a real practical example. Two important issues can be concluded from this section: WLAN is preferred for data transfer; given that IEEE's wireless networks have much faster speed and coverage area as compared to RFID transceivers\transponders technology. Yet, RFID technology is the best for data storage and locating positions of medical staff and patients as well.

The other point is that we need a RFID Transceiver and programmer embedded in a Biomedical Device for data acquisition and dissemination, and only a RFID Transceiver embedded in the doctor's wireless mobile device for obtaining the medical data. With the progress the RFID technology is currently gaining, it could become a standard as other wireless technologies (Bluetooth for example), and eventually manufacturers building them in electronic devices, biomedical devices for our case.

5. CLASSIFICATION OF USER AND DATA FOR OPERATION/TRANSACTION CONTROL

A hospital can be impacted by the corruption, unauthorized access, or theft of its data. A data security breach can impact organization's operations as well as causing large financial, legal implications. It can impact the personal privacy and public confidence in such an organization. With patient data in hospital, human lives could be at risk by unauthorized access, corruption, and modification of such a data.

An intelligent agent system is developed to check the access control from the users to the data stored in the database of a hospital. The intelligent agent system objective is to prevent the unauthorized observation of classified hospital data.

Discretionary Access Controls provide users with permits to access (allow) or disallow other users access to data items stored in a hospital. Such User or group of users with certain access permissions is allowed to access data items. It is possible that authorized users can then pass such data items to other users that may not have permission access to such a data. One way to restrict access to data items can be based an intelligent agent being capable to identity user/s data access level to which data can be provided. In this case, each data item contains metadata information about its security and privacy. An intelligent agent can then control data access of users by checking metadata information attached to data.

In such a case, a data item is provided to user/s after an intelligent agent checks its access permission. If an authorized user obtains a data item and passes it to an unauthorized user, then the unauthorized user will not be able to access that data item. The data permission is checked for each data item as soon as a user wishes to access a data item.

Therefore, each data item permits access privileges to their users based on the metadata stored with each data item. Hence access to a data item is left to the discretion of an intelligent agent and the metadata of that given data item. The intelligent agent then can provide access to authorized users based on the metadata values of a data item under their control without the intercession of other authorities such as a system administrator.

Using an intelligent agent provides a higher level of security to hospital data. As it is stated by Ferraiolo and Kuhn: "In many organizations, the end users do not 'own' the information for which they are allowed access. For these organizations, the corporation or agency is the actual 'owner' of system objects as well as the programs that process it" (Ferraiolo & Kuhn, 1992).

Intelligent agent access control based on metadata stored with data items can provide another level of security to the already existing Role-Based Access Control (RBAC).

Data access controls in organizations are determined by user roles. In such organizations data access control decisions for user access can be based on responsibilities and duties of user/s. In a hospital situation, the user role can be specified by the position of the user in the hospital such as doctor, nurse, administrator, and pharmacist. Therefore, the user role defines their data access based on organization's policy and functions of user/s. Users in such environment cannot pass their access permissions on to other users but they may be able to pass data they access to other users (Ferraiolo & Kuhn, 1992).

In such a case, it is assumed that user/s do not pass data to other users and that they are aware and follow the organizations security, privacy and government's security and privacy laws. In hospital, the data security and privacy associated with the diagnosis of ailments, treatment of disease, and the administering of medicine is of crucial importance (Ferraiolo & Kuhn, 1992).

Generally, the data security and privacy policies are set, controlled and maintained centrally by central security administration.

Each user or group of user in an organization is provided with access rights required for user/s to be able to access their required data and to perform their functions in the organization (Ferraiolo & Kuhn, 1992). The central security administration grant/revoke access to users based on policies provided to them from government or/and organizations laws and regulations.

In a hospital as an example, a doctor can provide prescriptions to patients or enters a diagnosis for a patient into the hospital database or access data related to the past admission and diagnosis of a patient and medication used etc. Such prescriptions can be provided to the patient and then passed to the pharmacist at the hospital but it cannot be passed to a nurse (Ferraiolo & Kuhn, 1992). However, a pharmacist cannot prescribe medication but can dispense prescription drugs. Our proposed intelligent agent system can restrict access to a data item based on the sensitivity measure (stored with each data item as represented by metadata) of the information contained with the data and the formal authorization (i.e. clearance) of user/s to access information of such sensitivity.

In such an environment data access policies provides the capability to authorize who can read what data and an unauthorized flow of information from a user with high level access to a user with a low level access is not possible. It is also possible to provide more constraints on who can read or both read and write/update data by adding a metadata to support such constraint on a data item. Therefore, each metadata attached to each role provides certain access and privileges to certain data items. Given the new proposed method of access control based on metadata stored the following benefits are obtained:

- The security, privacy, and confidentiality of data can be enforced further. For example, in a hospital environment a doctor could be provided with read/ write access to a prescription data whereas the pharmacist will have the read only access of prescriptions data.
- Only authorized users can modify data items. An unauthorized flow of information from a user with high-level access to a user with a low-level access is not possible.

There is a need to provide the minimum disruption when implementing this security and privacy control to an organization. Using intelligent agents, technologies, and metadata access control information for each data will minimize resources impact without needing to re-design databases in an organization such as a hospital. We can add extra information to each data item by adding metadata information to the attributes of each entity in relational-data bases and domains in classes in object-oriented databases.

Consider the simple relational database as shown below:

- Patient(PatientID, Name, Address, TelNo, InsuranceID)
- Insurance(InsuranceID, Type, InsuranceProviderID)
- InsuranceProvider(InsuranceProviderID, Name, Address, TelNo, FaxNo)
- Doctor(DoctorID, Name, OfficeNo, TelNo, PagerNo)
- PatientDoctor(PatientDoctorID, PatientID, DoctorID, VisitDate, Notes)

The meta-data information could be the value or degree of user roles and related policies for privacy and security for that data item. Metadata values can then be used for adaptation and implementation of access/operation performance identification with each data item in the above database. The meta-data values can be obtained from the knowledge workers of the organization based on organization policies, procedure and business rules as well as government requirements for data privacy and security. Table 3 shows the metadata values for table Patient attributes.

Now assume that the following domain metadata linguistic variables for the users (Docror, Nurse, Pharmesists etc..) of data in a given hospital as: TP = "top access user," MD = "medium access user," LO = "low access user" and ZE = "no access to data."

For example Table 4 shows the metadata value related to security data access control of several kind of users based on organization's security access policy.

The values are in the range of 0 to 70, where seventy indicates the metadata for a user of the hospital data that has top (full) access and zero indicates the metadata for a user that has no access to the data in the hospital. Note that other values are also possible. For simplicity assume that the linguistic terms describing the metadata for the attributes of entities in the above database have the values: TP = [35,..,70], MD = [25,..,37], LO = [15,..27], ZE = [17,..,0]

Based on each userID metadata value for each user attributes the membership of that attribute to each linguistic variable can be calculated. In this case study, Triangular fuzzy set was used to represent the data access classifications. The membership value of metadata for each user can be calculated for all these using the following formulas for calculation triangular fuzzy memberships:

$$m_A(x) = 0, \ x < a_1$$

$$m_A(x) = \frac{x - a_1}{a_2 - a_1}, \ a_1 \leq x \leq a_2$$

$$m_A(x) = \frac{a_3 - x}{a_3 - a_2}, \ a_2 \leq x \leq a_3$$

$$m_A(x) = 0, \ x > a_3$$

where x is metadata value for the attribute userID (e.g., DoctorID, NursID, PharmesistID, etc.) and a_1, a_2, and a_3 are the lower middle and upper bound values of the fuzzy set data access security classification. Now assume that metadata value based on organization policy for users are as shown in Table 3. Based on the metadata

Table 3. Metadata values for table patient attributes

Patient Attributes	Meta-data Value of data security access control access based on organization policy for patient data
PatientID	70
Name	50
Address	29
TelNo	15

Table 4. Metadata values for different user

userID	Meta-data value given base on organization policy for data access
DoctorID	52
NurseID	29
PharmacistID	20

value for each user the membership of each user to access and perform operation on data item can be calculated.

The degree of membership value of the attribute userID based on metadata from Table 4 can then be calculated as Table 5.

Now assume that the following access rights exist for each data item. NA = *"no access,"* RD = *"read access,"* WE = *"write access,"* RDWE =*"read and write access,"* DE = *"delete access,"* FA =*"Full access."*

Now the data items and users of data items can be classified and categorized into fuzzy sets (with membership value), a process for determining precise actions (access rights) to be applied must be developed. This task involves writing a rule set that provides an action for any data access classification and user classification that could possibly exist. The formation of the rule set is comparable to that of an expert system, except that the rules incorporate linguistic variables with which human are comfortable. We write fuzzy rules as antecedent-consequent pairs of If-Then statements. For example:

IF *Organizational_Data_Access_Classification* is TP and *User_Data_Access_ Classification* is TP Then *Level_ of_Data_Access_Manipulation is* FA

The overall fuzzy output is derived by applying the "max" operation to the qualified fuzzy outputs each of which is equal to the minimum of the firing strength and the output membership function for each rule.

Users' metadata and the metadata of each data item can be used to determine data access based on user security level and data security level for each data item. The precise actions that are allowed or not allowed on that data item by a given

Table 5. Fuzzy membership of metadata value of users as specified in Table 4

μ(USERID)	TP	MD	LO
μ(DoctorID)	0.85	0	0
μ(NurseID)	0	0.66	0
μ(PharmacistID)	0	0	0.71

user can now be determined. The role of the intelligent agent is to perform data access authorization base on requested data by a user and to allow/disallow access to the data and the operations that can be performed on the data. The knowledge base shown in Table 6 is used by the intelligent agent in this research study for its decision making.

5.1. Framework of User Data Access for Medical Data

The previous section (Practical Cases using RFID Technology) focused on how to design a wireless framework to reflect how patient's medical data can be managed efficiently and effectively leading to the elimination of errors, delays, and even paperwork. Similarly, this section will focus on the previously discussed framework from a security perspective, attempting to increase security and data integrity and user access control for:

- Acquisition of Patient's Medical Data.
- Doctors stimulating the patient's active RFID tag using their wireless mobile devices in order to acquire the medical data stored in it.

The third case study which is concerned about locating the nearest available doctor to the patients location is not discussed here.

The lower part of Figure 4 represents the physical (hardware) encryption layer. This part is divided into two sides. The left side demonstrates the case of a doctor

Table 6. Metadata values for table Patient data access

Meta-data Value based on organization policy for patient data				
μ(DoctorID)	FA	RD	WE	RDWE	DE
PatientID	Not allowed	Allowed	Allowed	Allowed	Not Allowed
Name	Allowed	Allowed	Allowed	Allowed	Not Allowed
Address	Allowed	Allowed	Allowed	Allowed	Not Allowed
TelNo	Allowed	Allowed	Allowed	Not Allowed	Not Allowed

acquiring patient's medical data via a passive RFID tag located in a band around the patient's wrist. The passive RFID tag contains only a very limited amount of information such as the patients name, date of admission to the hospital and above all his/her Medical Record Number (MRN), which will grant access to the medical record containing the acquired medical data and other information regarding the patient's medical condition. This process is implemented in the following steps, and involves two pairs of encryption and decryption. The first encryption occurs after the doctor stimulates the RFID passive tag to acquire the patient's MRN, so the tag will encrypt and reply back the MRN to the doctors PDA for example. Then the doctor will decrypt the MRN and use it to access the patient's medical record from the hospital's server.

Finally, the hospital server will encrypt and reply back the medical record, which will be decrypted once received by the doctor's PDA. This action is performed based on the assumption that the intelligent agent for data access control authorizes the doctor-based metadata attached to the DoctorID and the metadata attached to the patient data items, to access the patient data.

The right side of Figure 4 represents a similar case but this time using an active RF tag. This process involves only one encryption and decryption. The encryption happens after the doctor stimulates the active RFID tag using his PDA, which has an in-equipped RFID transceiver, so the tag replies with the medical data encrypted. Then the received data is decrypted through the doctor's PDA.

The upper part of Figure 4 represents the application encryption layer. Requiring the doctor to enter a pass-phrase to decrypt and then access the stored medical data. So whenever the doctor wants to access patient's medical data, he\she simply enters a certain pass-phrase to grant access to either wireless mobile device or a hospital server depend where the medical data actually resides. This is an extra security measure.

In conclusion securing medial data seems to be uncomplicated, yet the main danger of compromising such data comes from the people managing it, e.g. doctors, nurses, and other medical staff. For that, we have noted even though the transmitted medical data is initially encrypted from the source, doctors have to run application level encryption on their wireless mobile devices in order to protect this important data if the devices gets lost, left behind, robbed, etc. Nevertheless, there is a compromise. However, increasing security through using an intelligent agent that performs the required check and authorization as described above can improve data security in this situation. It is also possible to increase length of encryption keys. However, this action will decrease the encryption\decryption speed and causes unwanted time delays, whether we were using application or hardware level of encryption. As a result, this could delay medical data sent to doctors or on-line monitoring units.

Figure 4. Functional flow

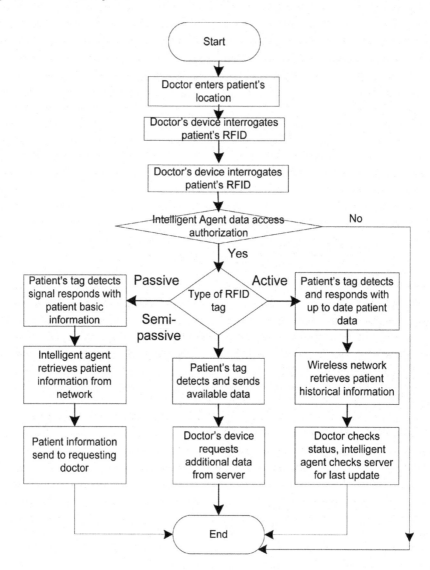

6. CONCLUSION

Managing patients' data wirelessly can prevent errors, enforce standards, make staff more efficient, simplify record keeping and improve patient care. This research in the wireless medical environment introduces new ideas in conjunction to what is already available in the RFID technology and wireless networks.

With the reduction in cost of Radio Frequency Identification (RFID) technology, it is expected the increased use of RFID technology in healthcare in monitoring patients and assisting in health care administration. An intelligent agent using fuzzy logic techniques is implemented for profile matching based on Mohammadian and Jentzsch (2008). A second intelligent agent system is developed for data/user access control and classification to improve the application of regulatory data requirements for security and privacy of data exchange.

ACKNOWLEDGMENT

The authors would like to acknowledge the initial research work performed on this project at the University of Canberra by MIT students. The authors would like also to acknowledge the research work on Data Classification that was performed initially by Masoud Mohammadian and Professor Dimitrios Hatzinakos at the University of Toronto and used in this research study. Part of the research study presented in this chapter is published in journal and conferences in the past few years. The reference to these publications is provided in this manuscript when appropriate.

REFERENCES

Angeles, R. (2007). An empirical study of the anticipated consumer response to RFID product item tagging. *Industrial Management & Data Systems, 107*(4), 461–583. doi:10.1108/02635570710740643

Balaji, P. G., & Srinivasan. (2010). Multi-agent system in urban traffic signal control. *IEEE Computational Intelligence Magazine, 5*(4), 43-51.

Bhuptani, M., & Moradpour, S. (2005). *RFID field guide - Deploying radio frequency identification systems*. Upper Saddle River, NJ: Prentice Hall.

Bigus, J. P., & Bigus, J. (1998). *Constructing intelligent software agents with java – A programmers guide to smarter applications*. New York, NY: Wiley.

Cline, J. (2007). *Growing pressure for data classification*. Retrieved from http://www.computerworld.com/action/article.do?articleId=9014071&command=view ArticleBasic

Do, H., & Rahin, E. (2002). Coma: A system for flexible combination of schema matching approaches. In *Proceedings of 28th Conference on Very Large Databases*, (pp. 610-621). San Francisco, CA: Morgan Kaufmann.

Doan, A.-H., Lu, Y., Lee, T., & Han, J. (2003). Profile-based object matching for information integration. *IEEE Intelligent Systems Magazine, 18*(5), 54–59. doi:10.1109/MIS.2003.1234770

Ferraiolo, D. F., & Kuhn, D. R. (1992). Role based access control. In *Proceedings of the 15th National Computer Security Conference*, (pp. 554-563). ACM.

Finkenzeller, K. (1999). *RFID handbook*. New York, NY: John Wiley and Sons Ltd.

Glover, B., & Bhatt, H. (2006). *RFID essentials*. New York, NY: O'Reilly Media.

Hedgepeth, W. O. (2007). *RFID metrics: Decision making tools for today's supply chains*. Boca Raton, FL: CRC Press.

Kowalke, M. (2006). RFID vs. WiFi for hospital inventory tracking systems. *TMCnet Wireless Mobility Blog*. Retrieved from http://blog.tmcnet.com/wireless-mobility/rfid-vs-wifi-for-hospital-inventory-tracking-systems.asp

McGraw, G. (2006). *Software security*. Reading, MA: Addison-Wesley.

Mickey, K. (2004). RFID grew in 2002. *Traffic World, 5*, 20–21.

Mohammadian, M., & Jentzsch, R. (2007). Intelligent agent framework for RFID. In *Web Mobile-Based Applications for Healthcare Management* (pp. 316–335). New York, NY: IRM Publishing. doi:10.4018/978-1-59140-658-7.ch014

Mohammadian, M., & Jentzsch, R. (2008). Intelligent agent framework for secure patient-doctor profilling and profile matching. *International Journal of Healthcare Information Systems and Informatics, 1*, 1–10.

Odell, J. (Ed.). (2000). *Agent technology*. OMG Document 00-09-01. OMG Agents Interest Group.

Pramatari, K. C., Doukidis, G. I., & Kourouthanassis, P. (2005). Towards 'smarter' supply and demand-chain collaboration practices enabled by RFID technology. In Vervest, P., Van Heck, E., Preiss, K., & Pau, L. F. (Eds.), *Smart Business Networks* (pp. 197–210). Berlin, Germany: Springer. doi:10.1007/3-540-26694-1_14

Qiu, R., & Sangwan, R. (2005). Toward collaborative supply chains using RFID. In *CIO Wisdom II: More Best Practices* (pp. 127–144). Upper Saddle River, NJ: Prentice-Hall.

Schuster, E. W., Allen, S. J., & Brock, D. L. (2007). *Global RFID: The value of the EPCglobal network for supply chain management*. Berlin, Germany: Springer.

Shaalana, K., El-Badryb, M., & Rafeac, A. (2004). A multiagent approach for diagnostic expert systems via the Internet. *Expert Systems with Applications, 27*(1), 1–10. doi:10.1016/j.eswa.2003.12.018

Shepard, S. (2005). *RFID: Radio frequency identification.* New York, NY: McGraw-Hill.

Tindal, S. (2008). One in ten RFID projects tag humans. *ZDNet Australia.* Retrieved from http://www.zdnet.com.au/news/hardware/soa/RFID-people-tagging-benefits-health-sector-/0,130061702,339285273,00.htm

Weinstein, R. (2005). RFID: A technical overview and its application to the enterprise. *IT Professional Magazine, 7*(3), 27–33. doi:10.1109/MITP.2005.69

Whiting, R. (2004). MIT = RFID + Rx. *Information Week, 988,* 16.

Wooldridge, M., & Jennings, N. (1995). Intelligent software agents: Theory and practice. *The Knowledge Engineering Review, 10*(2), 115–152. doi:10.1017/S0269888900008122

Zadeh, L. A. (1965). Fuzzy sets. *Information and Control, 8,* 338–352. doi:10.1016/S0019-9958(65)90241-X

Chapter 15
Application of Handheld Computing and Mobile Phones in Diabetes Self-Care

Abdullah Wahbeh
Dakota State University, USA

EXECUTIVE SUMMARY

Advances in technology have accelerated self-care activities, making them more practical and possible than before using these technologies. The utilization of new Health Information Technologies (HIT) is becoming more and more apparent in self-care. Many patients incorporate the use of PDAs in diabetes self-care (Forjuoh, et al., 2007; Jones & Curry, 2006). Mobile phones are used in diabetes self-management by diabetes patients (Carroll, DiMeglio, Stein, & Marrero, 2011; Faridi, et al., 2008; Mulvaney, et al., 2012). Also, reminders based on SMS cell phone text messaging are used to support diabetes management (Hanauer, Wentzell, Laffel, & Laffel, 2009). Given the current advances in the field of health care, health care technologies, and handheld computing, this case explores the possible primary usages of mobile phones, PDAs, and handheld devices in self-care management. More specifically, the case illustrates how such technologies can be used in diabetes management by patients and health care providers.

DOI: 10.4018/978-1-4666-2671-3.ch015

BACKGROUND

For people with chronic diseases like diabetes, technical convergence makes even more sense. With medications, pumps, glucose and pressure meters, insulin injections, and the need of health care providers to track and document different kind of signs, so patients with diabetes are able to welcome a bit of help from technology (Beckley, 2005).

Handheld computing has been utilized in four large clinics in a hospital located in a large university, multispecialty group practice associated with 186,000 member of Health Maintenance Organization (HMO) have employed the use of PDAs in diabetes self-care by patients with type 2 diabetes. The four clinics are affiliated with the Central Texas Primary Care Research Network which is a primary care practice based research network located in Temple, Texas within the Scott and White Health System of the Texas A&M Health Science Center College of Medicine (Forjuoh, Reis, Couchman, & Ory, 2008; Forjuoh, et al., 2007). A diabetes center in Boston, Massachusetts has used a computerized automated reminder diabetes system based on SMS cell phone text messing to support diabetes management (Hanauer, et al., 2009).

A family medicine clinic located at the college of medicine at Pennsylvania state university has assessed the use of a PDA based electronic management system in a primary care office (The family clinic). There were 58 patients and 1 physician. In addition, there was a control group of 115 patients seen by 1 of 5 other physicians. All patients were with type 2 diabetes (Jones & Curry, 2006). Two Community Health Centers (CHC) located at Connecticut have evaluates the impact of using mobile phones on type 2 diabetes patients' self-management. The clinics have similar demographic characteristics and they were randomly assigned for the intervention and control of thirty patients with type 2 diabetes (Faridi, et al., 2008). A University Medical Center has test the use of mobile phones to measure adolescent diabetes adherence for patients from a large academic diabetes clinic. Only patients with type 1 diabetes for at least one year are involved in the test (Mulvaney, et al., 2012). Diabetes clinics at the James Whitcomb Riley hospital for children, Indianapolis, Indiana have test the use of cell phone based glucose monitoring system for adolescent diabetes management by patients with type 1 diabetes for at least 1 year (Carroll, et al., 2011). The department of engineering science at university of Oxford in collaboration with e-San Ltd have developed a real time, mobile phone based telemedicine system to support patients with type 1 diabetes, the software system was implemented on a Motorola T720i phone and a One Touch Ultra blood glucose meter (Farmer, et al., 2005).

SETTING THE STAGE

Diabetes management is a complex and difficult. Previously, effective diabetes managements requires continual and demanding daily self-care behaviors and processes in different areas, such as testing and measuring glucose level, insulin injection, diet control, taking medications several times a day, seeking general information on diabetes from the libraries, calculating variable insulin dosage by estimating nutritional content of food, monitoring bodily symptoms and taking steps to feel normal again, exercise, and seeking specific information relating to own diabetes (Freund, Johnson, Silverstein, & Thomas, 1991; Hinder & Greenhalgh, 2012; Johnson, Silverstein, Rosenbloom, Carter, & Cunningham, 1986). Also, because of the difficulty of making lifestyle change, achieving effective management of diabetes has proven to be very difficult (Freund, et al., 1991; Johnson, et al., 1986).

Previously, diabetes patients deal with many of the previous tasks and behaviors such as glucose monitoring and diet control by recording all of the obtained results on a sheet of paper. Using a piece of paper, diabetes patients records all of the measurements taken, these measurements may be taken before and after primary meals and even before bedtime (Skyler, Lasky, Skyler, Robertson, & Mintz, 1978). However, this traditional paper medical record does little to help facilitating diabetes care management. (Smith, et al., 1998). Another utility that is used by diabetes patient for diabetes self-management is using paper diaries (Burke, et al., 2005). Using paper diaries, the patients are instructed to record all food intake and also record exercise (energy expenditure). The recording process may be extended to places, time, quantity eaten, and the target nutrient values. This process is tedious and time consuming process that is very hard to implement in some situations (Burke, et al., 2005).

Using such traditional methods for diabetes management requires literacy. In addition, using such tools requires patients to search for foods in a nutrient guide and calculate and record the content of foods eaten is time consuming. In addition, using papers makes it difficult for the clinician or researcher to determine when the diary was completed. Finally, Research focused on human memory reveals that memory recall is unreliable and that each step in the process of recalling information has the potential to introduce inaccuracy and bias (Burke, et al., 2005).

The advances in Information and Communication Technologies (ICT) have introduced new approaches that support health care delivery and patient education in diabetes case. The advent in Information Technology (IT) had a powerful influence through data collection, information sharing, streamlined process and many other ways (Wyne, 2008). Diabetes represents an ideal case for the incorporation of information and communication technologies in the provision of care. Diabetes is highly prevalent in managed care populations, frequently associated with comorbid conditions, requires multiple medications in its management, and requires monitoring of several measures of disease control. All of these factors combined make diabetes an opportune disease for the implementation of IT in managed care (Wyne, 2008). Handheld devices, mobile phones and PDAs represents the advances in ICT and considered as an effective tools for managing diabetes by patients (Carroll, et al., 2011; Hanauer, et al., 2009; Mulvaney, et al., 2012).

Several types of handheld devices exists, however the mostly used handheld devices include Palm OS-based PDAs, pocket PC, smart phones, and Blackberries (Lu, Xiao, Sears, & Jacko, 2005). Using these devices to achieve better diabetes self-care in patients with diabetes is becoming more and more important. Such devices allows patients to keep track of their appointments, store memos and messages, save phone numbers, keep track of tasks using features such as reminders and alarms, and act as a calculator (Forjuoh, et al., 2007). Also, these devices include address book, scheduler, to do list and memo function (Fischer, Stewart, Mehta, Wax, & Lapinsky, 2003). Also, some of the handheld devices are equipped with wireless capabilities such as Bluetooth (Istepanian, et al., 2009). Handheld devices are also customizable devices making them more intimate with diabetes self-care by expanding memories to help storing diabetes self-care activity monitoring software programs (Forjuoh, et al., 2007).

A password protected PDA preinstalled with Diabetes Pilot software (www.diabetespilot.com) is used by patients with diabetes to help in diabetes managements. Training on using the PDA with the installed software is done using one-on-one training session; a copy of a training manual is provided to patients; in addition, a one-week follow-up monitoring phone call and ongoing phone support by the research assistant. Training for the study is done on some of the capabilities of Diabetes Pilot; these capabilities include diet count, carbohydrate count, readings for blood sugar, duration and type of exercise, and medications (Forjuoh, et al., 2007). The Diabetes Pilot software is a tool developed by Digital Altitudes (Mount Prospect, IL) and designed in a way that help making diabetes management easier and more accurate than use of traditional paper logs. The software is developed and designed in a way the helps handling information in a faster and easier way for recording and reviewing. "Diabetes Pilot is capable of recording blood glucose measurements, insulin and other medication dosages and administration times, meals, exercise, test results, and other notes. Also, it is able to track intake of carbohydrates, calories, fat, protein, and fiber in the foods consumed using an integrated food database that contains information on thousands kind of foods." Diabetes Pilot is supported by some visualization capabilities that help visualizing trends in blood glucose using different graphs and reports format in addition to the ability to categorize records by the time of day or any other preferred system. It allows data to be transferred faster and easier (synchronized) to a desktop computer software package for further exploration, analysis and communication with others such systems (Forjuoh, et al., 2007).

A Novel Interactive Cell-phone technology for Health Enhancement (NICHE) aimed at enhancing self-management of type 2 diabetic patients was utilized by 15 patients (the intervention group which is exposed to the NICHE technology) with type 2 diabetes and compared by another 15 patients (the control group which is not exposed to NICHE) with the same type of diabetes who continued with their standard diabetes management. The system was employed with wireless biometric devices (glucometer and pedometer) in order to send clinical data to an online server, the online server then sends specific feedback to patients via cellular phone text messaging. The NICHE technology is an interactive informational feedback system, which utilizes wireless technologies in order to provide a tailored reminders and feedback based on the received data from the patients data, such reminders and feedback are sent to patients and providers via messages on cellular phones. Two Community Health Centers (CHC) nurse practitioners have received an extensive training sessions in the NICHE system. A one day training workshop was provided by the two nurses to the intervention patients, patients were taught how to use and utilize the NICHE technology for the management of type 2 diabetes. Patients were asked to measure glucose level once a day, wear their pedometers during the day and upload data onto the NICHE server daily (Faridi, et al., 2008).

A self-help software tool called Easy Health Diary based on smartphones was used for patients with Type 2 diabetes. The functionality of Easy Health Diary applies to three main aspects of diabetes management; these aspects include physical activity, nutrition, and healthy blood glucose values. The Easy Health Diary self-help tool had low technical thresholds and a highly usable design because it is targeted towards patients with diabetes who aged 50 years and more. Easy Health Diary allow the blood glucose levels and physical activity to be captured wirelessly using sensors, and it also allow nutrition data to be entered and registered through a simple user interface. In addition, the tool process and presents the data to the patients. The strategy followed for developing the software tool differentiates it from existing software. The strategy aims for an "easy way of interacting with the system, ideally in a "no-touch" manner as achieved with Easy Health Diary for wireless transfer of blood glucose values and step counts." Easy Health Diary requires as few physical interactions/finger touches as possible. "The tool has a very easy interface for data capture as well as highly intuitive and user-friendly output procedures, enabling both context awareness and self-adjusting capabilities." The Easy Health Diary self-help tool provides diabetes patients with both general and specific information about some of the health parameters to inspire and/or enlighten these patients to change to more healthy habits (Arsand, Varmedal, & Hartvigsen, 2007).

A diabetes monitoring system called HealthPia GlucoPack was developed by the HealthPia Incorporation located in Palisades Park, NJ. The system integrates a glucose monitoring system onto a conventional cell phone. The HealthPia Gluco-Pack diabetes monitoring system is equipped with a small blood glucose monitoring device integrated into the battery pack of a cell phone. The device is used to transmit self-monitoring data to a website for review and analysis. The device consists of several components that are integrated to achieve the overall goal of the monitoring system, these components include a strip sensor, analog circuit, microcontroller unit, communication interface, and phone input/output. Once the strip is inserted into the device a circuit is generated and passed through the measurement device, then it is converted into a voltage, amplified, and then sent into the microcontroller unit. The analog data obtained from the microcontroller unit are then converted into a digital data according to the measurement and temperature correction tables. These data are in turn sent to the specific phone input/output protocols. More specifically, the data is sent to the phone display as well as to a secure server through a cellular signal. "The software for the phone application is supported on many platforms, including BREW, J2ME, and WIPI." Data from the glucometer are sent to a server that from which patients, parents, and clinicians are allowed to see the blood glucose values in a number of different formats over the Web using a secure connection. Also, patients can use a mobile phone to discuss therapeutic options with health care provider (Carroll, et al., 2011; Carroll, Marrero, & Downs, 2007).

A fully automated, two-way text messaging system has been used to help encouraging more and more blood glucose monitoring in teens and young adults with diabetes using a Computerized Automated Reminder Diabetes System (CARDS). The proposed system utilizes the cell phones text messaging capabilities which is known as Short Messaging Service (SMS)—a well-known communication service among used by adults—to send and receive small snippets of data like blood glucose measurements. SMSs provide reminders for clinic visits, tuberculosis medication compliance, and diabetes monitoring in adults. The card system itself consists of a Web-based module and a messaging/reminder module designed to run autonomously. In addition, the system is capable of recording all processes and action in a log for later analysis. The system operates on an Apple Macintosh PowerBook laptop computer with 768 MB of memory. Patients logged in the system using a secure website via username and password. The CARDS site provided a customizable screen for patients to manage their schedule for reminder messages whether by time of day and day of week. The CARDS site allows for providing comment, edit, view, and print blood glucose diaries with a time and date stamp. CARDS system is able to send a reminder either by cell phone text message or by e-mail to check the blood glucose. If the CARDS system has no response from the patients within 15 min, a single repeat reminder from a set of existing reminders is sent until the patient submits the blood glucose level. Once blood glucose level is received, the CARDS system sends a positive feedback to the patients. On the other hand, if the blood glucose value received by the CRADS system is out of a specific range, the system sends a warning to the patient to "take appropriate action according to the healthcare team's recommendations and then recheck the blood glucose. Finally, any blood glucose values submitted by the patients using cell phone or e-mail could can be viewed immediately and printed (Hanauer, et al., 2009).

A mobile based remote patient monitoring system that help improving the level of blood pressure and actively engages patients in the process of care. The mobile-based blood pressure monitoring system is developed using different type of hard-ware including a Bluetooth-enabled home blood pressure monitor, a mobile phone used to send and receive the data, a centralized server for processing the data, a fax system aims at sending the physicians' reports, and a blood pressure alerting system. The blood pressure Tele-management system consists of the patient component and the physician-reporting and alerting component. The patient component is a data storage and decision support system. This component of the system consists of a "commercially available Bluetooth-enabled BP monitoring device and a dedicated, preprogrammed mobile phone." The mobile phone receives the reading from pa-tients at home and sends these reading wirelessly from the blood pressure monitor and then sends them securely to the server. The Bluetooth technology utilized in the system is a "universal, short-range, wireless data-transmission protocol operat-ing in the unlicensed 2.4-GHz frequency band." The Web server—the back end of the system—collects the results from patients and store them into a database and "applies a set of clinical rules on the BP monitoring schedule and BP alerts." The trigger event for these rules is carried out by the reporting and alerting component of the system. "The reporting and alerting system sends secure written progress and coaching messages automatically to the mobile phone after every reading." An automated voice messages sent to the patient's home phone when the system detect any non-adherence to the preset home blood pressure monitoring schedule or when the blood pressure readings that exceed a pre specified threshold values. In addition, the Tele-management system sends automated blood pressure alerts that popup on patients' mobile phones. The Tele-management system also allows the physicians to set and change the number of monitoring days per week and the threshold values for critical blood pressure alerts. Using the Tele-management system allows patients, physicians, and their assistants to request a fax report to be sent to a pre specified phone number of physicians. The person who sends such report has to enter a numeric user identification and password that are validated against the database before sending the report (Logan, et al., 2007).

A 3G Mobile Phone Application (MPA) is used to improve a self-management of individuals with Type 1 Diabetes Mellitus (T1DM). The application is made of five interfaces for the management of blood pressure, blood glucose, insulin dosage, physical activity, and food/drink intake. The application allows the patients to take notes, pressing a button in the case of emergency, transmit the patients' location immediately to an emergency call center. The data are stored on the mobile phone and are regularly wirelessly transmitted to the patient management unit located at the hospital Web server via the General Packet Radio Service (GPRS), the 3G network or WiFi networks. The architecture of the patient centric system consists of two units namely the patient unit and the patient management unit. The patient component consists of vital signals monitoring devices and a mobile phone to install the mobile MPA. Data from the monitoring devices and the information collected about food/drink intake, physical activity, insulin therapeutic scheme, and text notes are provided manually or automatically using interfaces by the patients who use the MPA. The MPA allows for the processing and presentation of the data to the user using the appropriate user interfaces. When patients feel unsecure, he has the ability to send data to the Web server in the patient management unit. In the case of dangerous metabolic condition, the MPA allows the patients to push a button on mobile equipped with a Global Positioning System (GPS) receiver, to transmit and locate his position to an emergency call center and to the attendant physician. Physicians are able to access the stored data using personal computer with Internet connection or via mobile phone through a secure connection. In addition, they have the ability to use a number of tools to visualize the data, create, edit or update the treatment and communicate with the patient by sending/receiving emails or comments to him. "The database of the PMU is designed on the basis of Health Level 7 (HL7) standard, in order to support the communication with the hospital information system." The MPA is designed with the following requirements, the need for diabetes self-management, personal use, and easy access to the MPA anytime and anywhere, large display units to be legible even by elder persons, and user-friendly interfaces. MPA runs on windows mobile phones and data entering is accelerated by using stylus (Mougiakakou, Kouris, Iliopoulou, Vazeou, & Koutsouris, 2009).

DESCRIPTION

Handheld devices, PDAs, and mobile phones have been used to assist self-care activities by diabetes patients and health care providers. However, these days adopting the PDAs for diabetes management is very rare, most of the patients and health care providers are using mobile phones more than PDAs for health care provision. Based on the review how handheld devices are used for diabetes management we found that 14 studies have adopt the use of mobile phones for diabetes management where only 5 studies have used PDA devices for the same purposes. Also, based on Tatara, Arsand, Nilsen, and Hartvigsen's (2009) review of handheld devices for diabetes managements, most of the application used for diabetes management for patients with either type 1 or type 2 diabetes are used on mobile phones, where 30 studies have adopt the use of mobile phones, also, 17 studies reviewed by Krishna and Boren (2008) adopt mobile phone for diabetes management. 9 studies adopt the use of PDAs, 17 studies adopt the use of personal computers, and only 3 studies adopt other devices for diabetes management (Tatara, et al., 2009). Also, as stated by Phillips, Felix, Galli, Patel, and Edwards (2010), the functionalities of mobile phones and smartphones are more than those found on the PDA devices even those PDA devices capable of making phone calls. Mobile phones and smart phones functionalities include voice, SMS, MMS, email, WAP Internet, wireless cellular broadband, audio, and video. On the other hand PDA devices functionality include voice, SMS, MMS, email, WAP Internet, and wireless cellular broadband (Phillips, et al., 2010). Based on the differences in functionalities between mobile phones and PDA devices and based on the number of studies that adopt mobile phones for diabetes management compared with those who adopt PDAs for the same purposes, we can see that PDAs are becoming an old technology and not widely used by health care providers for health care provision.

This section provides an overview of how PDAs and mobile phones are used in diabetes self-care and provide a description of case about using mobile phones in diabetes management. We starts by describing how PDAs are used and the major activities that are carried out using these old technologies, then we describe the adoption of mobile phones by health care providers and diabetes patient for the management of diabetes.

Personal Digital Assistant (PDA)

Personal Digital Assistant (PDA) devices are one of the handheld devices used for diabetes management by diabetes patients and by care providers. These devices are equipped with many different types of diabetes management software such as Diabetes Pilot (Forjuoh, et al., 2008; Forjuoh, et al., 2007) and Glycemic Index Meal Planner (Ma, et al., 2006), these software helps making diabetes management much more easier and more accurate than using traditional methods based on paper sheets (Skyler, et al., 1978) and paper diaries (Burke, et al., 2005). The PDA device allows data to be handled faster and make data reviewing and recording easier (Forjuoh, et al., 2007).

Diabetes patients use such PDAs devices equipped with diabetes management software to regularly enter data as they self-manage their diabetes (Forjuoh, et al., 2008). Diabetes patients provides data about the levels of blood glucose, insulin dosages, meals, exercises, test results, track intake of carbohydrates, calories, fat, protein, and fiber in the foods eaten using an integrated database (Forjuoh, et al., 2008; Forjuoh, et al., 2007; Rigla, et al., 2007). These devices have capabilities that allow diabetes patients to graph the entered data in order to visualize trends in blood glucose levels using different output formats (Forjuoh, et al., 2008, 2007). Also, using these devices, patients receive reminders from physicians about due or overdue diabetes guideline recommendations for better health care (Jones & Curry, 2006) and receive predefined alarm messages from doctors whenever recurrent out-of-range glucose values occurred (Rigla, et al., 2007).

Once all of the diabetes related information is provided by the patients, the PDA device allows for fast and easy transfer of data to a server equipped with complementary program for further analysis and communication with others such as one's health care provider (Forjuoh, et al., 2007). The privacy of data is assured by using a data encryption method before transmission using the secure socket layer secure protocol (Rigla, et al., 2007). Data sent by diabetes patients using PDA devices are analyzed by health care providers (Rigla, et al., 2007) to provide health related advices to the patients. Also, PDA devices allow physicians to help provides health-care to diabetes patients by recording all patients related data such as glycol-hemoglobin, hepatic enzymes, weight, systolic and diastolic blood pressure, and date of glucometer correlation (Jones & Curry, 2006). In addition, PDA devices are used to assist diabetes patients with self-monitoring of dietary intake (Fukuo, et al., 2009; Ma, et al., 2006). Diabetes patients use PDA devices to record daily dietary intake and meal starting times as soon as possible after eating (Fukuo, et al., 2009; Ma, et al., 2006) and allow them to selects the food item from a list of foods and drinks, which included the name, energy and amount of each item (Fukuo, et al., 2009). Using the PDA device, the patient can choose the type of the meal (breakfast, lunch, dinner, or snack), and then select the food group from a list and based on the selected list of food a glycemic index score or calories per serving is presented to the patients. Values presented to the patients help them better choosing foods that helps better management of diabetes (Ma, et al., 2006).

Mobile Phones

Mobile phones are another kind of hand held devices that is used in self-care management by diabetes patients. Mobile phones are equipped either with a software program such as Diabetes Partner (Årsand, Tufano, Ralston, & Hjortdahl, 2008) designed to help patients with diabetes managements (Mougiakakou, et al., 2009) or with a blood glucose meter (Carroll, et al., 2011, 2007; Farmer, et al., 2005; Istepanian, et al., 2009). For some of the mobile phones, a small blood glucose monitoring device is integrated into the battery pack of the mobile phone (Carroll, et al., 2007).

Sometimes, the two devices are connected via cables (Farmer, et al., 2005), where other are connected using Bluetooth technology (Istepanian, et al., 2009).

Mobile phones are used to alert the patients when the diabetes related measurements must be taken (Istepanian, et al., 2009). For example, some patients measure the blood sugar using a one touch glucose meter by following the instructions for blood glucose testing that are displayed on the phone once the diabetes software is activated (Farmer, et al., 2005) and the measures are transmitted via Bluetooth technology to a mobile phone (Farmer, et al., 2005; Istepanian, et al., 2009). Others measures their blood pressure levels and send these measurements to a mobile phone wirelessly from the blood pressure monitor (Logan, et al., 2007).

Some mobile devices are equipped with diabetes management software that allow capturing and displaying data about users' dietary habits, use of insulin, and blood glucose levels (Årsand, et al., 2008) where other software teach patients about the impacts of dietary on blood glucose levels, direct patients to generate higher-quality blood glucose and suggested therapy recommendations on health care provider prescribing behavior (Quinn, et al., 2008). Other mobile based diabetes management devices support diabetes patients in providing diabetes-related data such as injected insulin doses, blood glucose level, carbohydrates levels in food, well-being, and physical activities (Kollmann, Riedl, Kastner, Schreier, & Ludvik, 2007).

Other diabetes management devices consist of a strip sensor, microcontroller unit, analog circuit, communication interface, and phone input/output. When the patient insert the strip into the device a measure is obtained and passed through the measurement device, converted into a voltage, amplified, and then sent into the microcontroller unit. Analog data from the microcontroller unit are converted to digital data where these data are sent to the specific phone input/output protocols (Carroll, et al., 2007). Some devices consist of commercially available Bluetooth-enabled blood pressure monitoring device/one touch blood glucose meter and a dedicated, reprogrammed mobile phone that when the patient removed the test strip out of the blood glucose meter or measured the blood pressure, the patient's measured values are wirelessly, securely, and automatically sent to the patient's cell phone (Logan, et al., 2007; Quinn, et al., 2008).

When a measurement value is received by the mobile phone, the mobile application is triggered asking the patient to identify when the measurement was taken. When the patient specify the time for the measure, a feedback is provided to him/her based on the obtained measure. For example, if measurement (ex. blood glucose) level is above or below his/her target levels, the mobile phone give the patient real-time feedback on how to correct the measurement (blood glucose) level (Kollmann, et al., 2007; Quinn, et al., 2008). If no problems detected with the obtained measures, the mobile phone give the patient positive feedback. If the patient faces any problem, then he/she is provided with educational material specific to that issue (Quinn, et al., 2008).

Once the measurements are on the mobile phone they are remotely synchronized to a server using a cellular connection (Carroll, et al., 2011, 2007; Logan, et al., 2007) or using the General Packet Radio Service (GPRS) (Kollmann, et al., 2007) where the clinicians review these measures using a specially designed software program (Carroll, et al., 2011; Farmer, et al., 2005; Istepanian, et al., 2009). Such programs includes a predetermined prompting algorithm designed to identify blood glucose patterns that needed to be addressed to reduce potential acute and chronic problems (Carroll, et al., 2011). Depending on the quality of the transmitted data, patients might be telephoned or sent a text message by the health care providers to discuss recent blood glucose values, offer possible regimen adjustments, or suggest additional contacts (Carroll, et al., 2011).

The server send a summary of blood glucose results measured within the previous results to the patients and provide them with a reminder of overall progress which could then prompt attention to adjust the insulin dose (Farmer, et al., 2005). Also, the server provides patients and practitioners with details of the amalgamated readings and treatment recommendations (Istepanian, et al., 2009) and allow them and health care providers view the measured values in a number of formats over a secure Internet connection (Carroll, et al., 2007). Some server applies a set of clinical rules on the blood pressure monitoring schedule and blood pressure alerts based on the obtained measures (Logan, et al., 2007). The server sends a voice messages to the patients' phone when non adherence to the preset home blood pressure monitoring schedule is detected or when the blood pressure exceeds a pre specified threshold values (Logan, et al., 2007).

Implementing a Mobile-Based System for Diabetes Management by Both Diabetes Patients and Health Care Providers

Implementing a mobile-based system for diabetes management requires several kind of software and hardware that are integrated together to provide the optimal functionality and provide health care services in a perfect manner. The diabetes management system implemented in this case consist of a smart mobile phone capable of sending and receiving messages, has connectivity capability (Bluetooth, wireless, GPRS, and cable connectivity), capable of installing custom software. The system consist also of a one touch blood glucose and blood pressure meter, this devices is an integrated devices that is used for achieving two functionality using one device, the device is equipped with a Bluetooth, wireless, and cable connectivity capabilities.

In addition, the system consists of a diabetes management software; this software is to be installed on the smart mobile phone and has several capabilities with respect to diabetes; the capabilities of the software include receiving measures obtained from the blood glucose and pressure meter, recoding insulin injections, recording frequency and type of exercises, recording the amount and type of food consumed, capable of sending and receiving information to/from the centralized server at the health care provider location. Another important component of the system is a centralized server located at the health care provider location, the server is used to receive all of the information recorded by the patients, and health care providers access this information on the server anywhere, anytime for analysis and for providing useful advices to patients based on the received results. Finally, the last component of the system is specialized software installed on the centralized server, this specialized software is capable of analyzing the information obtained from the patients in different ways, and it is capable of sending several kinds of alerts and reminders based on the analyzed data. Figure 1 illustrates the major components of the diabetes management system and how it is implemented.

Figure 1. Implementing the diabetes management system

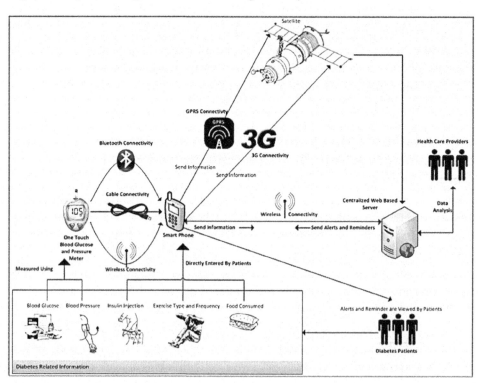

As shown in the figure, a mobile phone integrated with one touch glucose and blood pressure meter is provided to patients with diabetes, the integration between the two devices is done using a Bluetooth connectivity, cable connectivity, or wireless connectivity. A mobile based software that is designed to provide alerts and a reminder to the diabetes patients regarding the times that he/she have to measure the blood glucose and pressure levels is installed on the mobile phone. The mobile-based software is designed to send reminders to patients on a specific time interval times, more specifically, the software sends reminder before and after meals time and before going to bed.

Based on the preprogrammed reminders that are sent to the patient, he/she measure his/her blood glucose level and the blood pressure. Once these measurements are taken, they are transmitted to the mobile phone and they are automatically installed in the mobile phone using the mobile-based diabetes management software. Along with these measurements, the patient provides other measures such as the time of insulin dosages, the amount and type of food consumed, and whether any kind of exercise is done by the patient. Based on this information the patients can receive several kind of feedback that can help them to manage the diabetes disease and maintain good habits and help improve and enhance their daily life.

The mobile phone is synchronized with a central server located at the hospital, the synchronization between the mobile phone and the centralized server is done through using either a GPRS connection or 3G connection, or through a wireless connectivity connection. All the measurements taken by the patients are stored on the mobile phone and transferred on a daily basis to the central server using the mobile network either via General Packet Radio Services (GPRS) or using a wireless network or via a 3G/4G connection. The main server is equipped with special software that analyses these measurements. In addition, a health care provider reviews the measurement for each patient and provides some kind of feedback based on the measurements value. The health care providers can access these data using a personal computer within the hospital or in emerging situations and circumstances he/she can connect to the server at the hospital sing the Internet or via the General Packet Radio Services (GPRS) in order to obtain the latest data about his/her patients. The health care providers analyze the patients' information once every three days and send the patients several recommendations for adjustment to insulin doses, type of exercise, diet, and for better management of the disease based on the provided data. In addition, the patients can obtain advices from the health care providers about overcoming some obstacles faced by them and tips to maintain an appropriate level of activity in addition to different kind of physical activities that are good to better manage their diabetes. In addition, the patients can receive weekly charts, trends and reports about the blood glucose levels, blood pressure, and other important information that are important to the management of diabetes.

If a patient did not took the required measurements for the blood glucose level and blood pressure at the specified time intervals, the specialized software on the central server sends him/her a reminder to take the measures as soon as possible, such reminders appears as a pop up message on the mobile screen. If the patient did not adhere to the reminder message within 45 minutes, another alarm in the form of a text message using the Short Message Service (SMS) is sent to the patient phone to remind him/her about the measurements. In case of a measurement of blood glucose level and blood pressure that is lower than or greater than a pre-specified threshold, the central server sends alarms to the patient mobile along with a text message that contains some useful information that the patient should follow to adjust the level of sugar in blood or to control the blood pressure. On the other hand, if the blood glucose at an optimal level and the blood pressure is good then the centralized server sends an automated short message using the Short Message Service (SMS) informing the patient that no treatment changes are required.

In the case of dangerous conditions, the patients has the ability to use the mobile based software to send a preprogrammed alarm to the central server, which in turn and based on the patient location that is sent along with the patient alarm using the Global Positioning System (GPS) available on the mobile phone, find the nearest emergency center and send the patient location and an emergency message to the nearest health care center or hospital.

CURRENT CHALLENGES

Like any other technologies utilized for many different purposes, the use of mobile phones and other handheld devices have many challenges, these challenges are associated with the devices themselves, the way the devices are used for health care provision, and other challenges related to the entire system where these devices are used. Many of the challenges mentioned in this section are faced by a number of previous studies in the area of health care and self-care management by diabetes patients (Faridi, et al., 2008; Fischer, et al., 2003; Koch, 2010; Satyanarayanan, 1996).

The main challenge associated with the use of mobile phone for diabetes management is ease of use of the mobile phones itself and the use of the blood glucose and the blood pressure meters. In term of ease of use, diabetes patients using a mobile phone for diabetes management may suffers from the software used for the management process. The software might be designed in such a way that does not take into consideration ease of use by the patients, the software may consist of a lot of menus that patients have to navigate through in order to upload the glucose and blood pressure measurements and other diabetes related information. In addition, people have a problem with using such technologies for diabetes managements because they are not willing or have no intentions to use such new technologies, using mobile technologies for diabetes managements and health care required the patients to be literate in the area of technology and how to use such technologies.

Another challenge associated with the use of mobile phones for diabetes managements and for health care in general is the patients' confidentiality. Patients' information must be kept in a secure place preventing unauthorized use for such information by anybody other than the patients themselves and any health care provider responsible for those patients. In addition, the confidentiality of the patients while they are using the mobile phones for diabetes management is extremely serious and challenging concern. Along with these issues, ensuring and keeping the security tools and software working, correctly configured, and appropriately documented is another challenge that falls in the area of patients' confidentiality.

A third challenge faced by most health care providers who try to adopt the use of handheld devices and mobile phones for diabetes management is the cost associated with such use. Cost of using mobile phones for diabetes management tend to be high, such cost is not only related to the cost of mobile devices since these are used by patients for daily activity in the case health care providers does not offer the patients with the mobile phones. Other costs such as the cost of software used for diabetes managements, cost of the back end servers, cost of the upgrades required for the health care providers' network, the cost of mobile devices if they are provided by the health care provider, and finally the cost associated support are real challenges faced by health care providers.

Another challenge for using the handheld devices and mobile phones for diabetes managements is associated with the devices themselves. Mobile phones have limited displays that are problematic for people who have poor eyesight or cannot read small fonts. In addition, the limited displays result in making the patients spends a lot of time paging and navigating through tens of screens for the purposes of entering the data and obtaining information. In addition, mobile phones and handheld devices have limited and low processing power that can results in incomplete, unclear, and missing information. Handheld device and mobile phones are potential for security vulnerabilities. They are also easy to lose and forget. Finally, these devices have a short battery life depending on the actual usage of the device during the day; also, some of these devices suffer from the small amount of memory storage associated with these devices. The mobile device's connectivity is highly variable and changeable in terms of performance, dependability, and reliability, and this may be problematic for patients who are submitting their information using the mobile phone using either a wireless network or using GPRS services. This is because some places, buildings, or areas provide or are served by reliable and high bandwidth connectivity while other places may suffer from low bandwidth and unreliable connectivity.

SOLUTIONS AND RECOMMENDATIONS

Because of the previously mentioned challenges, that faces health care providers in general and the diabetes patents in specific, many patients are not willing to adopt the use of mobile phone devices for diabetes management and prefer using traditional methods such as piece of paper or a dietary paper to manage their diabetes.

However, there exists some suggestions to overcome most of the previously challenges rose by the use of mobile phones in diabetes managements. The ease of use of the mobile phones itself and the use of the blood glucose and the blood pressure meters can be solved by providing training sessions to the patients on how to use mobile devices, glucose meter, and blood pressure meter for diabetes managements. In addition, providing the patients with a manual bout using such devices may be helpful for overcoming such problem. Finally, the health care providers may take advantages from the mobile device itself by sending patients short messages using the SMS services about using such devices for diabetes managements. Ease of use problems faced by old people is solved as we move by time, because people becoming older in the future will be more responsive and aware of using such technology to meet the demands of handling age-related diseases and ill health.

The patients' confidentiality challenge can be solved indifferent way. One of solution to such problem is through user authentication using a password as a protection mechanism. In addition, health care providers can use some kind of identifiers such as an ID or last digits from the social security number as an identification method instead of using patients' name. In addition, the information stored on the mobile device by the patients can be protected by using the security features associated with these devices. As we know, different security mechanism can be found on mobile phones such as a four digits code or using patterns where the user draw a number of straight lines over some specific points to access the mobile device. Using these security mechanisms, the patients can access their information by unlocking the mobile phone using the specified access methods every time he/she wants to look at specific information or add new information.

Cost associated with the adoption of mobile phones for diabetes managements can be thought of being an advantage to health care providers since interventions using such technologies will help improve services provided to patients. Also, "cost return will occur through decreasing charting time, fewer errors, and more time left for patient care" (Fischer, et al., 2003). Finally, comparing such devices costs with other technologies, such as Personal Computers (PCs) and tablets, show that costs of mobile devices are less than PCs and tablets.

Challenges associated with mobile device itself can be solved by health care provider thorough looking for and comparing different mobile devices available in the market. As we know, advances in Information and Communication Technologies (ICT) in these days has results in mobile devices equipped with large screens, touching capabilities, larger memory storage, expansion slot for memory, and several kind of ports to connect almost any kind of devices to these mobile phones. Therefore, careful selection of the most appropriate device may solve much of the challenges related to the mobile devices. Other problems such as losing the device or forgetting it may be overcome by the patients themselves once they get used to these devices for diabetes management. Finally, the problem associated with short battery life can be solved by making patients charging their devices on a daily bases and this is not going to be problematic, because patients are used to charge their mobile phones almost daily before using such devices for self-care.

REFERENCES

Årsand, E., Tufano, J. T., Ralston, J. D., & Hjortdahl, P. (2008). Designing mobile dietary management support technologies for people with diabetes. *Journal of Telemedicine and Telecare, 14*(7), 329–332. doi:10.1258/jtt.2008.007001

Arsand, E., Varmedal, R., & Hartvigsen, G. (2007). *Usability of a mobile self-help tool for people with diabetes: The easy health diary*. Retrieved from http://munin.uit.no/bitstream/handle/10037/2762/paper_1.pdf?sequence=3

Beckley, E. T. (2005). Wellness goes wireless. *DOC News, 2*(6), 7.

Burke, L. E., Warziski, M., Starrett, T., Choo, J., Music, E., & Sereika, S. (2005). Self-monitoring dietary intake: Current and future practices. *Journal of Renal Nutrition, 15*(3), 281–290. doi:10.1016/j.jrn.2005.04.002

Carroll, A. E., DiMeglio, L. A., Stein, S., & Marrero, D. G. (2011). Using a cell phone–based glucose monitoring system for adolescent diabetes management. *The Diabetes Educator, 37*(1), 59–66. doi:10.1177/0145721710387163

Carroll, A. E., Marrero, D. G., & Downs, S. M. (2007). The HealthPia GlucoPack™ diabetes phone: A usability study. *Diabetes Technology & Therapeutics, 9*(2), 158–164. doi:10.1089/dia.2006.0002

Evangelista, L. S., & Shinnick, M. A. (2008). What do we know about adherence and self-care? *The Journal of Cardiovascular Nursing, 23*, 250–257.

Faridi, Z., Liberti, L., Shuval, K., Northrup, V., Ali, A., & Katz, D. L. (2008). Evaluating the impact of mobile telephone technology on type 2 diabetic patients' self-management: The NICHE pilot study. *Journal of Evaluation in Clinical Practice, 14*(3), 465–469. doi:10.1111/j.1365-2753.2007.00881.x

Farmer, A., Gibson, O., Hayton, P., Bryden, K., Dudley, C., Neil, A., & Tarassenko, L. (2005). A real-time, mobile phone-based telemedicine system to support young adults with type 1 diabetes. *Informatics in Primary Care, 13*(3), 171–178.

Fischer, S., Stewart, T. E., Mehta, S., Wax, R., & Lapinsky, S. E. (2003). Handheld computing in medicine. *Journal of the American Medical Informatics Association, 10*(2), 139–149. doi:10.1197/jamia.M1180

Forjuoh, S. N., Reis, M. D., Couchman, G. R., & Ory, M. G. (2008). Improving diabetes self-care with a PDA in ambulatory care. *Telemedicine and e-Health, 14*(3), 273-279.

Forjuoh, S. N., Reis, M. D., Couchman, G. R., Ory, M. G., Mason, S., & Molonket-Lanning, S. (2007). Incorporating PDA use in diabetes self-care: A central Texas primary care research network (CenTexNet) study. *Journal of the American Board of Family Medicine, 20*(4), 375–384. doi:10.3122/jabfm.2007.04.060166

FreeDictionary. (2012). *Diabetes management.* Retrieved 05, 2012, from http://medical-dictionary.thefreedictionary.com/knowledge%3A+diabetes+management

Freund, A., Johnson, S. B., Silverstein, J., & Thomas, J. (1991). Assessing daily management of childhood diabetes using 24-hour recall interviews: Reliability and stability. *Health Psychology, 10*(3), 200. doi:10.1037/0278-6133.10.3.200

Fukuo, W., Yoshiuchi, K., Ohashi, K., Togashi, H., Sekine, R., & Kikuchi, H. (2009). Development of a hand-held personal digital assistant–based food diary with food photographs for japanese subjects. *Journal of the American Dietetic Association, 109*(7), 1232–1236. doi:10.1016/j.jada.2009.04.013

Hanauer, D. A., Wentzell, K., Laffel, N., & Laffel, L. M. (2009). Computerized automated reminder diabetes system (CARDS): E-mail and SMS cell phone text messaging reminders to support diabetes management. *Diabetes Technology & Therapeutics, 11*(2), 99–106. doi:10.1089/dia.2008.0022

Hinder, S., & Greenhalgh, T. (2012). This does my head in: Ethnographic study of self-management by people with diabetes. *BMC Health Services Research, 12*, 83. doi:10.1186/1472-6963-12-83

Istepanian, R. S. H., Zitouni, K., Harry, D., Moutosammy, N., Sungoor, A., Tang, B., & Earle, K. A. (2009). Evaluation of a mobile phone telemonitoring system for glycaemic control in patients with diabetes. *Journal of Telemedicine and Telecare, 15*(3), 125–128. doi:10.1258/jtt.2009.003006

Johnson, S. B., Silverstein, J., Rosenbloom, A., Carter, R., & Cunningham, W. (1986). Assessing daily management in childhood diabetes. *Health Psychology, 5*(6), 545. doi:10.1037/0278-6133.5.6.545

Jones, D., & Curry, W. (2006). Impact of a PDA-based diabetes electronic management system in a primary care office. *American Journal of Medical Quality, 21*(6), 401–407. doi:10.1177/1062860606293594

Koch, S. (2010). Healthy ageing supported by technology-A cross-disciplinary research challenge. *Informatics for Health & Social Care, 35*(3-4), 81–91. doi:10.3109/17538157.2010.528646

Kollmann, A., Riedl, M., Kastner, P., Schreier, G., & Ludvik, B. (2007). Feasibility of a mobile phone–based data service for functional insulin treatment of type 1 diabetes mellitus patients. *Journal of Medical Internet Research, 9*(5). doi:10.2196/jmir.9.5.e36

Krishna, S., & Boren, S. A. (2008). Diabetes self-management care via cell phone: A systematic review. *Journal of Diabetes Science and Technology, 2*(3), 509.

Logan, A. G., McIsaac, W. J., Tisler, A., Irvine, M. J., Saunders, A., & Dunai, A. (2007). Mobile phone-based remote patient monitoring system for management of hypertension in diabetic patients. *American Journal of Hypertension, 20*(9), 942–948. doi:10.1016/j.amjhyper.2007.03.020

Lu, Y. C., Xiao, Y., Sears, A., & Jacko, J. A. (2005). A review and a framework of handheld computer adoption in healthcare. *International Journal of Medical Informatics, 74*(5), 409–422. doi:10.1016/j.ijmedinf.2005.03.001

Ma, Y., Olendzki, B. C., Chiriboga, D., Rosal, M., Sinagra, E., & Crawford, S. (2006). PDA-assisted low glycemic index dietary intervention for type II diabetes: A pilot study. *European Journal of Clinical Nutrition, 60*(10), 1235–1243. doi:10.1038/sj.ejcn.1602443

Mougiakakou, S. G., Kouris, I., Iliopoulou, D., Vazeou, A., & Koutsouris, D. (2009). Mobile technology to empower people with diabetes mellitus: Design and development of a mobile application. In *Proceedings of Information Technology and Applications in Biomedicine*. IEEE Press. doi:10.1109/ITAB.2009.5394344

Mulvaney, S. A., Rothman, R. L., Dietrich, M. S., Wallston, K. A., Grove, E., Elasy, T. A., & Johnson, K. B. (2012). Using mobile phones to measure adolescent diabetes adherence. *Health Psychology, 31*(1), 43. doi:10.1037/a0025543

Phillips, G., Felix, L., Galli, L., Patel, V., & Edwards, P. (2010). The effectiveness of m-health technologies for improving health and health services: A systematic review protocol. *BMC Research Notes, 3*(1), 250. doi:10.1186/1756-0500-3-250

Quinn, C. C., Clough, S. S., Minor, J. M., Lender, D., Okafor, M. C., & Gruber-Baldini, A. (2008). WellDoc™ mobile diabetes management randomized controlled trial: Change in clinical and behavioral outcomes and patient and physician satisfaction. *Diabetes Technology & Therapeutics, 10*(3), 160–168. doi:10.1089/dia.2008.0283

Rigla, M., Hernando, M. E., Gómez, E. J., Brugués, E., García-Sáez, G., & Torralba, V. (2007). A telemedicine system that includes a personal assistant improves glycemic control in pump-treated patients with type 1 diabetes. *Journal of Diabetes Science and Technology, 1*(4), 505.

Satyanarayanan, M. (1996). *Fundamental challenges in mobile computing.* Retrieved from http://www.cs.cmu.edu/~coda/docdir/podc95.pdf

Skyler, J. S., Lasky, I. A., Skyler, D. L., Robertson, E. G., & Mintz, D. H. (1978). Home blood glucose monitoring as an aid in diabetes management. *Diabetes Care, 1*(3), 150–157. doi:10.2337/diacare.1.3.150

Smith, S. A., Murphy, M. E., Huschka, T. R., Dinneen, S. F., Gorman, C. A., & Zimmerman, B. R. (1998). Impact of a diabetes electronic management system on the care of patients seen in a subspecialty diabetes clinic. *Diabetes Care, 21*(6), 972–976. doi:10.2337/diacare.21.6.972

Tatara, N., Arsand, E., Nilsen, H., & Hartvigsen, G. (2009). A review of mobile terminal-based applications for self-management of patients with diabetes. In *Proceedings of eHealth, Telemedicine, and Social Medicine.* IEEE Press. doi:10.1109/eTELEMED.2009.14

Wikipedia. (2012). *Mobile phone.* Retrieved from http://www.wikipedia.org

Wu, S., Chaudhry, B., Wang, J., Maglione, M., Mojica, W., & Roth, E. (2006). Systematic review: Impact of health information technology on quality, efficiency, and costs of medical care. *Annals of Internal Medicine, 144*(10), 742–752.

Wyne, K. (2008). Information technology for the treatment of diabetes: Improving outcomes and controlling costs. *Journal of Managed Care Pharmacy, 14*(2), 12.

ADDITIONAL READING

Carroll, A. E., Marrero, D. G., & Downs, S. M. (2007). The HealthPia GlucoPack™ diabetes phone: A usability study. *Diabetes Technology & Therapeutics, 9*(2), 158–164. doi:10.1089/dia.2006.0002

Ferrer-Roca, O., Cardenas, A., Diaz-Cardama, A., & Pulido, P. (2004). Mobile phone text messaging in the management of diabetes. *Journal of Telemedicine and Telecare, 10*(5), 282–285. doi:10.1258/1357633042026341

Istepanian, S. R., Zitouni, K., Harry, D., Moutosammy, N., Sungoor, A., Tang, B., & Earle, K. A. (2009). Evaluation of a mobile phone telemonitoring system for glycaemic control in patients with diabetes. *Journal of Telemedicine and Telecare, 15*(3), 125–128. doi:10.1258/jtt.2009.003006

Voice, U. M. (2011). *Study finds mobile phone technology helps patients manage diabetes.* Retrieved from http://umvoice.com/2011/12/study-finds-mobile-phone-technology-helps-patients-manage-diabetes/

KEY TERMS AND DEFINITIONS

Diabetes Management: Diabetes management is the extent of understanding conveyed about diabetes mellitus, its treatment, and the prevention of complications (FreeDictionary, 2012).

Health: Care Providers: A health care provider is any person who helps in identifying or preventing or treating illness or disability.

Health Information Technologies (HIT): HIT provides the umbrella framework to describe the comprehensive management of health information across computerized systems and its secure exchange between consumers, providers, government and quality entities, and insurers. Health information technology (HIT) is in general increasingly viewed as the most promising tool for improving the overall quality, safety and efficiency of the health delivery system (Wu, et al., 2006).

Mobile Phones: A mobile phone (also known as a cellular phone, cell phone, and a hand phone) is a device that can make and receive telephone calls over a radio link whilst moving around a wide geographic area. It does so by connecting to a cellular network provided by a mobile phone operator, allowing access to the public telephone network (Wikipedia, 2012).

Self-Care: Self-care refers to specific behaviors that individuals initiate and perform on their own behalf, with the intention of improving health, preventing disease, or maintaining their well-being (Evangelista & Shinnick, 2008).

Chapter 16
Mobile Device Application in Healthcare

Sandeep Lakkaraju
Dakota State University, USA

Santhosh Lakkaraju
Dakota State University, USA

EXECUTIVE SUMMARY

Clinical practitioners need to have the right information, at the right time, at the right place, which is possible with mobile healthcare information technology. This chapter will help in understanding the need for mobile device usage across six different roles in healthcare: physicians, nurses, administrative staff, pharmaceutical staff, emergency staff, and patients. Research indicates that even in this advancing digital age, there are more than 98,000 deaths because of preventable medical errors. This can be abated with proper utilization of mobile devices in the healthcare sector. Utilization of technology in the process of sharing information may help in improving the decision making, and thereby reducing the medical errors and costs involved. This chapter illustrates the implementation and the application of mobile devices in healthcare from six different user perspectives, and summarizes the advantages, challenges, and solutions associated with mobile information technology implementation in healthcare.

DOI: 10.4018/978-1-4666-2671-3.ch016

BACKGROUND

According to June 2011 statistics, United States of America (USA) has a population of about 310 million people, and there are about 327.5 million wireless subscriber connections, i.e. about 1.02 wireless users per person across USA (U.S. Wireless Quick Facts, 2011). This is a huge network and accessing it can help the healthcare practitioners to offer faster healthcare services. Mobile technology can help in solving multiple health problems worldwide (Waegemann & Tessier, 2002). Rapid growth in mobile users (CTIA, 2008) every year stands as a proof that mobile technology has a lot to offer to the healthcare industry. Many nations across the world have identified the usefulness of these mobile devices, and have applied in various general and emergency cares (Ammenwerth, Gräber, Herrmann, Bürkle, & König, 2003; Haux, 2006). The large-scale adoption of mobile technology is taking technology adoption in healthcare on to a whole new level. Research indicates that mobile devices have direct impact on the process of offering care (Burley & Scheepers, 2002). These mobile devices possess various characteristics that can help users to efficiently document ever changing patient's health condition, allows easy browsing through the records, efficiently maintaining daily schedules, offering software's for almost anything, and clinical information capturing. Any new applications (related to the healthcare) installed into those mobile devices may result in fruitful results in the process of offering care by the healthcare organizations. Utilization of technology in the process of sharing information may help in improving the decision making time, and thereby reducing the medical errors and costs involved (Kinkade & Verclas, 2008). Proper training provided by the hospital staff to the patients before their discharge on how to use their mobile devices (shown in Table 1) to access their health related information and other usage, will help in significantly improving the delivery of quality care. Available mobile devices, technologies used by them, and their applications in healthcare are shown in Table 1.

SETTING THE STAGE

Several different groups of healthcare professional work together in a hospital organization for providing patient care. In this chapter, we focus on the workflows of administrative staff, nurses, physicians, pharmaceutical staff, patient/users, and emergency staff. Let us consider a sample patient workflow in a hospital scenario as shown in the Figure 1. A typical patient workflow may start with a request from a patient for an appointment with a physician. In other cases, it may start by the emergency staff that might find the patient in an emergency situation and is in need

Table 1. Mobile devices in healthcare (Lakkaraju & Moran, 2011)

Available Mobile Devices	Technologies used	Use in Healthcare
PDAs	Apps, Wi-Fi, WAP	(Baumgart, 2005; Fischer, Stewart, Mehta, Wax, & Lapinsky, 2003; Lapinsky, et al., 2001; Lapinsky, Mehta, Varkul, & Stewart, 2000)
Laptop/PCs/ Tablets	Wi-Fi, Bluetooth, 802.11n	(Ping, et al., 2009; Weitzel, Smith, Deugd, & Yates, 2010; Weitzel, Smith, Lee, Deugd, & Helal, 2009)
Mobile Phones	Apps, Wi-Fi, WAP, NFC, Display Technologies, SMS/ MMS, Bluetooth, GPS	(Ivanov, Gueorguiev, Bodurski, & Trifonov, 2010; Marcus, et al., 2009; Wang, Tsai, Liu, & Zao, 2009)
Pico Projectors	Display Technologies	(Inami, Kawakami, Sekiguchi, & Yanagida, 2000; Vijayaraghavan, Parpyani, Thakwani, & Iyengar, 2009)
Bodily Wearable Sensors	GPS, Wi-Fi, WAP	(Espinoza, Garcia-Vazquez, Rodriguez, Andrade, & Garcia-Pena, 2009; Trossen & Pavel, 2007)

of immediate care. The administrative staff (front desk staff) may check for the patient's status, whether he/she is a returning patient or a new one. If the patient is a new comer, his/her demographic information (like the patient's medical history details, social history, etc.) will be entered into the patient management system (any electronic system that may be accessed using a computer on wheels, laptop, etc.). Once the patient is registered, the patient will be given an appointment based on the physician's availability. The patient's record will be forwarded to the physician for pre-checkup analysis. At the appointment time, a clinical staff (nurse) will accompany the patient to visit the physician where the physician will evaluate the patient's current condition. Based on the diagnosis information, the patient may be given a prescription of drugs, or he/she may be suggested to admit into the hospital for further diagnosis, and the patient's record will be updated. Based on the physician's prescription, the patient may visit the pharmacy store to get the drugs. The pharmacy store may check the patient's identification and compare patient's prescription details with the details obtained from the physician, and will hand over the drugs. If the patient is required to be admitted into the hospital for further diagnosis, the patient will be allotted into a ward under supervision of a nurse, where the patient's record will be further updated on a timely basis.

Based on this basic workflow (shown in Figure 1), the participants of a regular hospital process can be divided into mainly six categories as shown in Figure 2. It includes: Physicians, Nurse, Administrative Staff, Emergency Staff, Pharmaceutical Staff, and Patient. Each of these participants of the current workflow (administrative staff, patient, physician, nurse, emergency staff, and pharmaceutical staff) may have to use a health record as common means of source for reference. If they are using

Figure 1. Basic workflow in a hospital organization

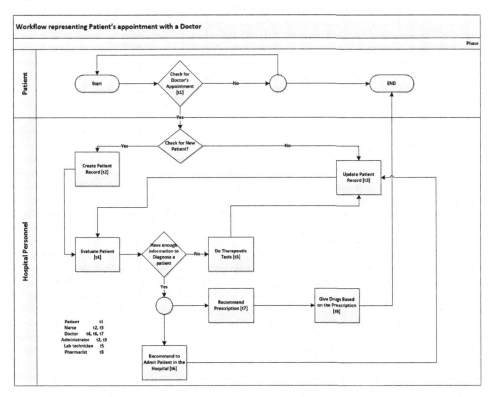

a paper-based record, it would be a cumbersome process to store, update the record, retrieve, and search for information in the health record, and also to carry it between each department. Each of these activities can be easily performed with an electronic health record, where the electronic health record will use electronic devices as medium. These devices can be any of the PDAs, laptops, computers on wheels, mobile phones, projectors, bodily wearable sensors, etc. The advantages of utilizing these mobile devices in a healthcare scenario, and the role of these devices in each of these actor's (administrative staff, patient, physician, nurse, emergency staff, and pharmaceutical staff) day to day activities is discussed in detail in a case to case basis. Analyzing the role of mobile technology in each of these below cases may help in understanding the role of mobile technologies in a healthcare scenario as a whole.

Figure 2. Role-based mobile device usage

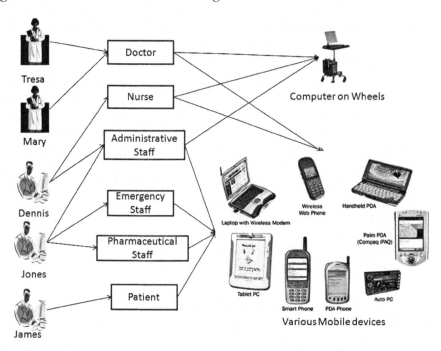

CASE DESCRIPTION

Each of the six cases where mobile devices can be used in a healthcare organization is discussed below in detail.

Case 1: Application of Mobile Devices in Admission and Patient Registration Workflows

The admission and patient registration process is typically the first component of a patients care workflow. The patient's source of entry may vary based on the situation he/she is in, i.e. a patient may be picked up by the emergency staff, or came for a general checkup or for a major operation. Whatever the reason may be, the process of admitting into the hospital is a must. The administrative staff (front desk staff) check for the patient's status, whether he/she is a returning patient or a new one. If the patient is a new comer, the administrative staff will have to document his/her demographic information (like the patient's medical history details, social history, etc.) into a medical record, which will be regularly needed by any authorized hospital personnel dealing with the concerned patient. The medical records are traditionally saved in paper-based formats and when such a record is 'regularly needed' by many authorized hospital personnel, having such important information on a paper is not a feasible, permanent, secure, and safe solution. Thus, many organizations are moving on to 'electronic health records.' Implantation of RFID chips and tags into patient's body can be considered as an example for integrating mobile technology into healthcare (Edwards, 2009; Halamka, 2007; Versel, 2011). These RFID chips contains a 16 digit encrypted code which will be linked to an electronic health record residing on a secured website that records a particular patient's information (Halamka, 2007). RFID chips records each of the patient's movements in an emergency department, notifying real time updates about patient's to the concerned physicians and nurses on their mobile devices. These implanted RFID chips can also be used for patient identification purposes (Campbell, 2011). Campbell (2011) indicates that XECAN RFID technology will help the administrative staff in identifying the patient, 'placing the patient in the EMR daily schedule queue,' opening the patient's treatment plan, and also provides the patient navigation system. XECAN indicates that their XECAN RFID technology will improve the patient's safety by reducing the 'wrong patient and treatment errors' (Campbell, 2011). Halamka (2007) indicates that these RFID chips may be very helpful for those whose injury makes them 'non-communicative.' The patient's insurance details can be validated and dealt with either through tablet PCs or through smart phones with usage of mobile applications such as 'CSC mobile insurance solutions' (CSC, 2010). Mobile device usage by the administrative staff saves ample of time in conducting administrative functions. The time spent on chart handling, searching missing charts, new patient chart generation, lab result handling can be minimized, thereby reducing the overall organizational paper usage resulting in fewer personnel to deal with the documents. Table 2 indicates the mobile functions that can be executed using the mobile devices by the administrative staff as a part of their daily activities.

Case 2: Application of Mobile Devices in Nursing Workflows

Among all the personnel at the hospitals, nurses are considered as primary staff that will have frequent encounters with the patients. In order to act based on the situation, they need to have right information about the right person at the right time and this process to have right information may often be a hard task with the paper-based records. It would not only be hard to search for appropriate paper forms in their repository, but is also a cumbersome process to search for the required information in the papers. Mobile devices with proper software can help nurses to overcome such cumbersome processes by allowing them to access accurate data much more easily and effectively, thereby eliminating costly errors and saving time which in turn may allow them to spend more time on patients rather than searching for information in the papers. Mobile devices will not only help nurses in dealing

Table 2. Mobile functions by administrative staff

Administrative Staff Activities	Description	Mobile functions	Mobile Devices/ Applications
Inspect the patient's status	whether he/she is a returning patient or a new patient	Search engine usage, Rule based personalization, Browse FAQs, etc.	Wi-Fi enabled PDA's or Portable Mobile devices equipped with compatible mobile applications like RFID readers (Campbell, 2011)
Validate patient's insurance	patient's insurance details will be validated	Expert systems, discussions with insurance agents, browsing clinical repositories, etc.	Wi-Fi enabled PDA's or Portable Mobile devices equipped with compatible mobile applications like CSC mobile insurance solutions (CSC, 2010)
Schedule an appointment	Intimate patient and physician about appointment	Electronic publishing, scheduling	Wi-Fi enabled PDA's or Portable Mobile devices equipped with compatible mobile applications like RFID readers can place the patients on treatment list (Halamka, 2007)
Calculate insurance deductibles	calculate the deductibles and update patient's record with their deductable information	knowledge-based system, calculation software's, etc.	Wi-Fi enabled PDA's or Portable Mobile devices equipped with compatible mobile applications like CSC mobile insurance solutions (CSC, 2010)

with paper-based records, but also help them to communicate effectively. These mobile devices with features like calling, e-mail, and chatting can allow nurses to communicate with their fellow nurses and practitioners. Nurses may utilize mobile devices to maintain to do lists, calendars, address book, memo pads, etc. They also use these devices to refer for clinical guidance, to verify for medication information, to go through the lab reports of the patients, and to update the progress notes of the patients. Through mobile devices, nurses can browse through the Internet for electronic accessing of medical diagnosis information, or for any clinical guidance (Newbolt, 2003; Rosenthal, 2003; Stroud, Erkel, & Smith, 2005). Table 3 indicates the mobile functions that can be executed using the mobile devices by the nursing staff as a part of their daily activities.

Research indicates that of all the available mobile devices (tablet PCs, Computers on Wheels (COW), ergonomic COWs, Laptops, PDAs, palmtops, and mobile phones), PDAs are the mostly used mobile devices by the nurses (Ondash, 2004). Computer on wheels and ergonomic COWs can be placed in the nurse stations where these nurses will update the patient records and any information about the patient.

Table 3. Mobile functions by nursing staff

Nursing Activities	Description	Mobile functions	Mobile Devices/Applications
Inspect the patient's health condition	Check for patient's health condition	Visualization, Search engine usage, Rule based personalization, Browse FAQs, etc.	Wi-Fi enabled PDA's or Portable Mobile devices equipped with compatible mobile applications like Nursing central, Johns Hopkins Guides, Nurses' Handbook of Health Assessment etc. (Barlett, Auwaerter, & Pham, 2012; Weber, 2009)
Diagnose the patient	Actions that require support from the nurse	Expert systems, browsing clinical data repositories, discussions with physicians and fellow nurses, case based reasoning, etc.	Wi-Fi enabled PDA's or Portable Mobile devices equipped with compatible mobile applications like Diseases and Disorders, Davis's Laboratory and Diagnostic Tests etc. (Leeuwen, Poelhuis-Leth, & Bladh, 2011; Sommers, 2010)
Treatment	Perform treatment based on patient's health condition	Electronic publishing, browse through nurse's knowledge repositories, etc.	Wi-Fi enabled PDA's or Portable Mobile devices equipped with compatible mobile applications like Davis's Laboratory and Diagnostic Tests etc. (Leeuwen, et al., 2011)
Evaluating the patient	Based on the treatment, examining the improvements in patient's health condition	Evidence based systems, Decision support systems, etc.	Wi-Fi enabled PDA's or Portable Mobile devices equipped with compatible mobile applications like Nursing central, Evidence Central, Nurses' Handbook of Health Assessment, Nurses Pocket Guide, RNotes etc. (Doenges, Moorhouse, & Murr, 2010; Myers & Newman, 2007; Weber, 2009)

Also they may retrieve any information about patients from these COWs. But this process of utilizing COWs that are placed in the nursing stations will need nurses to travel. Research indicates that lesser the time nurses spent on traveling will increase the amount of time they spend on patients (Ulrich, Zimring, Quan, Joseph, & Choudhary, 2004). This can be achieved through other portable mobile devices such as PDAs, laptops, tablet PCs, palm tops, and mobile phones. Most of the available literature on application of mobile devices in healthcare indicates that of all the mobile devices available, role of PDAs has been predominant (Dee, Teolis, & Todd, 2005; Gururajan & Murugesan, 2005; Stroud, Smith, & Erkel, 2009). Nurses may use these portable mobile devices (discussed earlier) as bed side mobile devices to update patient information while taking care of the patients, to check for physician's suggestions about a particular patient and to validate and verify the drugs to be used on a patient, etc. With proper built-in functions, a mobile device can allow physicians to provide online transcriptions, which can be viewed and used by nurses on their mobile devices in the process of attending patients, in turn improving care towards the patients, and thereby improving the patient satisfaction. This is only possible by mobile devices as with paper transcriptions, nurses may have to spend more time searching for transcriptions and for appropriate information on the transcriptions. Time for location of charts can be minimized by using electronic medical records on mobile devices, which allow more time to be spent with the needy. They may also use their mobile devices to access the blood test results, administer the electronic prescriptions, drug dose calculations, and for any other clinical support from online or from other clinicians from other groups. Mobile devices also have the capability to alert the nurses of any abnormal conditions in the reports. Below are the steps to implement mobile devices across nursing staff.

1. Examine the existing work practices of the nursing staff.
2. Identify the existing infrastructure (wireless or wired or paper-based) used by the nursing staff in the process of documenting patient information while offering bedside care and offering therapy counseling to the patients.
3. Evaluate the need to repair or replace the existing infrastructure.
4. Conduct cross-functional meetings with the Information Technology (IT) personnel (who develops the needed infrastructure), higher management (who will finance the project), and the nursing staff (who will be using the infrastructure) to make them understand the need for this wireless infrastructure.
5. Once there is support (financially and morally) from the higher management, conduct meetings with the nursing staff and the IT personnel to identify the needs and design a mobile wireless infrastructure based on the needs of the nurses.
6. After the design is ready, implement the project in a big bang, phased, or parallel approach.
7. Following the implementation, conduct the training sessions for the nursing staff across the organization to make them accustomed to the new infrastructure. Along with these training sessions, Hospital Management should also consider the process of offering the much-needed IT support to the nursing staff even after the training.

Case 3: Application of Mobile Devices in Physician Workflows

Clinical practitioners need to have the right information, at the right time, at the right place; which is possible by mobile healthcare. According to a report by Institute of Medicine (IOM) in 2000, 'about 44,000 to 98,000 people are dying in United States of America just because of medical errors,' which shocked the healthcare organizations (Kohn, Corrigan, & Donaldson, 2000). With the use of proper alert mechanisms in the healthcare organizations, these medical errors can be prevented. With the ever growing volume of information, practitioners need to have access to 'right information at the right place at the right time' (Lakkaraju & Moran, 2011), which is possible by mobile devices. Physicians may use mobile devices such as tablet PCs, computers, Computers on wheels, Pico projectors, PDAs, and smart phones. Based on the research statistics provided by the 'Manhattan Research,' the percentage of physicians in USA using a smart phone may rise from 64% to 81% by the year 2012 (iHealthBeat, 2009). Physicians may use their mobile devices for comparative effectiveness research about drugs and treatments, to access patient health information through EHRs and PHRs, to provide electronic transcriptions to nurses, to write electronic prescriptions, to review drug alerts and perform drug dose calculations, evaluate the blood test results, for online reference to the clinical information, to maintain contact with their fellow practitioners, etc. With these mobile devices in place, practitioners will no longer have to run to the clinical libraries to check peer reviewed articles on critical ailments, but may use their mobile devices (like laptops, tablets, etc.) to browse through the online medical databases such as Medline, Pub Med, etc. The mobile functions that can be executed using the mobile devices by the practitioners as a part of their daily activities can be found in Table 4. The computers, and computers on wheels, may act as more like a static mobile devices that are connected to the Internet, which can be used for Web-based content referencing about clinical information, to participate in Web conferences (audio and video), to refer for patient information, etc. Whereas the tablet PCs, PDAs, Pico projectors, and smart phones allows the practitioners to conduct all the above mentioned activities (of computers) along with many other while on the move. Even the images such as endoscopic images and X-Rays can be reviewed in their mobile devices while on the go or even at their homes. Pico projectors are handheld devices, which run on batteries that can help the practitioners to project the images, videos, and electronic documents over any surfaces. There may be issues in the process of utilizing these Pico projectors with regards to the lighting around the surface, and sometimes volume and battery issues. These are embedded and are made available in wide variety of devices like smart phones, mp3 players, etc. Among the tablet PCs, 'Apple iPads' have their own mark. After its release, about 30% of the practitioners have bought and have made 'Apple iPads' one of their working devices. Compared to PDAs, tablet PCs like 'Apple iPads, Android tablets, etc' are attracting more and more physicians because of their size, easiness in access to the data, visibility, and more importantly for their availability of 'applications' popularly known as 'Apps.' MobiHealthNews 2010 (Dolan, 2010) report indicates that there are about 9,000 apps for smart phones and tablet PC users. By mid 2012, it is expected that there will be 'more than 13,000 apps' just for the users using 'Apple devices.' Various types of Apps available for practitioners include: clinical reference apps, diagnostic apps, public health apps, Tele-health apps, disease management apps, etc. Practitioners using the disease management apps indicate that these disease management apps have the capability to improve patient-physician communications. Healthcare practitioners may also use these mobile devices for note taking purposes while attending the patients. They may record, type, or shoot (capture through cameras) the patient behavior in particular cases. Physicians may also utilize the dictation applications available in various mobile devices and thereby save them in the database for future usage. The mobile functions that can be executed using the mobile devices by the physicians as a part of their daily activities can be found in Table 4.

Mobile devices also allow the practitioners to 'follow' their fellow practitioners through social networking sites. According to a research by Frost & Sullivan research and consulting firm, although 90% of the physicians have notably browsed a social networking site, only less than 10% of them have used these social networking sites

Table 4. Mobile functions by physicians

Physician Activities	Description	Mobile functions	Mobile Devices/Applications
Inspect the patient's health condition	Check for patient's health condition	Visualization, Search engine usage, Browse through patient records, etc.	Wi-Fi enabled PDA's or Portable Mobile devices equipped with compatible mobile applications like Epocrate, etc. (Epocrates, 2012)
Diagnose the patient	Actions that require support from the physician	browsing clinical data repositories, discussions with fellow physicians and nurses, case based reasoning, etc.	Wi-Fi enabled PDA's or Portable Mobile devices equipped with compatible mobile applications like Skyscape Medical Resources, etc. (Skyscape, 2012; Hirsch & Gandolf, 2011)
Treatment	Perform treatment based on patient's health condition	Check online clinical databases, physician's knowledge repositories, etc.	Wi-Fi enabled PDA's or Portable Mobile devices equipped with compatible mobile applications like Medscape, Medical Resources, etc. (Skyscape, 2012; WebMD, 2012)
Evaluating the patient	Based on the treatment, examining the improvements in patient's health condition	Evidence based systems, Decision support systems, etc.	Wi-Fi enabled PDA's or Portable Mobile devices equipped with compatible mobile applications like Epocrates Essentials Delux, Skyscape, etc. (Epocrates, 2012; Skyscape, 2012)
e-Prescribing	Ordering electronic prescriptions to the patients	Browsing through knowledge repositories for appropriate drugs, use prescription software's, etc	Wi-Fi enabled PDA's or Portable Mobile devices equipped with compatible mobile applications like Lexicomp, Micromedex Drug Information, Epocrates Essentials, etc. (Epocrates, 2012; Lexicomp, 2012; Reuters, 2012)
Clinical documenting	Document patient's health condition through dictations, etc	Use dictation software's through mobile devices, etc	Wi-Fi enabled PDA's or Portable Mobile devices equipped with compatible mobile applications like Medical Encyclopedia, Evidence Central, etc. (Unbound Evidence, 2011; University of Meryland, 2009)

for professional use. Another survey by QuantialMD reports that of all the available social networking sites, practitioners have been professionally active mainly in many physician communities. Nancy Fabozzi, an expert at 'Frost and Sullivan consulting firm' indicates that this increase in usage of social networking sites is a result of increase in smart phone usage among the practitioners (Hirsch & Gandolf, 2011).

Below steps will help to understand the process of implementing mobile devices across practitioners:

1. Examine the existing work practices of the physicians.
2. Identify the existing infrastructure (wireless or wired) used by the physicians in the process of offering care.
3. Evaluate the need for improvement in the existing infrastructure.
   a. If there is any wireless infrastructure, is there any need to repair or replace the existing infrastructure?
   b. If there is no wireless infrastructure, identify the needs of practitioners and thereby follow the below steps to develop a wireless infrastructure which can accommodate mobile devices.
4. Conduct cross-functional meetings with the Information Technology (IT) personnel (who develops the needed infrastructure), higher management (who will finance the project), and the practitioners (who will be using the infrastructure) to make them understand the need for this wireless infrastructure.
5. Once there is support (financially and morally) from the higher management, conduct meetings with the practitioners and the IT personnel to identify the needs and design a mobile wireless infrastructure based on the needs of the practitioners.
6. After the design is ready, implement the project in any of the below approaches:
   a. In a big bang approach: this involves strict time frames (i.e. the project should be completed in a fixed amount of time), the changed system or proposed system will be implemented all over the organization at the same time,
   b. In a phased approach: this involves implementing the proposed system change across various sectors of an organization at varied times. Here the organizations may prioritize the sectors that can be changed,
   c. In a parallel approach: this involves implementing a change across an existing system. This process will involve parallel execution of both the existing system and the new system for some days and once the members of that organization get used to the new system, the old system may be terminated.

7. Following the implementation, conduct the training sessions for the practitioners across the organization to make them accustomed to the new infrastructure. These training sessions will not only help them in understanding how to utilize the mobile devices but will also help to reduce the resistance of the practitioners towards the new system.

8. Along with these training sessions, Hospital Management should also consider the process of offering the much needed IT support to the practitioners. This IT support should be made available to the practitioners even after the training sessions.

Case 4: Application of Mobile Devices in Pharmacy Workflows

According to Jill Haug, PharmD, pharmacists are "medication theory experts" (Feature, 2008, p. 11). The role of pharmacy is crucial in the process of dispensing drugs, answering medication related questions to the patients and providing counseling to the patients about the drugs about their usage etc. In the process of addressing the growing cost issues and rapid increase in the volume of data issues, pharmacy has moved towards information technology applications adoption. With the paper-based prescriptions the pharmacists may have had hard time in understanding the physician's writing (Stross, 2012), leading to electronic prescriptions. Mobile devices such as Computers on Wheels, PDAs, smart phones, laptops, and tablet PCs are being used by the pharmacy staff for tasks ranging from clinical documentation to e-prescribing, out of which tablet PCs are suggested to be the most suitable and adoptable devices for pharmacy staff (Fahrni, 2009; Krogh, Rough, & Thomley, 2008; McCreadie & McGregory, 2005). With the usage of these mobile devices, pharmacists can employ decision support systems and evidence support systems using which they may examine the drug-drug interactions, drug-allergy interactions for any evidence of alerts in turn acting as a re-verification process of the provider's recommendation for drugs (Saverno, et al., 2011). These automated examinations by the software will reduce the medication therapy errors, thereby improving the patient care. Research indicates that PDAs have been widely used across man pharmacists (Bosinski, Campbell, & Schwartz, 2004; Clark & Klauck, 2003; Ford, Illich, Smith, & Franklin, 2006; Fox, Felkey, Berger, Krueger, & Rainer, 2007). A mobile device with certain applications (apps) and application packages can assist the pharmacist in performing his various activities such as: (1) order verification: this process may further involve re-validating the drugs proposed by the practitioner as soon as they are entered into the system, and thereby sorting the orders based on their priority; (2) results viewing: patient data can be used through the system for any further consultation suggestions; (3) decision support for drug suggestions: this may involve suggesting the drug dosage to a patient based on his/her personal details such as height, age, etc., examine drug-drug and drug-allergy interactions with respect to the patient; and (4) order dispensing: based on the automated suggestions from the mobile device, the pharmacist can maintain the medication level thereby preventing any wastage and maintaining only needed medication. Adopting mobile technology into pharmacy, there are many mobile applications available across various mobile operating systems (iOS, Android OS, and Blackberry OS) for various pharmacy stores: Walgreens (WalgreensCo, 2012), CVS pharmacy (Perez, 2012), Micro Medex (Reuters, 2012), etc. Various pharmaceutical apps across multiple mobile operating systems such as Lexi-Comp (Lexicomp, 2012), Epocrates (Epocrates, 2012), OTC guide (http://www.otcguide.net), etc. can be used on their mobile devices by the pharmacists using which they can access Internet for referencing guidelines on medication use and medication therapy suggestions. As there are no proper guidelines and restrictions on the app markets, there are multiple apps available in the app stores leaving a challenging task to choose one. Overall, pharmacists can use their mobile devices as drug encyclopedia for accurate, fast, and easy access of patient records, prescriptions, and to browse other pharmaceutical information on Web by installing various applications on their mobile devices (Editor, 2011; PepeNavas Melara, 2012). The mobile functions that can be executed using the mobile devices by the pharmaceutical staff as a part of their daily activities can be found in Table 5.

Below steps will help in understanding the process of implementing mobile devices across pharmaceutical staff.

1. Examine the existing work practices of the pharmaceutical staff.
2. Identify the existing infrastructure (wireless or wired or paper-based) used by the pharmaceutical staff in the process of dealing with the prescriptions.
3. Evaluate the need for improvement in the existing infrastructure and identify the need to repair or replace the existing infrastructure.
4. Conduct cross-functional meetings with the Information Technology (IT) personnel (who develops the needed infrastructure), higher management (who will finance the project), and the pharmaceutical staff (who will be using the infrastructure) to make them understand the need for this wireless infrastructure.
5. Once there is support (financially and morally) from the higher management, conduct meetings with the pharmacy staff and the IT personnel to identify the needs and design a mobile wireless infrastructure based on the needs of the pharmaceutical staff.
6. After the design is ready, implement the project in any of the below approaches:
   a. In a big bang approach: this involves strict time frames (i.e. the project should be completed in a fixed amount of time), the changed system or proposed system will be implemented all over the organization at the same time,

Table 5. Mobile functions by pharmaceutical staff

Pharmaceutical Activities	Description	Mobile functions	Mobile Devices/Applications
Evaluate the Prescription	Check for drugs	Visualization, Search engine usage, Rule based personalization, Browse drugs, etc.	Wi-Fi enabled PDA's, tablet PCs, or smart phones equipped with compatible mobile applications as discussed by Saverno et al. (2011), Epocrates, Lexicomp, etc. (Epocrates, 2012; Lexicomp, 2012)
Identify the patient	Actions that involve evaluating patient's identification	data mining, search engine usage, rule based personalization etc.	Wi-Fi enabled PDA's, tablet PCs, or smart phones equipped with compatible mobile applications like RFID readers (Campbell, 2011)
Dispense drugs	Dispense the drugs based on the prescription	Enter the dispensed drug information into the mobile system	Wi-Fi enabled PDA's, tablet PCs, or smart phones equipped with compatible mobile applications like Lexicomp, Micromedex Drug Information, Epocrates Essentials etc. (Epocrates, 2012; Lexicomp, 2012; Reuters, 2012)
Counseling the patient	counsel the patients about the drug usage, and drug related allergies	Provide mobile counseling through electronic mail, electronic social sites, calls, etc.	Wi-Fi enabled PDA's, tablet PCs, or smart phones equipped with compatible websites like PharmQD (www.pharmQD.com), etc., mobile devices equipped with apps like Epocrates (Epocrates, 2012), Lexicomp (Lexicomp, 2012), etc.

b. In a phased approach: this involves implementing the proposed system change across various sectors of an organization at varied times. Here the organizations may prioritize the sectors that can be changed,

c. In a parallel approach: this involves implementing a change across an existing system. This process will involve parallel execution of both the existing system and the new system for some days and once the members of that organization get used to the new system, the old system may be terminated.

7. Following the implementation, conduct the training sessions for the pharmaceutical staff across the organization to make them accustomed to the new infrastructure. Along with these training sessions, Hospital Management should also consider the process of offering the much-needed IT support to the pharmacy staff. This IT support should be made available to the practitioners even after the training sessions.

Case 5: Application of Mobile Devices for Patient Empowerments

Healthcare is all about delivering excellent care to the patients. The role of patients in healthcare is as important as any other healthcare staff (admission staff, nursing staff, physicians, emergency staff, and pharmacy staff), and they have to play an equal role in getting safer care by actively participating in the healthcare reform (OrthoInfo, 2002). Patients may use their mobile devices to retrieve, browse and update their current health conditions in the PHRs (Landro, 2010). They are flexible enough to make a physician appointment using electronic mail, messaging, and calls. The flexibility for the patient to update his/her current health conditions such as bodily temperatures, blood sugar levels and other vital conditions through their smart phones, tablet PCs and other mobile devices can help the physician to understand the patient's situation way before he/she reaches a hospital, and further can help the patient to keep track of his/her health conditions and sometimes it can even reduce the consultation time (Landro, 2010). The mobile devices are flexible enough to obtain the updated handy e-prescription, preorder the specified drugs from drug stores and pick them up with no wait time (Smith, 2009). The mobile functions that can be executed using the mobile devices by the patients as a part of their daily activities can be found in Table 6.

Recent advances in research on patient's perception on the use of mobile technology revealed the following facts: Patients may use mobile technology to a) access, retrieve and update their vital health conditions on the PHR/EHR, b) to obtain health related suggestions from the physician about their diabetic or ulcerative colitis conditions, c) enhanced portable mobile equipment can provide additional comfort to the patients and helps the physicians to provide efficient and effective patient care. The patients can make appointments, and can keep updated about their health conditions, refill, and referral requests. They may act as interactive communication channel between patients, and any of the physicians, nurses, pharmacy staff, and administrative staff. Patients may also use their Wi-Fi enabled PDA's, tablet PCs, or smart phones to participate in any online forums to discuss about their health conditions and read about any of those who might have experienced the same condition before through Web forums like AARDA (2009), Patients Like Me (Haywood, et al., 2004), etc. Another form of mobile devices used by patients include the use of bodily wearable sensors, which may help the hospital staff to keep track of the patient's health conditions and helps the physicians to provide enhanced care (Mcfadden & Indulska, 2004). Bodily wearable sensors may be considered as a 'wearable computer system' capable of capturing crucial indications based on the patient's health condition and thereby reporting to the concerned hospital staff (example: emergency staff) (Crilly & Muthukkumarasamy, 2010; Ooi, et al., 2005; Stanford,

Table 6. Mobile functions by patients

Patient Activities	Description	Mobile functions	Mobile Devices/ Applications
Browse EHRs, and other appointments	Check for his/her health records, meetings, appointments with physicians, etc.	Visualization, Search engine usage, Browse e-mails, calendars, etc.	Wi-Fi enabled PDA's, tablet PCs, or smart phones equipped with compatible applications like Capzule (Webahn, 2012), WebMD (WebMD, 2012), etc.
Contact the practitioners, pharmaceutical staff, administrative staff, etc.	Contact any of the hospital staff for more information on their drugs, or appointments, etc.	Make calls, discussions with fellow patients, physicians, nurses, pharmacy staff, etc.	Wi-Fi enabled PDA's, tablet PCs, or smart phones equipped with compatible applications like Patient (Mayo Clinic, 2012), Kaiser Permanente (Kaiser Permanente, 2012), etc
Use bodily wearable sensors	These may help the hospital people to keep track of patient's health condition even when they are at home	Keep practitioners updated with the patient information even when the patient is at his/her home, etc.	(Konstantas, 2007; Laerhoven, et al., 2004; Ooi, Culjak, & Lawrence, 2005)
Participate in online health forums	Use online forums to discuss with fellow patients about any treatments	Browsing, search-engine usage, participate in online health forums, etc.	Wi-Fi enabled PDA's, tablet PCs, or smart phones equipped with compatible Web forums like AARDA (AARDA, 2009), Patients-LikeMe (Haywood, Haywood, & Jeff, 2004), etc.

2002). Patients may use variety of bodily wearable sensors which will be in continuous 'physical contact,' and these may be designed as apparels, coats, glasses, belts, etc. (Ooi, et al., 2005). Monitoring health at home is being considered as one of the solutions to address care for ever growing population and their health needs and limited availability of human and financial resources is forcing towards the need for home monitoring of health (Korhonen, Pärkkä, & Van Gils, 2003; Stanford, 2002; Winters, Wang, & Winters, 2003).

Some steps to consider in the implementation of mobile devices for patients use include:

1. Identify the mobile device required to be used by the patient (whether it is bodily wearable sensor, mobile device, laptop, etc.).
2. Make the patient understand about the need for the device and the functionalities of the device.
3. Based on the mobile device used by the patient, install the required software in that mobile device. For example, install any hospital software which may be

used by the patient to input any of the patient health (temperature, BP monitoring, etc.) information based on which the healthcare organizations may send text messages, or electronic mails, or place calls to the patient about the steps the patient may need to take.

4. Once the device is installed, train the patient on how to use the system. For example, train the patient on how to use bodily wearable sensors, healthcare software's installed in their mobile devices.

5. In addition, the hospital personnel may have to educate the patients about the existing mobile applications and recommend some of the best medical and health related applications using which the patients may remain healthy. For example: 'Lose IT' – iphone app, 'Cardio Trainer + Racing' – Android app, 'Cure with diet' – Blackberry app, etc.

6. Patients may be trained on how to use their mobile devices to check for and set reminders for appointments, use electronic prescriptions, understand physician/nurse/pharmacist recommendations through e-mails, calls, etc.

Case 6: Application of Mobile Devices in ER Workflows

Emergency staff requires most factual, and precise information about the patient (who is in the emergency situation), failing to which may lead to drastic situations (Holzman, 1999). It is one of the crucial areas where there is high need for mobile device application, and research indicates that emergency department's physicians are the most frequent users of the mobile devices in healthcare (Hussain, 2011). Traditional method of using paper-based system in such emergency situations can be critical, and most of the information may be either not be entered at all, or remain inaccurate. Some of the crucial information required by the emergency staff involved in an emergency situation may include (but not limited to) a) being able to perform patient diagnostics (ex: based on coding like triage, etc.), b) being able to document the situational information and patient behavior, c) being able to retrieve proper first aid information and other necessary clinical information that is appropriate for that particular emergency situation, and d) being able to identify any healthcare facilities or hospitals that are available nearby. It would be often not possible to perform all of these actions without proper information technology enabled devices. Information should be mobile and readily available for the emergency staff, and this can be achieved through utilizing mobile devices. Some of the mobile devices used by the emergency staff may broadly involve belted tablet PCs, belted computers, belted laptops, PDAs, bodily wearable sensors, and smart phones. Along with these regular mobile devices, they also may utilize the mobile devices that have integrated video taking capability for situation surveillance. Some of the prominent research indicates utilization of 'belted' tablet PCs, laptops, and computers installed on the emergency vehicles (Anantharaman & Swee Han, 2001; Holzman, 1999). The mobile functions that can be executed using the mobile devices by the emergency staff as a part of their daily activities can be found in Table 7.

Emergency department staff may implant RFID chips into the patient which may not only allow the physicians to know about the patient's whereabouts but also allows the hospital staff to identify the patient and extract his/her health records; this RFID technology also assists the physicians by recording patient behavior in an emergency situation and allowing them (physicians) to revisit the patient's behavior at a later time (Halamka, 2007; Versel, 2011). As any small information in an emergency situation can remain critical and may be required afterwards, documenting situational information either through documents, audio, or video can be very helpful in the later treatments. Pattath et al. (2006)discussed about how visualization on handheld devices can be effective in offering later treatments. The emergency staff may also use bodily wearable sensors for situational awareness in the process of offering care by the first responder. The emergency staff may use these mobile phones to notify the hospital staff of arrival time of an emergency vehicle to the hospital, so that the hospital staff may be ready; also, the hospital staff may use the Global Positioning System (GPS) feature present in the bodily wearable sensors and determine the first responder's position. The emergency staff may use these mobile devices, and belted computer systems to request for suggestions in the process of providing first aid to the patients in an emergency situation (Anantharaman & Swee Han, 2001).

OVERALL ADVANTAGES WITH THESE NEW TECHNOLOGIES

Some of the advantages of Mobile device usage in Health Care Industry may include:

- **Ease of Access:** Accessing appropriate data timely and enable the providers and staff to have an increased decision making capabilities. A provider looking at a patient's diagnosis and medication history in the exam room can have a better scope for better prognosis (HIMSS, 2011; Mcalearney, Sc, Medow, & Ph, 2004).
- **Flexibility/Portability:** Mobile devices can be easily carried and can be used for data access from any distant location. Mobile devices are a flexible alternative for porting the information to a new device or sharing it with multiple devices. Mobile devices demand lesser resources and maintenance comparatively (HIMSS, 2011; Mcalearney, et al., 2004; Prestigiacomo, 2011).

Table 7. Mobile functions by emergency staff

Emergency Staff Activities	Description	Mobile functions	Mobile Devices/Applications
Inspect the patient's condition	Check for patient's health condition in that emergency situation	Visualization, Search engine usage, Rule based personalization, Browse FAQs, etc.	Utilizing RFID technology for recording patient behavior in an emergency situation (Halamka, 2007; Versel, 2011)
Diagnose the patient	Actions that require support from the emergency staff	Expert systems, data mining, discussions with physicians, nurses, and fellow staff, case based reasoning, etc.	Wi-Fi enabled PDA's, smart phones, and tablet PCs equipped with compatible mobile applications like Diseases and Disorders, Davis's Laboratory and Diagnostic Tests etc. (Leeuwen, et al., 2011; Sommers, 2010)
Treatment	Perform treatment based on patient's health condition	browse through emergency knowledge repositories, etc.	Refer through emergency knowledge repositories utilizing 'belted' tablet PCs, laptops, and computers installed on the emergency vehicles (Anantharaman & Swee Han, 2001; Holzman, 1999)
Evaluating the patient	Based on the treatment, documenting the patient's health condition	Evidence based systems, Decision support systems, etc.	Wi-Fi enabled PDA's, tablet PCs, or smart phones equipped with compatible mobile applications like RFID readers (Halamka, 2007)

- **Information Privacy:** Patients will feel more comfortable sharing private information at a Kiosk or an information station rather than sharing it with the staff (McAlearney, Schweikhart, & Medow, 2004).
- **Improved Emergency Assistance:** Interfacing various sensors and devices directly to a mobile device can improve emergency assistance. For example, A patients heart pace monitor connected to a mobile device can send an emergency signals to get help immediately.
- **Smoother and quieter work place:** These new technologies will help to run the offices smoother and quieter, which the sick patients may greatly appreciate.
- **Easily understandable prescriptions:** Prescription writings and transcription writings can be readable, avoiding multiple revisits to practitioners for clarification.
- **Organizational Policies:** Although there is wide usage of mobile devices in healthcare, 2011 HIMSS Mobile Technology Survey (HIMSS, 2011) there are only 38% of organizations that have policies administering the mobile device usage in healthcare, where as the remaining 72% have no strategies at all.

- **Information Flow:** Information flow can be organized into a set of loosely coupled continuous steps with usage of multiple mobile devices as a single system. For example, a day to day patient visit and steps involving in the Information flow:
  - A front desk assistant provides the patient with a tablet or Kiosk to gather patient demographics and Insurance information.
  - An exam room nurse will update the patient's vitals, previous diagnosis and medication history directly from the equipment attached.
  - A physician looking at the information from the previous steps can examine the patient and create an electronic prescription based current diagnosis.
  - The prescription details were sent to the pharmacy, patient's mobile device, and the database.
  - The visit ends with patients and hospitals mobile devices updated with a recall date and remainders.
- **Improving decision-making ability:** Improved use of mobile devices can improve accessibility of accurate patient information, thereby enhancing the physician's ability to take efficient decisions in the process of offering care. Research indicates that 'mobile Clinical Decision Support Systems (CDSS) on handheld computers support physicians in delivering appropriate care to their patients' (Kubben, et al., 2011).
- **Promising Future:** With recent advances in technology like cloud computing, the number of mobile devices accessing the data and there ease of access is skyrocketing.
- **Reduce Medication errors:** These mobile devices can reduce medical and data entry errors which often happen with the healthcare service providers (Burley & Scheepers, 2002; Prestigiacomo, 2011).

ISSUES WITH MOBILE DEVICES AND RECOMMENDATIONS

Disadvantages of Mobile device usage in Health Care Industry:

- **Complexity:** Mobile devices can be complex to use for some patients and hospital staff. Troubleshooting simple issues like resource overloading or device locks can be a hassle for some of the users (Wu, Li, & Fu, 2011).

Recommendation: Mobile devices can be designed with a better and simpler User Interface.

- **Information Security:** Not all mobile devices come with built in support for encrypting the data that should be transmitted. Mobile devices are susceptible to attack on data integrity. Including highly efficient encryption algorithms can make the devices slower and inefficient (Gururajan & Murugesan, 2005).

Recommendation: Recent advances in the technology provide an undeniable vision that mobile devices are becoming faster and more efficient periodically.

- **Increased Setup/Maintenance Cost:** Cost of implementing and maintaining the organizational mobile framework will be much higher than the alternatives. Considering the fact that advances in mobile technologies are recent and it is still a little far behind being proprietary, the cost of setting up and maintaining can be increased in the initial period of time.

Recommendation: Benefits outweigh this disadvantage and the rate at which technology is advancing can clearly show us that the costs can go down in the time to come.

- **Low Bandwidth/Lower network speed:** Mobile devices comparatively have a lower bandwidth for data transfer which the data transfers lower and less efficient. The rate at which the data can be transferred or accessed can vary depending on many factors like type of carrier, signal strength and number of connected users (Kinkade & Verclas, 2008).

Recommendation: Dedicated network and bigger wireless bandwidth can be purchased at a price, which can make the process efficient and provides faster alternative.

- **Maintenance Overhead:** Technically sound maintenance personnel are needed to maintain and trouble shoot the day-to-day problems. More skilled professionals will be needed at site to trouble shoot emergency backups and recoveries.
- **User interface:** Because of their smaller sizes, improperly designed user interfaces may result in hindering the mobile device usage by the staff and even patients. Poor user interfaces are deteriorating the extensive use of mobile devices by the patients (Weitzel, et al., 2010).

Recommendation: Cross-functional meetings (with both the IT personnel and the end users of the system, who are essentially hospital staff, patients, etc.) have to be conducted in the process of developing the user interfaces of these mobile devices.

- **Reliability on the system:** The mobile systems may be slow because of the hardware or software issues.

Recommendation: Regular software and hardware updates are recommended to avoid the system from becoming outdated and slow.

- **Hospital staff resistance:** They may tend to use other methods than the proposed mobile devices (such as paper-based methods) for data collection, but they have to be later on entered into an electronic device leading to time consumption (Rosenthal, 2003).

Recommendation: Healthcare organizations should encourage every staff member across the organization to use mobile device for their practices, which will improve their perception towards mobile devices thereby lowering the resistance.

- **Mobile device could be a distraction:** Users may use these mobile devices for other purposes rather than for health related uses (Räisänen, Oinas-Kukkonen, Leiviskä, Seppänen, & Kallio, 2010).

Recommendation: Restricting some websites to be used in a work location and allowing only those data repositories to be accessed which involves healthcare related databases, etc.

- Computers on Wheels may be left in their hallway where nurses and practitioners often move around (Timmons, 2003).

Recommendation: They should be placed at one place, which will save some room in the hallways and will allow the practitioners and nurses to find them at single place rather than searching for where they are residing.

- The user's lack of awareness on the increasing use mobile technology in the health sector is acting as a potential barrier between the patients and health service providers.

Recommendation: To improve the awareness of these mobile devices across the users in healthcare sector (administrative staff, nurses, physicians, pharmaceutical staff, emergency staff, and patients), they have to be educated about the mobile device importance and have to be properly trained.

Lastly, the hospital organizations may also have to consider below mobile related issues:

- Availability of number of applications (apps) for that particular mobile device will depend on the operating system on which that device is working on. For example, availability of Apps for 'Apple' operating systems differs from Android and Blackberry operating systems (Dolan, 2010).
  - Is there any data plan required by the carrier? What are the contracts required with a carrier provider? i.e. for example, in the cases where the mobile devices may require data plans from Verizon wireless or AT&T, etc.
  - Does that mobile device follow HIPAA guidelines for smart phones?
  - Some mobile devices may need memory cards, extension cords, extended batteries, etc.
  - Multiple wireless technologies may be required i.e. Bluetooth, WAN, LANS, which may further involve cost factors?
  - Which mobile system will comply with your organization's goals?

REFERENCES

AARDA. (2009). *American autoimmune related diseases association autoimmunity forum*. Retrieved from http://www.aarda.org/forum2/

Ammenwerth, E., Gräber, S., Herrmann, G., Bürkle, T., & König, J. (2003). Evaluation of health information systems—Problems and challenges. *International Journal of Medical Informatics, 71*(2-3), 125–135. doi:10.1016/S1386-5056(03)00131-X

Anantharaman, V., & Swee Han, L. (2001). Hospital and emergency ambulance link: Using IT to enhance emergency pre-hospital care. *International Journal of Medical Informatics, 61*(2-3), 147–161. doi:10.1016/S1386-5056(01)00137-X

Barlett, J. G., Auwaerter, P. G., & Pham, P. (2012). *Johns Hopkins guides*. Baltimore, MD: Johns Hopkins Medicine.

Baumgart, D. C. (2005). Personal digital assistants in health care: Experienced clinicians in the palm of your hand? *Lancet, 366*(9492), 1210–1222. Retrieved from http://www.ncbi.nlm.nih.gov/pubmed/16198770 doi:10.1016/S0140-6736(05)67484-3

Bosinski, T. J., Campbell, L., & Schwartz, S. (2004). Using a personal digital assistant to document pharmacotherapeutic interventions. *American Journal of Health-System Pharmacy, 61*(9), 931–934.

Burley, L., & Scheepers, H. (2003). Emerging trends in mobile technology development: From healthcare professional to system developer. *International Journal of Healthcare Technology and Management*, *5*(3-5), 179–193. doi:10.1504/IJHTM.2003.004125

Campbell, S. (2011). XECAN and trimble partner to deliver thingmagic powered RFID oncology solution providing direct interface to EMR. *EMR Daily News*. Retrieved from http://emrdailynews.com/2011/09/28/xecan-and-trimble-partner-to-deliver-thingmagic-powered-rfid-oncology-solution-providing-direct-interface-to-emr/

Clark, J. S., & Klauck, J. A. (2003). Recording pharmacists' interventions with a personal digital assistant. *American Journal of Health-System Pharmacy*, *60*(17), 1772–1774. Retrieved from http://www.ncbi.nlm.nih.gov/pubmed/14503114

Crilly, P., & Muthukkumarasamy, V. (2010). Using smart phones and body sensors to deliver pervasive mobile personal healthcare. In *Proceedings of the 2010 Sixth International Conference on Intelligent Sensors Sensor Networks and Information Processing*, (pp. 291-296). IEEE Press.

CSC. (2010). CSC mobile insurance. *Insurance Solutions*. Retrieved from http://assets1.csc.com/insurance/downloads/mobile_insurance_solutions.pdf

Dee, C. R., Teolis, M., & Todd, A. D. (2005). Physicians' use of the personal digital assistant (PDA) in clinical decision making. *Journal of the Medical Library Association*, *93*(4), 480–486. Retrieved from http://www.pubmedcentral.nih.gov/articlerender.fcgi?artid=1250324&tool=pmcentrez&rendertype=abstract

Doenges, M. E., Moorhouse, M. F., & Murr, A. C. (2010). Nurse's pocket guide. *F.A. Davis Company*. Retrieved from http://www.unboundmedicine.com/products/nurses_pocket_guide

Dolan, B. (2010). Number of smartphone health apps up 78 percent. *MobiHealthNews*. Retrieved from http://mobihealthnews.com/9396/number-of-smartphone-health-apps-up-78-percent/

Editor, A. (2011). App wrap. *Pharmacy Times*. Retrieved from http://www.pharmacytimes.com/publications/career/2011/PharmacyCareers_Spring2011/AppWrap

Edwards, J. (2009). PositiveID deal advances use of micrchip implants in Florida health system. *CBS News*. Retrieved from http://www.cbsnews.com/8301-505123_162-42843647/positiveid-deal-advances-use-of-microchip-implants-in-florida-health-system/

Epocrates. (2012). *Epocrates*. Retrieved from http://itunes.apple.com/us/app/epocrates/id281935788?mt=8

Espinoza, A., Garcia-Vazquez, J. P., Rodriguez, D. M., Andrade, A. G., & Garcia-Pena, C. (2009). Enhancing a wearable help button to support the medication adherence of older adults. *Web Congress*, 3-7.

Fahrni, J. (2009). *Tablet PCs in pharmacy practice*. Retrieved from http://www.jerryfahrni.com

Feature, S. (2008). Medication therapy management in pharmacy practice: core elements of an MTM service model (version 2.0). *Journal of the American Pharmacists Association, 48*(3), 341–353. Retrieved from http://www.ncbi.nlm.nih.gov/pubmed/16295642 doi:10.1331/JAPhA.2008.08514

Fischer, S., Stewart, T. E., Mehta, S., Wax, R., & Lapinsky, S. E. (2003). Handheld computing in medicine. *Journal of the American Medical Informatics Association, 10*(2), 139–149. Retrieved from http://www.pubmedcentral.nih.gov/articlerender.fcgi?artid=150367&tool=pmcentrez&rendertype=abstract doi:10.1197/jamia.M1180

Ford, S., Illich, S., Smith, L., & Franklin, A. (2006). Implementing personal digital assistant documentation of pharmacist interventions in a military treatment facility. *Journal of the American Pharmacists Association, 46*(5), 589–593. doi:10.1331/1544-3191.46.5.589.Ford

Fox, B. I., Felkey, B. G., Berger, B. A., Krueger, K. P., & Rainer, R. K. (2007). Use of personal digital assistants for documentation of pharmacists' interventions: A literature review. *American Journal of Health-System Pharmacy, 64*(14), 1516–1525. Retrieved from http://www.ncbi.nlm.nih.gov/pubmed/17617503 doi:10.2146/ajhp060152

Gururajan, R., & Murugesan, S. (2005). *Wireless solutions developed for the Australian healthcare: A review*. Retrieved from http://portal.acm.org/citation.cfm?id=1084254

Halamka, J. D. (2007). A chip in my shoulder. *Life as a Healthcare CIO*. Retrieved from http://geekdoctor.blogspot.com/2007/12/chip-in-my-shoulder.html

Haux, R. (2006). Health information systems - Past, present, future. *International Journal of Medical Informatics, 75*(3-4), 268–281. Retrieved from http://www.ncbi.nlm.nih.gov/pubmed/16169771 doi:10.1016/j.ijmedinf.2005.08.002

Haywood, J., Haywood, B., & Jeff, C. (2004). *Patients like me*. Retrieved from http://www.patientslikeme.com

HIMSS. (2011). *HIMSS mobile technology survey*. Retrieved from http://www.longwoods.com/blog/wp-content/uploads/2012/04/HIMSS-Mobile-Technology-Survey-FINAL-Revised-120511-Cover.pdf

Hirsch, L., & Gandolf, S. (2011). Nothing personal, but doctors still fear social media in physician marketing. *Healthcare Success*. Retrieved from http://www.healthcaresuccess.com/blog/physician-marketing/nothing-personal-but-doctors-still-fear-social-media-in-physician-marketing.html

Holzman, T. G. (1999). Computer-human interface solutions for emergency medical care. *Interaction, 6*(3), 13–24. doi:10.1145/301153.301160

Hussain, I. (2011). Emergency room doctors number one consumers of mobile, pathologists last, per report of physician mobile use. *iMedicalApps: Moible Medical App Reviews & Commentary by Medical Professionals*. Retrieved from http://www.imedicalapps.com/2011/04/doctors-consumers-mobile-use/

iHealthBeat. (2009). More physicians use smartphones, PDAs in Clinical care. *California HealthCare Foundation*. Retrieved from http://www.ihealthbeat.org/Articles/2009/1/6/More-Physicians-Use-Smartphones-PDAs-in-Clinical-Care.aspx

Inami, M., Kawakami, N., Sekiguchi, D., & Yanagida, Y. (2000). Visuo-haptic display using head-mounted projector. In *Proceedings IEEE* [IEEE Press.]. *Virtual Reality (Waltham Cross), 2000*, 233–240.

Ivanov, I. E., Gueorguiev, V., Bodurski, V., & Trifonov, V. (2010). Telemedicine and smart phones as medical peripheral devices (computational approaches). In *Proceedings of the 2010 Developments in Esystems Engineering*, (pp. 3-6). IEEE Press.

Kaiser Permanente. (2012). *Kaiser Permanente: On the go? Use our mobile app to stay connected*. Retrieved from http://mydoctor.kaiserpermanente.org/ncal/facilities/region/santarosa/area_master/members/mobile_app.jsp

Kinkade, S., & Verclas, K. (2008). Wireless technology for social change: Trends in mobile use by NGOs authors. *Communication, 2*(2), 1–59.

Kohn, L. T., Corrigan, J., & Donaldson, M. S. (2000). To err is human: Building a safer health system. *Medicine, 6*, 287.

Konstantas, D. (2007). An overview of wearable and implantable medical sensors. *Yearbook of Medical Informatics*. Retrieved from http://www.ncbi.nlm.nih.gov/pubmed/17700906

Korhonen, I., Pärkkä, J., & Van Gils, M. (2003). Health monitoring in the home of the future. *IEEE Engineering in Medicine and Biology Magazine, 22*(3), 66–73. doi:10.1109/MEMB.2003.1213628

Krogh, P. R., Rough, S., & Thomley, S. (2008). Comparison of two personal-computer-based mobile devices to support pharmacists' clinical documentation. *American Journal of Health-System Pharmacy, 65*(2), 154–157. doi:10.2146/ajhp070177

Kubben, P. L., Van Santbrink, H., Cornips, E. M. J., Vaccaro, A. R., Dvorak, M. F., Van Rhijn, L. W., et al. (2011). An evidence-based mobile decision support system for subaxial cervical spine injury treatment. *Surgical Neurology International, 2,* 32. Retrieved from http://www.pubmedcentral.nih.gov/articlerender.fcgi?artid=30 86168&tool=pmcentrez&rendertype=abstract

Laerhoven, K. V., Lo, B. P. L., Ng, J. W. P., Thiemjarus, S., King, R., Kwan, S., et al. (2004). Medical healthcare monitoring with wearable and implantable sensors. *UbiHealth Workshop*. Retrieved from http://www.healthcare.pervasive.dk/ ubicomp2004/papers/final_papers/laerhoven.pdf

Lakkaraju, S., & Moran, M. (2011). A framework to investigate the role of mobile technology in the healthcare organizations. In *Proceedings of MWAIS*. MWAIS.

Landro, L. (2010). How life's details help patients. *The Wall Street Journal: The Informed Patient*. Retrieved from http://online.wsj.com/article/SB100014240527 4870396000457542753154448678.html

Lapinsky, S., Mehta, S., Varkul, M., & Stewart, T. (2000). Qualitative analysis of handheld computers in critical care. In *Proceedings of the AMIA Symposium*, (p. 1060). AMIA.

Lapinsky, S. E., Weshler, J., Mehta, S., Varkul, M., Hallett, D., & Stewart, T. E. (2001). Handheld computers in critical care. *Critical Care (London, England), 5*(4), 227–231. Retrieved from http://www.pubmedcentral.nih.gov/articlerender.fcgi?art id=37409&tool=pmcentrez&rendertype=abstract doi:10.1186/cc1028

Leeuwen, A. M. V., Poelhuis-Leth, D. J., & Bladh, M. L. (2011). Davis's laboratory and diagnostic tests. *F.A. Davis Company*. Retrieved from www.unboundmedicine. com/products/davis_labs_diagnostic_tests

Lexicomp. (2012). *Lexicomp*. Retrieved from http://itunes.apple.com/us/app/lexi-comp/id313401238?mt=8

Marcus, A., Davidzon, G., Law, D., Verma, N., Fletcher, R., Khan, A., & Sarmenta, L. (2009). Using NFC-enabled mobile phones for public health in developing countries. In *Proceedings of the 2009 First International Workshop on Near Field Communication*, (pp. 30-35). IEEE Press.

Mayo Clinic. (2012). *MayClinic app for patients: Patient app*. Retrieved from http://www.mayoclinic.org/mayo-apps/

Mcalearney, A. S., & Medow, M. A. (2004, March). Handheld computers in clinical practice: Implementation strategies and challenges. *Leadership*, 1–68.

McAlearney, A. S., Schweikhart, S. B., & Medow, M. A. (2004). Doctors' experience with handheld computers in clinical practice: qualitative study. *BMJ (Clinical Research Ed.)*, *328*(7449), 1162. doi:10.1136/bmj.328.7449.1162

McCreadie, S. R., & McGregory, M. E. (2005). Experiences incorporating tablet PCcs into clinical pharmacists' workflow. *Journal of Healthcare Information Management*, *19*(4), 32–37. Retrieved from http://www.ncbi.nlm.nih.gov/pubmed/16266030

Mcfadden, T., & Indulska, J. (2004). Context-aware environments for independent living. *Science*, 1–6. Retrieved from http://archive.itee.uq.edu.au/~pace/publications/public/mcfadden-era2004.pdf

Myers, M., & Newman, M. (2007). The qualitative interview in IS research: Examining the craft. *Information and Organization*, *17*(1), 2–26. doi:10.1016/j.infoandorg.2006.11.001

Newbolt, S. K. (2003). New uses for wireless technology. *Nursing Management*, *22*, 22–32. doi:10.1097/00006247-200310002-00006

Ondash, E. (2004). Nurses choose PDAs over other mobile information technologies. *AMN Healthcare, Inc.* Retrieved from http://www.nursezone.com/nursing-news-events/devices-and-technology/Nurses-Choose-PDAs-Over-Other-Mobile-Information-Technologies_24474.aspx

Ooi, P., Culjak, G., & Lawrence, E. (2005). Wireless and wearable overview: Stages of growth theory in medical technology applications. In *Proceedings of the International Conference on Mobile Business ICMB05*, (pp. 528-536). IEEE Press.

OrthoInfo. (2002). *Patients have important role in safer health care*. Retrieved from http://orthoinfo.aaos.org/topic.cfm?topic=A00271#Additional Information

Pattath, A., Bue, B., Jang, Y., Ebert, D., Zhong, X., Ault, A., & Coyle, E. (2006). Interactive visualization and analysis of network and sensor data on mobile devices. In *Proceedings of the 2006 IEEE Symposium on Visual Analytics and Technology*, (vol. 9, pp. 83-90). IEEE Press.

PepeNavas Melara. (2012). Drug encyclopedia download review. *The Drugs Encyclopedia*. Retrieved from http://medical.appdownloadreview.com/online/drugs-encyclopedia

Perez, J. (2012). *myCVS on the go*. Retrieved from http://www.cvs.com/promo/promoLandingTemplate.jsp?promoLandingId=mobile-apps

Ping, A., Wang, Z., Shi, X., Deng, C., Bian, L., & Chen, L. (2009). Designing an emotional majormodo in smart home healthcare. In *Proceedings of the 2009 International Asia Symposium on Intelligent Interaction and Affective Computing*, (pp. 45-47). IEEE Press.

Prestigiacomo, J. (2011). Mobile healthcare anywhere: A proliferation of mobile devices means specific wireless challenges for healthcare organizations. *Healthcare Informatics, 28*(3), 34, 36.

Räisänen, T., Oinas-Kukkonen, H., Leiviskä, K., Seppänen, M., & Kallio, M. (2010). Managing mobile healthcare knowledge: Physicians' perceptions on knowledge creation and reuse. In *Proceedings of Health Information Systems: Concepts, Methodologies, Tools, and Applications*, (pp. 733-749). IEEE.

Reuters, T. (2012). Micromedex drug information. *Thomson Reuters*. Retrieved from http://healthcare.thomsonreuters.com/micromedexMobile/

Rosenthal, K. (2003). Touch vs. tech: Valuing nursing specific PDA software. *Nursing Management, 34*(7). doi:10.1097/00006247-200307000-00017

Saverno, K. R., Hines, L. E., Warholak, T. L., Grizzle, A. J., Babits, L., & Clark, C. (2011). Ability of pharmacy clinical decision-support software to alert users about clinically important drug-drug interactions. *Journal of the American Medical Informatics Association, 18*(1), 32–37. Retrieved from http://www.ncbi.nlm.nih.gov/pubmed/21131607 doi:10.1136/jamia.2010.007609

Skyscape. (2012). *Skyscape medical resource*. New York, NY: Skyscape, Inc.

Smith, S. D. (2009). E-prescribing 101. *Minnesota Medicine*. Retrieved from http://www.minnesotamedicine.com/PastIssues/PastIssues2009/January2009/QualityRoundsJanuary2009.aspx

Sommers, M. S. (2010). Diseases and disorders. *F.A. Davis Company*. Retrieved from http://www.unboundmedicine.com/products/diseases_disorders

Stanford, V. (2002). Using pervasive computing to deliver elder care. *IEEE Pervasive Computing / IEEE Computer Society [and] IEEE Communications Society*, *1*(1), 10–13. doi:10.1109/MPRV.2002.993139

Stross, R. (2012). Chicken scratches vs. electronic prescriptions. *The New York Times*. Retrieved from http://www.nytimes.com/2012/04/29/business/e-prescriptions-reduce-errors-but-their-adoption-is-slow.html

Stroud, S. D., Erkel, E. A., & Smith, C. A. (2005). The use of personal digital assistants by nurse practitioner students and faculty. *Journal of the American Academy of Nursing Management*, *17*(2), 67–75. doi:10.1111/j.1041-2972.2005.00013.x

Stroud, S. D., Smith, C. A., & Erkel, E. A. (2009). Personal digital assistant use by nurse practitioners: A descriptive study. *Journal of the American Academy of Nurse Practitioners*, *21*(1), 31–38. Retrieved from http://www.ncbi.nlm.nih.gov/pubmed/19125893 doi:10.1111/j.1745-7599.2008.00368.x

Timmons, S. (2003). Nurses resisting information technology. *Nursing Inquiry*, *10*(4), 257–269. Retrieved from http://www.ncbi.nlm.nih.gov/pubmed/14622372 doi:10.1046/j.1440-1800.2003.00177.x

Trossen, D., & Pavel, D. (2007). Sensor networks, wearable computing, and healthcare applications. *IEEE Pervasive Computing / IEEE Computer Society [and] IEEE Communications Society*, *6*, 58–61. doi:10.1109/MPRV.2007.43

Ulrich, R. S., Zimring, C., Quan, X., Joseph, A., & Choudhary, R. (2004). The role of the physical environment in the hospital of the 21st century: A once-in-a-lifetime opportunity. *Environment*. Retrieved from http://scholar.google.com/scholar?hl=en&btnG=Search&q=intitle:The+role+of+the+physical+environment+in+the+hospital+of+the+21st+century:+a+once-in-a-lifetime+opportunity#0

Unbound Evidence. (2011). Evidence central. *Wiley Blackwell*. Retrieved from www.unboundmedicine.com/products/evidence_central

University of Maryland. (2009). Medical encyclopedia. *Maryland Medical Systems*. Retrieved from itunes.apple.com/us/app/medical-encyclopedia/id313696784?mt=8

U.S. Wireless Quick Facts. (2011). *CTIA consumer info*. Retrieved from http://www.ctia.org/consumer_info/index.cfm/AID/10323

Versel, N. (2011). Emergency room patients tracked with RFID tags. *Information Week Healthcare*. Retrieved from http://www.informationweek.com/news/healthcare/EMR/231901224

Vijayaraghavan, K., Parpyani, K., Thakwani, S. A., & Iyengar, N. C. S. N. (2009). Methods of increasing spatial resolution of digital images with minimum detail loss and its applications. In *Proceedings of the 2009 Fifth International Conference on Image and Graphics*, (pp. 685–689). IEEE Press.

Waegemann, C. P., & Tessier, C. (2002). Documentation goes wireless: A look at mobile healthcare computing devices. *Journal of American Health Information Management Association, 73*(8), 36–39.

WalgreensCo. (2012). *Walgreens mobile*. Retrieved from http://www.walgreens.com/topic/apps/learn_about_mobile_apps.jsp

Wang, M.-Y., Tsai, P. H., Liu, J. W. S., & Zao, J. K. (2009). Wedjat: A mobile phone based medicine in-take reminder and monitor. In *Proceedings of the 2009 Ninth IEEE International Conference on Bioinformatics and BioEngineering*, (pp. 423-430). IEEE Press.

Web, M. D. (2012). WebMD for android, iphone, and ipad. *WebMD.com*. Retrieved from http://www.webmd.com/webmdapp

Webahn, I. (2012). *Capzule-PHR*. Retrieved from http://capzule.com/

Weber, J. R. (2009). Nurses' handbook of health assesment. *Lippincott Williams & Wilkins*. Retrieved from http://www.unboundmedicine.com/products/nurses_handbook_health_assessment

Weitzel, M., Smith, A., Deugd, S. D., & Yates, R. (2010). A web 2.0 model for patient-centered health informatics applications. *Computer, 43*(7), 43–50. doi:10.1109/MC.2010.190

Weitzel, M., Smith, A., Lee, D., Deugd, S., & Helal, S. (2009). Participatory medicine: Leveraging social networks in telehealth solutions. *Lecture Notes in Computer Science, 40*. Retrieved from http://portal.acm.org/citation.cfm?id=1575560

Winters, J. M., Wang, Y., & Winters, J. M. (2003). Wearable sensors and telerehabilitation. *IEEE Engineering in Medicine and Biology Magazine, 22*(3), 56–65. doi:10.1109/MEMB.2003.1213627

Wu, I.-L., Li, J.-Y., & Fu, C.-Y. (2011). The adoption of mobile healthcare by hospital's professionals: An integrative perspective. *Decision Support Systems, 51*(3), 587–596. doi:10.1016/j.dss.2011.03.003

Chapter 17
Clinical Decision Support System for Diabetes Prevention:
An Illustrative Case

Sarin Shrestha
Dakota State University, USA

EXECUTIVE SUMMARY

Millions of people around the world have diabetes. It is the seventh leading cause of death in US. An advancement of technologies may serve as the backbone for controlling diseases. Computerizing healthcare is expected to be one of the powerful levers essential for significant transformation in the quality and cost of delivering healthcare. Data management and technology is essential for providing the ability to exchange data and information at the right place in the right time to the right people in the healthcare process, to enable informed decision-making, and to achieve better health outcomes. Clinical Decision Support System (CDSS) provides guidance specific to the patient, including importing/entering patient data into the CDSS application and providing relevant information like lists of possible diagnoses, drug interaction alerts, or preventive care reminders to the practitioner that assists in their decision-making. This chapter has focuses on the use of CDSS for diabetes prevention.

DOI: 10.4018/978-1-4666-2671-3.ch017

BACKGROUND

Healthcare is a global issue that consumes a large percentage of the capital of our society (Chignell, Yesha, & Lo, 2010). Healthcare systems are struggling all around the world to maintain patient needs, improve the quality of care and reducing costs. At the same time, more data is being captured and stored around healthcare processes in the form of Electronic Health Records (EHR), medical imaging databases, health insurance claims, disease registries, and clinical trials. There is a need of federal legislation for not only to store these data in an electronic format but also use it in significant ways.

There has been a trend towards bigger databases with real-time updating, data analytics and visualization tools. These tools are being applied in extensive areas with examples including in search engine, and engineering design. Furthermore, with plethora of information and embracement of evidence-based medicine, healthcare professionals are finding themselves suffering from information overload (Ely, et al., 2002). Therefore, with this massive amount of data, and requirement of clinical decision making under time pressure, health care is a domain where extensive use of Information Systems tools can be particularly helpful (Chignell, et al., 2010). Data management and technology is essential for providing the ability to exchange data and information between associates in healthcare processes, to enable informed decision making, and to achieve better health outcomes (Loo & Lee, 2001).

Diabetes is the seventh leading cause of death in the United States (CDC, 2011; NDIC, 2011). In order to spread awareness of the disease and its preventive measures, the International Diabetes Federation (IDF) engages millions of people worldwide in diabetes advocacy and awareness (IDF, 2011) "*14 November is marked as a World Diabetes Day*" and is a global diabetes awareness campaign, led by the IDF..

More than 346 million people around the world have diabetes, and the number of diabetes patients is increasing significantly (WHO, 2011). In last 30 years, the frequency of diabetes in the US has increased fivefold, and it is estimated that about 21.4 million people will have diabetes in the U.S. by 2025 (King, Aubert, & Herman, 1998). About 3.4 million people died due to consequences of high blood sugar in 2005, and World Health Organization (WHO) projects that death due to diabetes will double by 2030. The medical cost for diabetes was 116 billion dollars in 2007 alone in United States (NDIC, 2011). The American Diabetes Association (ADA) projected the national costs of diabetes in the USA for will be increasing to $192 billion in 2020 (WHO/IDF, 2006). The medical expenses for people with diabetes are twice that of people without diabetes (CDC, 2011). Despite these enormous expenses in diabetes care, control of blood glucose is extremely poor, in general, in patient populations.

The control of blood glucose level to avoid or delay the development of diabetes related complication heavily relies on patient behavior and proper guidance from the health professionals (Dagogo-Jack, 2002). The flow of information between the patient, doctor, and information management may be achieved by IT elements such as, Internet, computer, electronic equipments, data mining and health analytics. Health Information Technology (HIT) provides the path for knowledge and safety, information about patient conditions, treatments and other significant characteristics, reminder to provider about the point of care of important quality steps (DORR, et al., 2007). In addition, the concepts of health-care analytics and pre-analytics bring further promise. Despite the well-recognized potential of IT in management of chronic diseases such as diabetes, there is little schematic evaluation of current impact on health care system (Eldar, 2002).

Computerizing healthcare is expected to be one of the powerful levers essential for significant transformation in the quality and cost of delivering healthcare. The management of chronic diseases such as diabetes heavily relies on flow of information between patients and healthcare providers. Thus, advancement of technologies may serve as the backbone for controlling diseases. Even though there is a massive gap between the guidelines and care of patients, the evidence shows that enhancing methodology and providing priority may assist in the reduction of the gap (O'Connor, 2003). Several promising efforts have been initiated for the implementation of information technology in diabetes management from late 1970s. The efforts are projected in the area of telemedicine, electronic records and decision support (Bellazzi, 2008).

SETTING THE STAGE

A nationwide audit assessing 439 quality indicators found that US adults receive only about half of recommended care (McGlynn, et al., 2003). American Institute of Medicine published a study titled "*To Err is Human: Building a Safer Health System*" in 1999, which reports significant increase in medical errors. The report was based upon analysis of numerous studies by a variety of institutions and concludes that on account of medical errors, between 44,000 to 98,000 people die every year (Kohn, Corrigan, & Donaldson, 1999). The errors that occur frequently during the course of providing health care services are incorrect medical dosage, surgical injuries, improper transfusions, mistaken patient identities, and many more. The high error rates with serious consequences are most likely to occur in operation theaters, intensive care units, and in emergency services.

Most of the medical errors arise due to human factors and these severe mistakes can be avoided with faster, comprehensive, and more accessible patient documentation. Many healthcare organizations have started to appreciate the fact that deploying information technology terminals in field of medicine can increase patient safety and reduce medical errors. The new technologies are providing opportunities to make healthcare more efficient through better communications and access (Abraham, Watson, & Boudreau, 2008).

Artificial Intelligence in Medicine (AIM) and Medical Informatics are few examples of new disciplines that have emerged which made scientists, doctors and physicians appreciate the potential of IT (Information Technology) to support information management within health care organizations (Coiera, 1997; Altman, 1997). In recent years, systematic application of science based practice in medicine such as evidence based medicine (Sacket, Straus, Richardson, Rosenberg, & Haynes, 2000), and knowledge translation where knowledge about best practice is put into action. The evidence based medicine can be implemented by computerized guidelines which are form of clinical decision support system (Leong, Kaiser, & Miksch., 2007). However, it is not easy to assimilate evidence-based practices into clinical workflow. Clinical Decision Support System (CDSS) can be implemented using a variety of platforms, for e.g., Internet-based, local personal computer, or a handheld device. Clinical Decision Support systems are a potential way for delivering the precise information to the right person at proper time, but this requires careful design of the interactions required for selecting and displaying information (Graham, Chignell, & Takeshita, 2002).

A Decision Support System (DSS) is an interactive computer based systems which consist of inputs, user knowledge and expertise, output, and decision making that assist decision makers to utilize data, models, solvers, and user interfaces to solve problems (Loo & Lee, 2001; Sprague, 1980). DSS which are based on the intelligent agent and perform intellectual decision making are known as Intelligent Decision Support Systems (Aronson & Turban, 1998). Clinical Decision Support System (CDSS) is any system that takes input as information about clinical situation, and produces as output inferences that can assist practitioners in their decision making and that would be judged as "intelligent" by program users (Musen, 1997). The useful characteristics of the patient are made available to clinicians for further examination through the use of specific CDSS (Hunt, Haynes, Hanna, & Smith, 1998). CDSS does not make decisions but supports diagnostic decisions of health professionals. It is viewed as information technology, defined as mechanisms to execute desired information handling in the organization (Avgerou & Cornford, 1993).

To address the deficiencies in healthcare, organizations are gradually moving to clinical decision support systems, which provide clinicians with patient-specific assessments or recommendations to assist in clinical decision making (Hunt, et al., 1998). CDSS can help investigate the queries related to patient's medical history and best cure available for specific medical case. CDSS has the ability to synthesize and amalgamate patient information, perform complex evaluations, and present the results to clinicians in practice (Hunt, et al., 1998). Therefore, providing healthcare professional with improved access to health information, at the appropriate time, could enhance the patient care. The information recipients include patients, clinicians and others involved in patient care delivery. CDSS also provides additional assistance in recommending appropriate drug doses or providing immunization reminders.

There are vast amount of research studies on the decision support systems in healthcare (Bell, et al., 2010; Cercone, An, Li, Gu, & An, 2011; Co, et al., 2010; O'Connor, et al., 2011). Coiera (2003) illustrated that expert systems, or knowledge based systems are most widely used for decision making in clinical setting. Moreover, such system can be applied into number of tasks such as assisting in diagnosis, therapy planning, and image finding and interpretation. There are several decision support tools that are available to health professional, and these studies seek how available support is employed. Hunt et al. (1998) conducted systematic review on clinical decision support system, and concluded that such system are useful in preventive measure, but have little effects on diagnosis. Moreover, Hunt et al. (1998) stated that usage of decision support on clinical setting must be further studied. Garg et al. (2005) performed a systematic review, and report that clinical decision support have positive impacts on physician but impact on patients is still unclear. Kawamoto, Houlihan, Balas, and Lobach (2005) performed systematic review of 70 randomized controlled trial for identifying critical success factor clinical decision support system. They found four features that should be available in such system are as provide decision automatically on the routine of physician workflow, deliver decision making at the required time without any delay, provide feasible recommendation and it usage computer for suggesting decision.

CASE DESCRIPTION: DIABETES

"Diabetes mellitus" normally referred as diabetes, is a chronic disease in which a person has high blood sugar, either because the body does not produce enough insulin, or because cells do not respond to the insulin that is produced (Shoback, 2011). Insulin is very essential for human body to be able to use glucose for energy. When we eat food, the body breaks down the food into glucose, a form of sugar, which is needed for our everyday life. Insulin takes the sugar from the blood into the cells for growth and energy. When glucose builds up in the blood instead of going into cells, it can lead to serious complications. The symptoms of diabetes are frequent urination (polyuria), increased thirst (polydipsia), and increased hunger (polyphagia). Before developing diabetes, people usually have pre-diabetes. It is a condition where blood glucose levels are higher than normal but not high enough for a diagnosis of diabetes. The three main types of Diabetes Mellitus (DM) are:

- **Type 1 DM:** It is a type of diabetes, which arises due to failure of insulin production from the body. The patient with Type 1 DM requires injecting insulin to survive. It is also called Insulin-Dependent Diabetes Mellitus (IDDM) or juvenile diabetes. This diabetes is usually diagnosed in children and young adults, even though disease onset can occur at any age. About 5% of the people with diabetes have this type of disease (NDIC, 2011). There is not any known way to prevent type 1 diabetes. Numerous clinical trials for preventing Type 1 DM are in progress currently or are being planned.
- **Type 2 DM:** This is a most common type of diabetes. It is also called Noninsulin-Dependent Diabetes Mellitus (NIDDM) or adult onset diabetes. It is a type of diabetes that arises due to insulin resistance, a condition in which the cells fail to use insulin properly. Type 2 DM is associated with obesity, family history of diabetes, older age, history of gestational diabetes, impaired glucose metabolism, physical activity, and many more.
- **Gestational diabetes:** It is a condition when pregnant women, who have never had diabetes before, have a high blood glucose level during pregnancy. It may also lead to development of type 2 DM. It is caused when the body of a pregnant woman does not produce enough insulin required during pregnancy, leading to increased blood sugar levels. There is about 2% - 10% of chances of occurring this disease during pregnancies and may recover or may disappear after the delivery (DiabeticsAnonymous) (CDC, 2011). This gestational diabetes is treatable but requires cautious medical supervision. Approximately 35% - 65% of affected women may develop Type 2 DM in next 10-20 years (CDC, 2011).

Other forms of diabetes mellitus include congenital diabetes that is due to genetic defects of insulin secretion, cystic fibrosis-related diabetes, steroid diabetes induced by high doses of glucocorticoids, pancreatic diseases and several forms of monogenic diabetes.

Over time, diabetes can damage the heart, kidneys, eyes, blood vessels, and nerves. Diabetes leads to improved rates of micro vascular disease such as retinopathy, renal disease, neuropathy, stroke, and disability and a reduced life expectancy of 7 to 8 years (Harris, 1995).

- Diabetes increases the risk of heart disease and stroke. The risk of stroke is 2 to 4 times higher than adults with diabetes. It is also the leading cause of kidney failure. Approximately 10-20% of patient with diabetes die because of kidney failure.

- Diabetic retinopathy is a critical cause of blindness. It occurs as an effect of continuing accumulation which results in damages to the small blood vessels in the retina that leads to blindness. After 15 years of diabetes, about 2% of the people become blind, and about 10% develop severe visual impairment. About 4.2 million people with diabetes aged 40 years or older had diabetic retinopathy in 2005-2008 (CDC, 2011).
- Diabetic neuropathy is damage to the nerves and affects up to 60%-70% of patient with diabetes. Even though many different problems can occur as a result of diabetic neuropathy, common symptoms are tingling, pain, numbness, or weakness in the feet and hands (CDC, 2011).
- Combined with reduced blood flow, neuropathy in feet increases the chance of foot ulcers and eventual limb amputation.
- The overall risk of dying among people with diabetes is at least double the risk of their peers without diabetes.

The diabetic patient gets treated either taking insulin or oral medication or both to control the glucose level. According to 2007-2009 National health interview survey, among adults with diagnosed diabetes either type 1 or type 2, 12% take insulin only, 58% take oral medication only, 14% take both insulin and oral medication, or 16% do not take either insulin or oral medication (CDC, 2011) (see Figure 1).

A Systematic approach for the development of clinical decision support systems is necessary for an effective design and implementation of medical information system. The common function of a CDSS is to provide guidance with patient specific information includes the knowledge base and communication mechanism. It includes importing or entering patient data into the CDSS application and providing relevant information like lists of possible diagnoses, drug interaction alerts, or preventive care reminders to the clinician. For instance, healthcare practitioners enters patient data and prescriptions into the system and receive prompt feedback about clinically imperative information that may improve their prescribing decision (Doolan, Bates, & James, 2003; Wears & Berg, 2005). CDSS provides support to the health professionals at different stages in the care process, from preventive care through diagnosis and treatment to monitoring and follow-up (Berner, 2009).

Use of CDSS for Diabetes Prevention

When any patient gets treated, the doctors/clinicians need to make sure that they should identify the patients with diabetes. Large pool of people around the world have diabetes and still not yet been diagnosed. Prior to treating any patient, screen-

Figure 1. Adult percentage data on diabetic patient receiving treatment with insulin/ oral medication, US 2007-2009

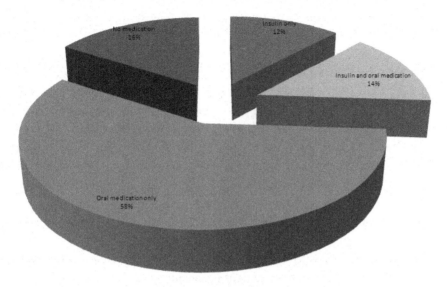

Source: 2007–2009 National Health Interview Survey

ing process for diabetes should be carried out. Electronic health records has made it very easy to work on a prevention program on diabetes which can constantly provide screening for high risk patients and can identify those patients which have moved from high risk to pre-diabetes and pre-diabetes to diabetes. Healthcare professionals, doctors, and clinicians needs to be more cautious to identify those who have undiagnosed diabetes. In addition, special attention should be provided to those who are at high risk of developing diabetes and importantly to those who have pre-diabetes.

There are not only two types of patient in regard to diabetes. Those who have it and those who do not, but there are two more kind. There are patients who are at high risk of diabetes and there are patients who have pre-diabetes.

The prevention program on diabetes starts by identifying these groups (Holly, 2010):

1. Patients who have diabetes.
2. Patients who do not have diabetes.
3. Patients who have pre-diabetes.
4. Patients who are at high risk for diabetes.
5. Patients who are of an age that they should be screened for diabetes even though they are not at high risk of diabetes or have pre-diabetes.

315

Lab Test on Diagnosis of Diabetes and Pre-Diabetes

An outline of laboratory test to diagnose diabetes are described below (Holly, 2010; NDIC, 2008; WHO/IDF, 2006):

1. **Lab Test by Fasting blood glucose:** A patient has fasting blood glucose value greater than 100 mg/dl and less than or equal to 125 mg/dl on two different instances is considered to have pre-diabetes and if the value is greater than or equal to 126 mg/dl, then the patient is considered to have diabetes.
2. **Lab Test by Random blood glucose:** A patient has a random blood glucose value greater than 140 mg/dl and less than or equal to 199 mg/dl, the patient is considered to have pre-diabetes and if the value is greater than or equal to 200 mg/dl the patient is considered to have diabetes.
3. **2-hour Glucose tolerance test:** A patient has a 2-hour Glucose Tolerance Test with a value greater than 140 mg/dl and less than or equal to 199 mg/dl, the patient is considered to have pre-diabetes and if the value is greater than or equal to 200 mg/dl, then the patient is considered to have diabetes.
4. **Hemoglobin A1C test**: A patient has HgbA1C value ranges in between 5.5% to 6.5% on two different days, the patient is considered to have pre-diabetes and if the value ranges greater than or equal to 6.5%, then the patient is considered to have diabetes.

The CDSS based healthcare system provides instant response on patient diabetic condition by providing appropriate recommendations, including drug adjustments and change in life styles. CDSS is designed to work as an alert system for estimating diabetic condition and checking doses of medication. If the patient's data meets the criteria of diabetes, that patient record is stored in the diabetes database. The system maintains a prescription check master and verifies whether the patient has a problem which is a contradicted with the prescribed medication. If a problem exists, an alert is sent to healthcare professionals (Matsumura, et al., 2009).

CDSS generates messages being specific to patient, for example:

*   If the patient's fasting blood glucose level is between 100 mg/dl and 126 mg/dl, and random blood glucose level is between 140 mg/dl and 199 mg/dl; a message is sent to the patient signifying that it is a case of pre-diabetes and system generates dates for appointments to consult with the doctor.
*   If the patient's data synchronizes with the condition of diabetes such as the patient's fasting and random glucose value is equal to more than 126 mg/dl and 200 mg/dl, respectively; an alert is generated signifying that the patient is diabetic and message is sent to the patient to ensure appropriate action

to change the lifestyle, suggest for medical therapy and generates appointments to consult the doctor. If, the patient is admitted in the hospital, the system checks the dose of each medication according to a patient's medical history. When the dosage is over-prescribed, an alert is sent to the healthcare practitioners.

The healthcare professionals are able to download patient specific data from the system which are represented in a graphical format. This would draw attention towards the abnormal results of a patient and facilitates practitioners for more detailed discussion. CDSS initiates information technology into clinical settings in a way that supports interaction between the patient and healthcare professional and educates patients about their risk factors and encourages behavior change patients (Carroll, et al., 2002).

Screening for Insulin Resistance

Insulin resistance is an important risk factor for diabetic patient and cardiovascular disease (DeFronzo & Ferrannini, 1991). Insulin is produced by the pancreas and is needed by the body to regulate the level of glucose in the blood. Human body requires a balanced amount of glucose and that glucose comes from the food that we eat. This is where insulin comes into play; it allows body to store glucose so that it can be used when needed. When a person has more glucose in blood then needed at the time, insulin moves blood sugar into the liver and into muscles. It signals the liver to stop making sugar or glucose out of the protein and carbohydrates. Normally, in this type of situation, the liver and muscles do not respond to insulin. This is called insulin resistance, and is the forerunner to Type 2 diabetes. Some of the contributing cases to insulin resistance are age, obesity, genetics, and a sedentary life style. In order to identify insulin resistance and to take steps to reverse it and to prevent the development of diabetes, health care professionals should estimate the risk of insulin resistance.

HDL-to-Triglyceride ratio, fasting insulin, Homeostasis Model Assessment (HOMA) are all used to predict insulin sensitivity (McAuley, et al., 2001). Additionally, a healthcare professional can calculate numerical scores for above prediction which indicates the presence of insulin resistance in human body.

- **HDL/Triglyceride ratio:** If the value of this ratio is greater than 2, it signify the patient body is insulin resistance. It results when the cholesterol is checked (Holly, 2010). According to Luz, Favarato, Junior, Lemos, and Chagas (2008) study, the ratio of HDL to triglycerides was found to be an influential factor of extensive coronary disease (Luz, et al., 2008). The patient portal is updated in the system with indication of risk of diabetes, so further steps must be taken to prevent it.

- **HOMA-IR:** This HOMA-IR is associated with high risk of diabetes and this score is based on a mathematical equation which is calculated with a fasting insulin level and a fasting blood sugar (Matthews, et al., 1985; Wallace, Levy, & Matthews, 2004). When the value of this ratio is above 2; it is signifying of the presence of insulin resistance (Holly, 2010). In this case, patient portal is updated with indication of insulin resistance and a message is sent to the patient requesting to consult doctor soon.

- **Cardio Metabolic Risk Syndrome:** Previously it is referred as Syndrome X, Insulin Resistance Syndrome or Metabolic Syndrome. The presence of the Cardio metabolic Risk Syndrome is indication of the presence of insulin resistance. Metabolic syndrome is caused by various factors such as excessive weight, physical inactivity or smoking (Cathy, 2010). A provider can routinely assess the presence of this condition with standards published by both the World Health Organization and the ATP-III. ATP is an Adult Treatment Panel, a third report of the expert panel on detection, evaluation, and treatment of high blood cholesterol in adults. About 64 million people meet the condition for the metabolic syndrome, thus representing a large number of people potentially at risk for diabetes (Ford, Giles, & Dietz, 2002). In addition, an update is done automatically to the patient portal and sets up further appointments with health specialist and list of medications are provided.

- **Fasting Insulin Level:** When high insulin is present in the fasting state, it is indicative of insulin resistance which results in increased insulin levels to compensate for the liver and muscles decreased response to insulin. Furthermore, system automatically setups future appointment with doctors and sends message to the patient. In McAuley et al. (2001) study, fasting insulin alone was accurate in predicting insulin resistance.

A healthcare professional enters the patient ID in the system and the patient portals pop-up and also investigates the alerts concerning the patients and displays the message (Matsumura, et al., 2009). If a patient has insulin resistance and does not yet have diabetes, system sends an alert message regarding the steps to be taken on time to lose weight, exercise, stop smoking, reduce stress, and get proper sleep in order to delay or avoid diabetes.

Five Components of Diabetes Prevention

The five major components of Diabetes Prevention are dietary management, exercise, monitoring health status, medical therapy, and education. The patients with a low risk of diabetes exhibits:

- Have a low body mass index.
- Consume a diet high in cereal fiber and polyunsaturated fat.
- Quit Smoking.
- Consume a diet low in trans-fatty acids.
- Engage in physical activity for at least 30 minutes each day.
- Do not consume more than 5 grams of alcohol per day.
- Drink more water (see Figure 2).

We may reduce the risk of developing diabetes, by 58% through the modest weight loss (Holly, 2010; DPPRG, 2002; Tuomilehto, et al., 2001). The study of National Institutes of Health supported by Centers for Disease Control and Prevention showed that making some behavior changes, such as improving food choices and increasing physical activity to at least 150 minutes per week helped participants lose 5 to 7 percent of their body weight (CDC, 2012).

Figure 2. Five components of diabetes prevention

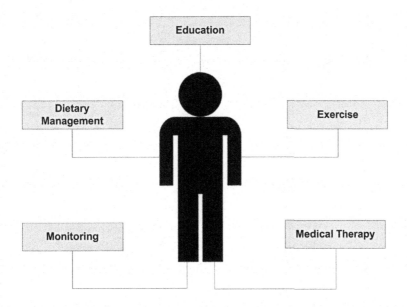

The increased physical activity that raises fitness levels can help to lower cholesterol, lower blood pressure, reduce the risk of heart attack and stroke, relieve stress, and improve the quality of life by strengthening the heart, muscles, and bones. System sets up an automated email and messages to patients at high risk of diabetes and pre-diabetic patient that provides knowledge on nutrition management, daily exercise, health monitoring on a timely basis (see Figure 3).

Summary

Even though it is possible to live productively with diabetes, it is better for the patient to know their risk of developing diabetes and to take steps to delay or prevent it. The primary care providers should be committed to quality care of those with diabetes, identifying those at increased risk of diabetes, and identifying those who have pre-diabetes. The commitment should extend to teaching the latter two groups how to avoid or delay the onset of diabetes. A prevention program on diabetes is electronically deployed and makes it easy to constantly perform these tasks with every patient seen in a primary care practice.

The main aim of the CDSS is to facilitate practitioners/patients and display patient specific information in a format that they could understand and alert clinicians as required. The CDSS is a specific tool used by clinicians in diabetes clinics

Figure 3. Diabetes screening and prevention chart

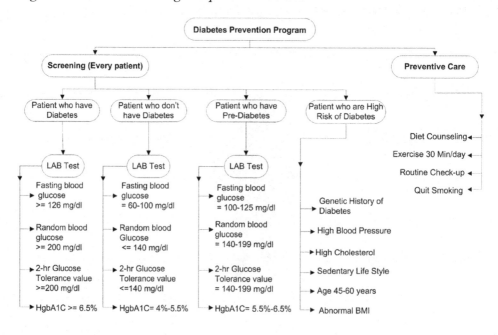

to facilitate patients understanding of their condition. CDSS would act both as an educating and motivating tool for patients in addition to providing a means of bringing quality care to patients.

The examples of CDSS interventions are (HIMSS, 2011):

- Instant Alerts
- Care Plans and Protocols
- Parameter Guidance
- Smart Documentation Forms
- Relevant Patient Data Summary
- Multi-patient Monitors and Dashboards
- Predictive Analytics
- Expert Workup Advisors (see Table 1).

CHALLENGES AND SOLUTION

Clinical decision support systems do not always results in improved clinical practice. However, in a recent systematic review of computer based systems, 66% improved clinical practice (Hunt, et al., 1998). Relatively, sound scientific evidence is available to explain why systems succeed or fail (Kaplan, 2001; Kanouse, Kallich, & Kahan, 1995). The acceptance of a CDSS program requires support from all levels of the organization. High-level executives must support the change and approve resources and medical leadership must understand the value of resulting changes. Although diabetes management through Information System has been found to be beneficial through different studies, but there is still research lacking in different aspects. The research of Nijland (2009) showed that 44 percentages of the patients are very inactive in using Internet for diabetes management. Moreover, research of Mollon (2008) showed that only 60% are interested to use technological intervention. It means remaining patients are still facing difficulty in using technological intervention for the diabetes care.

Hence, future research must focus on these issues and try to devise the framework that is effective and easy to use by healthcare professioanls as well as patients. In another instant, we have different methods of intervention such as telephone, Internet, telemedicine, and all these means of intervention may not have the same effect to all class of people. We have very few study which evaluate the effectiveness of different alternatives of intervention. In the study of Hanauer, Wentzell, Laffel, and Laffel (2009), they found that intervention through mobile phone short messaging service has greater output than intervention through email. There may be a need to

Table 1. Use of CDSS for diabetes prevention

Clinical Process	CDSS – IT implications	Description
Monitoring patient for Diabetes – Lab Test	• Patient's portal updated • Alert message send to Patient • Sets up future appointment with doctor	Performing lab test on diagnosis and update the patient portals with report. An alert message is send to the patient signifying they are at high risk or have pre-diabetes or diabetes with appropriate action to change the lifestyle & suggest for medical therapy. System also sets up future appointments to consult with doctor.
Screening for Insulin Resistance	• Alert message send to patient	If a patient has an indication of insulin resistance, system sends an alert message to patient regarding the steps to be taken on time to lose weight, exercise, stop smoking, reduce stress, and get proper sleep in order to avoid diabetes.
See alerts before treating any patient	• Enter Patient's ID & Patient's portal pops-up	A clinician enters the patient ID in the system and the patient portals pop-up and investigates the alerts concerning the patients before examining.
Monitoring medication dose & Synchronization	• Checks dose for medication • Synchronize medication	Monitors the medication dose prescribed and if over prescribed sends alert message to clinicians. Prompts an alert to the clinicians when the medication is not synchronized for the patient as indicated.
Medication/Test Reminder	• Reminds clinicians for medication dose • Reminds clinicians for remaining test	Clinicians are reminded for medication dose in appropriate time by beeping. Clinicians are reminded by sending messages for remaining test.
Demographic view of patient data	• Download Patient specific medical data • Graphical view of data to observed abnormality	Display patient specific data as well as the demographic view to observe the abnormality and if serious concerns, consult with senior doctors
Assist clinicians in making decisions	• Pops-up messages	System helps doctors and clinicians in making decision by providing various suggestions specific to the patient medical problems
Educate patient with high risk of diabetes and pre-diabetes	• Alert messages • Alert emails	System sets up an automated email and messages to patients that provide knowledge on nutrition management, daily exercise, health monitoring on a timely basis.

investigate the model that employ combined intervention methods, and intervention is given according to matching class group.

Numerous research is being conducted for usage of information care for diabetes management, and it has rising scope with development of new technology and methodology. The future study on diabetes managemenr will focus on two types of intervention for diabetes management: long term intervention and short term intervention. Long term intervention will redesign the whole process of diabetes care and will mainly focus on continuous communication between health care providers, communication between the health care providers and patients, and in decision making (Bellazzi, 2008). The first initiation is done in Italy by the social and healthcare information systems of the Lombardia and Veneto regions. They are trying to connect general practitioners, hospitals, and pharmacies in a single, distributed, regional health care delivery network (Bellazzi, 2008).

By recent advancement in technology, IS tools can be efficiently employed to redesign the methodology of diabetes care. The new and efficient way of communication between the diabetes patient and health care provider can be initiated by using facilities provided by IS. Not only this, healthcare providers can integrate, and central system can be built that assist in decision making, automating the communication with patient, and many more. It is also true that the model of diabetes care by employing Information System is not in fully capable phase. An extensive research is needed to install the system into large scale, and capability that IT can provide for chronic diseases care should be coined. Moreover, outcomes of articles review showed that focus is projected only in the post-diabetes care, but according to statistics of NDIC about 35% of US adults of age 20 years or more have pre-diabetes (NDIC, 2011). Therefore, usage of high level IS techniques such as pre-analytics has become urgent in order to take care of pre-diabetes.

The adoption and impact of CDSS has been uneven; some clinical organizations have achieved marked reductions in adverse events, improvements in quality metrics and cost savings, while others have had poor acceptance or unintended consequences, or have avoided implementation. CDSS should not be thought of as the only tool available to solve the organization's problems. There are limitations to its interventions too. CDSS implementation is not stand-alone; it must be paired with other communications and decision-making. The capabilities of CDSS integrate evaluation, treatment, and consultation by maximizing the quality and safety lowering the cost. The ability to manage health records electronically has resulted in improved quality of patient care, increased physician and patient satisfaction, and increased operational efficiencies. CDSS should be carried out as a mean to support a decision and not to force it, and it must allow providers the ability to make their own judgments. However, when electronic health records and computerized clinical decision-support systems apprehends great promise as interventions that will defeat challenges for improving evidence-based health care delivery.

REFERENCES

Abraham, C., Watson, R. T., & Boudreau, M. (2008). Ubiquitous access: On the front lines of patient care and safety. *Communications of the ACM, 51*(6), 95–99. doi:10.1145/1349026.1349045

Altman, R. B. (1997). Informatics in the care of patients: Ten notable challenges. *The Western Journal of Medicine, 166*(2), 118–122.

Aronson, J., & Turban, E. (1998). *Decision support systems and intelligent systems.* Upper Saddle River, NJ: Prentice Hall.

Avgerou, C., & Cornford, T. (1993). *Developing information systems: Concepts, issues and practise.* Basingstroke, UK: Macmillan.

Bell, L. M., Grundmeier, R., Localio, R., Zorc, J., Fiks, A. G., & Zhang, X. (2010). Electronic health record-based decision support to improve asthma care: A cluster-randomized trial. *Pediatrics, 125*(4), E770–E777. doi:10.1542/peds.2009-1385

Bellazzi, R. (2008). Telemedicine and diabetes management: Current challenges and future research directions. *Journal of Diabetes Science and Technology, 2*(1), 98–104.

Berner, E. S. (2009). *Clinical decision support systems: State of the art.* Rockville, MD: Agency for Healthcare Research and Quality.

Carroll, C., Marsden, P., Soden, P., Naylor, E., New, J., & Dornan, T. (2002). Involving users in the design and usability evaluation of a clinical decision support system. *Computer Methods and Programs in Biomedicine, 69*, 123–135. doi:10.1016/S0169-2607(02)00036-6

Cathy, H. (2010). *Cadiometabolic risk management: Addressing metabolic syndrome.* Health Dialog.

CDC. (2011). *National diabetes fact sheet, 2011.* Atlanta, GA: U.S. Department of Health and Human Services, Centers for Disease Control and Prevention.

CDC. (2012). *National diabetes prevention program.* Retrieved from http://www.cdc.gov/diabetes/prevention/about.htm

Cercone, N., An, X., Li, J., Gu, Z., & An, A. (2011). Finding best evidence for evidence-based best practice recommendations in health care: The initial decision support system design. *Knowledge and Information Systems, 29*(1), 159–201. doi:10.1007/s10115-011-0439-8

Chignell, M., Yesha, Y., & Lo, J. (2010). *New methods for clinical decision support in hospitals.* Paper presented at the 2010 Conference of the Center for Advanced Studies on Collaborative Research. Toronto, Canada.

Co, J. P. T., Johnson, S. A., Poon, E. G., Fiskio, J., Rao, S. R., & Van Cleave, J. (2010). Electronic health record decision support and quality of care for children with ADHD. *Pediatrics, 126*(2), 239–246. doi:10.1542/peds.2009-0710

Coiera, E. (1997). Artificial intelligence in medicine. In *Guide to Medical Informatics, the Internet and Telemedicine.* London, UK: Arnold.

Coiera, E. (2003). *Guide to health Informatics.* London, UK: Arnold.

Dagogo-Jack, S. (2002). Preventing diabetes-related morbidity and mortality in the primary care setting. *Journal of the National Medical Association, 94*(7), 549–560.

DeFronzo, R., & Ferrannini, E. (1991). Insulin resistance: A multifaceted syndrome responsible for NIDDM, obesity, hypertension, dyslipidemia, and atherosclerotic cardiovascular disease. *Diabetes Care, 14,* 173–194. doi:10.2337/diacare.14.3.173

DiabeticsAnonymous. (2012). *Types of diabetes.* Retrieved May 7, 2012, from http://www.diabeticsanonymous.org/types.html

Doolan, D., Bates, D., & James, B. (2003). The use of computers for clinical care: A case series of advanced US sites. *Journal of the American Medical Informatics Association, 10,* 94–107. doi:10.1197/jamia.M1127

Dorr, D., Bonner, L. M., Cohen, A. N., Shoai, R. S., Perrin, R., Chaney, E., & Young, A. S. (2007). Informatics systems to promote improved care for chronic illness: A literature review. *Journal of the American Medical Informatics Association, 14*(2), 156–163. doi:10.1197/jamia.M2255

DPPRG. (2002). Diabetes prevention program research group: The diabetes prevention program: Reduction in the incidence of type 2 diabetes with lifestyle intervention or metformin. *The New England Journal of Medicine, 346,* 393–403. doi:10.1056/NEJMoa012512

Eldar, R. (2002). Health technology: Challenge to public health. *Croatian Medical Journal, 43*(4), 470–474.

Ely, J., Osheroff, J., Ebell, M., Chambliss, M., Vinson, D., Stevermer, J., & Pifer, E. (2002). Obstacles to answering doctors' questions about patient care with evidence: Qualitative study. *British Medical Journal, 324*(7339), 710. doi:10.1136/bmj.324.7339.710

Ford, E., Giles, W., & Dietz, W. (2002). Prevalence of the metabolic syndrome among U.S. adults: Findings from the third national health and nutrition examination survey. *Journal of the American Medical Association, 287,* 356–359. doi:10.1001/ jama.287.3.356

Gardner, D. G. (Ed.). (2011). *Greenspan's basic & clinical endocrinology* (9th ed.). New York, NY: McGraw Hill Medical.

Garg, A. X., Adhikari, N. K. J., McDonald, H., Rosas-Arellano, M. P., Devereaux, P. J., & Beyene, J. (2005). Effects of computarized clinical decision support system on practitioner performance and patients outcomes. *Journal of the American Medical Association, 293*(10), 1223–1238. doi:10.1001/jama.293.10.1223

Graham, M., Chignell, M., & Takeshita, H. (2002). *Design of documentation for handheld ergonomics: Presenting clinical evidence at the point of care.* Paper presented at the 20th Annual International Conference on Computer Documentation. Toronto, Canada.

Hanauer, D. A., Wentzell, K., Laffel, N., & Laffel, L. M. (2009). Computerized automated reminder diabetes system (CARDS): E-mail and SMS cell phone text messaging reminders to support diabetes management. *Diabetes Technology & Therapeutics, 11*(2), 99–106. doi:10.1089/dia.2008.0022

Harris, M. (1995). *Summary in diabetes in America* (2nd ed.). Bethesda, MD: National Institute of Diabetes and Digestive and Kidney Diseases, National Institutes of Health.

HIMSS. (2011). *Improving outcomes with clinical decision support: An implementer's guide* (2nd ed.). Chicago, IL: HIMSS.

Holly, J. L. (2010). *The importance and content of a diabetes prevention program (DPP).* Chicago, IL: Healthcare Information and Management Systems Society (HIMSS).

Hunt, D., Haynes, R., Hanna, S., & Smith, K. (1998). Effects of computer based clinical decision support systems on physician performance and patient outcomes: A systematic review. *Journal of the American Medical Association, 280*(15), 1339–1346. doi:10.1001/jama.280.15.1339

IDF. (2011). *About world diabetes day.* Retrieved from http://www.idf.org/world-diabetesday/about

Kanouse, D. E., Kallich, J. D., & Kahan, J. P. (1995). Dissemination of effectiveness and outcomes research. *Health Policy (Amsterdam)*, *34*(3), 167–192. doi:10.1016/0168-8510(95)00760-1

Kaplan, B. (2001). Evaluating informatics applications - Some alternative approaches: Theory, social interactionism, and call for methodological pluralism. *International Journal of Medical Informatics*, *64*(1), 39–55. doi:10.1016/S1386-5056(01)00184-8

Kawamoto, K., Houlihan, C. A., Balas, E. A., & Lobach, D. F. (2005). Improving clinical practice using decision support systems: A systematic review of trials to identify features critical to success. *British Medical Journal*, *330*(7494). doi:10.1136/bmj.38398.500764.8F

King, H., Aubert, R., & Herman, W. (1998). Global burden of diabetes, 1995-2025. *Diabetes Care*, *21*, 1414–1431. doi:10.2337/diacare.21.9.1414

Kohn, L. T., Corrigan, J. M., & Donaldson, M. S. (1999). *To err is human: Building a safer health system*. Washington, DC: National Academy Press.

Leong, T.-Y., Kaiser, K., & Miksch, S. (2007). Free and open source enabling technologies for patient-centric, guideline-based clinical decision support: A survey. *Yearbook of Medical Informatics*, *207*, 74–86.

Loo, G. S., & Lee, P. C. H. (2001). *A soft systems methodology model for clinical decision support systems (SSMM-CDSS)*. Paper presented at the 12th International Workshop on Database and Expert Systems Applications. Munich, Germany.

Luz, P. L. D., Favarato, D., Junior, J. R. F.-N., Lemos, P., & Chagas, A. C. P. (2008). High ratio of triglycerides to HDL-cholesterol predicts extensive coronary disease. *Clinics (Sao Paulo, Brazil)*, *63*(4), 427–432. doi:10.1590/S1807-59322008000400003

Matsumura, Y., Yamaguchi, T., Hasegawa, H., Yoshihara, K., Zhang, Q., Mineno, T., & Takeda, H. (2009). Alert system for inappropriate prescriptions relating to patients' clinical condition. *Methods of Information in Medicine*, *48*(6), 566–573. doi:10.3414/ME9244

Matthews, D., Hosker, J., Rudenski, A., Naylor, B., Treacher, D., & Turner, R. (1985). Homeostasis model assessment: Insulin resistance and beta-cell function from fasting plasma glucose and insulin concentrations in man. *Diabetologia*, *28*, 412–419. doi:10.1007/BF00280883

McAuley, K. A., Williams, S. M., Jim, I., Mann, D., Walker, R. J., & Lewis-Barned, N. J. (2001). Diagnosing insulin resistance in the general population. *Diabetes Care*, *24*(3), 460–464. doi:10.2337/diacare.24.3.460

McGlynn, E. A., Asch, S. M., Adams, J., Keesey, J., Hicks, J., DeCristofaro, A., & Kerr, E. A. (2003). The quality of health care delivered to adults in the United States. *The New England Journal of Medicine, 348*(26), 2635–2645. doi:10.1056/ NEJMsa022615

Mollon, B., Holbrook, A. M., Keshavjee, K., Troyan, S., Gaebel, K., Thabane, L., & Perera, G. (2008). Automated telephone reminder messages can assist electronic diabetes care. *Journal of Telemedicine and Telecare, 14*, 32–36. doi:10.1258/ jtt.2007.070702

Musen, M. A. (1997). Modelling of decision support. In Bemmel, J. H. V., & Musen, M. A. (Eds.), *Handbook of Medical Informatics* (pp. 1–26). Berlin, Germany: Springer-Verlag.

NDIC. (2008). *Diagnosis of diabetes.* Washington, DC: U.S. Department of Health and Human Services, National Institutes of Health.

NDIC. (2011). *National diabetes statistics, 2011.* Retrieved from http://diabetes. niddk.nih.gov/DM/PUBS/statistics/

Nijland, N., Seydel, E. R., Gemert-Pijnen, J. E. W. C. V., Brandenburg, B., Kelders, S. M., & Will, M. (2009). Evaluation of an internet-based application for supporting self-care of patients with diabetes mellitus type 2. In *Proceedings of the 2009 International Conference on eHealth, Telemedicine, and Social Medicine,* (pp. 46-51). IEEE.

O'Connor, P. (2003). Setting evidence-based priorities for diabetes care improvement. *International Journal for Quality in Health Care, 15*(4), 283–285. doi:10.1093/ intqhc/mzg062

O'Connor, P. J., Sperl-Hillen, J. M., Rush, W. A., Johnson, P. E., Amundson, G. H., & Asche, S. E. (2011). Impact of electronic health record clinical decision support on diabetes care: A randomized trial. *Annals of Family Medicine, 9*(1), 12–21. doi:10.1370/afm.1196

Sacket, D. L., Straus, S. E., Richardson, W. S., Rosenberg, W., & Haynes, R. B. (2000). *Evidence based medicine: How to practice & teach EBM.* New York, NY: Churchill Livingstone.

Sprague, R. H. (1980). A framework for the development of DSS. *Management Information Systems Quarterly, 4*(4), 1–26. doi:10.2307/248957

Tuomilehto, J., Lindstrom, J., Eriksson, J. G., Valle, T. T., Hamalainen, H., & Ilanne-Parikka, P. (2001). Finnish diabetes prevention study group: Prevention of type 2 diabetes mellitus by changes in lifestyle among subjects with impaired glucose tolerance. *The New England Journal of Medicine, 344*, 1343–1350. doi:10.1056/NEJM200105033441801

Wallace, T., Levy, J., & Matthews, D. (2004). Use and abuse of HOMA modeling. *Diabetes Care, 27*, 1487–1495. doi:10.2337/diacare.27.6.1487

Wears, R., & Berg, M. (2005). Computer technology and clinical work: Still waiting for Godot. *Journal of the American Medical Association, 293*(1261), 1–3.

WHO. (2011). *Diabetes*. Retrieved April 2, 2012, from http://www.who.int/media-centre/factsheets/fs312/en/

WHO/IDF. (2006). *Definition and diagnosis of diabetes mellitus and intermediate hyperglycemia*. Geneva, Switzerland: World Health Organization.

KEY TERMS AND DEFINITIONS

Clinical Decision Support Systems (CDSS): Any system that takes input as information about clinical situation, and produces as output inferences that can assist practitioners in their decision-making.

Diabetes Mellitus (DM): A chronic disease in which body fails to convert glucose (sugar) to energy.

Electronic Health Records (EHR): A systematic collection of patient health information in an electronic form.

Health Information Technology (HIT): Organizing medical information through computerized systems which involves the secure exchange of health information between patient, providers, and insurers.

Insulin Dependent Diabetes Mellitus (IDDM): A type of diabetes that arises due to failure of insulin production from the body and requires injecting insulin to survive.

Non-Insulin Dependent Diabetes Mellitus (NIDDM): Most common type of diabetes that arises due to a condition in which the cells fail to use insulin properly.

Pre-Diabetes: A condition where blood glucose levels are higher than normal but not high enough for a diagnosis of diabetes.

Compilation of References

AARDA. (2009). *American autoimmune related diseases association autoimmunity forum*. Retrieved from http://www.aarda.org/forum2/

Abell, D. (1997, Autumn/Fall). What makes a good case?. *European Case Clearing House*, 4-7.

Abraham, C., Watson, R. T., & Boudreau, M. (2008). Ubiquitous access: On the front lines of patient care and safety. *Communications of the ACM, 51*(6), 95–99. doi:10.1145/1349026.1349045

Adair, J. (2005). *How to grow leaders: The seven key principles of effective leadership development*. London, UK: Kogan Page.

Agarwal, R., Gao, G., DesRoches, C., & Jha, A. K. (2010). The digital transformation of healthcare: Current status and the road ahead. *Information Systems Research, 21*(4), 796–809. doi:10.1287/isre.1100.0327

AHCA. (2010). *Legal agreements for participation in the FHIN*. Florida Legal Work Group Memorandum. Retrieved November 14, 2011 from http://ahca.myflorida.com/schs/AdvisoryCouncil/AC061710/TabD-UpdateOnLegalWorkGroup.pdf

AHCA. (2011). *State health information exchange cooperative agreement program strategic and operational plans*. State Health Information Exchange Cooperative Agreement Program. Retrieved November 14, 2011 from http://www.fhin.net/pdf/floridaHie/StrategicandOperationalPlansApproved.pdf

AHIMA. (2005). Update: Maintaining a legally sound health record – Paper and electronic. *Journal of American Health Information Management Association, 76*(10), 64A–L.

AHIMA. (2010a). *Managing the transition from paper to EHRs*. Retrieved October 31, 2011, from http://library.ahima.org/xpedio/groups/public/documents/ahima/bok1_048418.hcsp?dDocName=bok1_048418

AHIMA. (2010b). *Information security—An overview*. Retrieved October 31, 2011, from http://library.ahima.org/xpedio/groups/public/documents/ahima/bok1_048962.hcsp?dDocName=bok1_048962

Ajzen, I., & Fishbein, M. (1980). *Understanding attitudes and predicting social behavior*. Englewood Cliffs, NJ: Prentice Hall.

Al-Gahtani, S. S. (2001). The applicability of TAM outside North America: An empirical test in the United Kingdom. *Information Resources Management Journal, 14*(3), 37–46. doi:10.4018/irmj.2001070104

Compilation of References

Altman, R. B. (1997). Informatics in the care of patients: Ten notable challenges. *The Western Journal of Medicine, 166*(2), 118–122.

American Telemedicine Association. (2011). *Removing medical licensure barriers: Increasing consumer choice, improving safety and cutting costs for patients across America.* Retrieved November 15, 2011, from http://www.fixlicensure.org

American Telemedicine Association. (2012). *American telemedicine association.* Retrieved from http://www.americantelemed.org/i4a/pages/index.cfm?pageid=1

Ammenwerth, E., Gräber, S., Herrmann, G., Bürkle, T., & König, J. (2003). Evaluation of health information systems—Problems and challenges. *International Journal of Medical Informatics, 71*(2-3), 125–135. doi:10.1016/S1386-5056(03)00131-X

Anantharaman, V., & Swee Han, L. (2001). Hospital and emergency ambulance link: Using IT to enhance emergency pre-hospital care. *International Journal of Medical Informatics, 61*(2-3), 147–161. doi:10.1016/S1386-5056(01)00137-X

Angeles, R. (2007). An empirical study of the anticipated consumer response to RFID product item tagging. *Industrial Management & Data Systems, 107*(4), 461–583. doi:10.1108/02635570710740643

Apple Inc. (2012). *Apple - FaceTime.* Retrieved from http://www.apple.com/mac/facetime/

Arnst, C. (2006, July 17). The best medical care in the US: How veteran affairs transformed itself and what it means for the rest of us. *Business Week,* 50–56.

Aron, R., Dutta, S., Janakiraman, R., & Pathak, P. A. (2011). The impact of automation of systems on medical errors: Evidence from field research. *Information Systems Research, 22*(3), 429–446. doi:10.1287/isre.1110.0350

Aronson, J., & Turban, E. (1998). *Decision support systems and intelligent systems.* Upper Saddle River, NJ: Prentice Hall.

Arsand, E., Varmedal, R., & Hartvigsen, G. (2007). *Usability of a mobile self-help tool for people with diabetes: The easy health diary.* Retrieved from http://munin.uit.no/bitstream/handle/10037/2762/paper_1.pdf?sequence=3

Årsand, E., Tufano, J. T., Ralston, J. D., & Hjortdahl, P. (2008). Designing mobile dietary management support technologies for people with diabetes. *Journal of Telemedicine and Telecare, 14*(7), 329–332. doi:10.1258/jtt.2008.007001

Ash, J. S., Sittig, D. F., Dykstra, R., Campbell, E., & Guappone, K. (2009). The unintended consequences of computerized provider order entry: Findings from a mixed methods exploration. *International Journal of Medical Informatics, 78*(S1), S69–S76. doi:10.1016/j.ijmedinf.2008.07.015

Assimacopoulos, A., Alam, R., Arbo, M., Nazir, J., Chen, D., Weaver, S., … Ageton, C. (2008, October). A brief retrospective review of medical records comparing outcomes for inpatients treated via telehealth versus in-person protocols: Is telehealth equally effective as in-person visits for treating neutropenic fever, bacterial pneumonia, and infected bacterial wounds?. *Telemedicine and e-Health,* 762-768.

Attewell, P. (1992). Technology diffusion and organizational learning: The case of business computing. *Organization Science, 3*(1), 1–19. doi:10.1287/orsc.3.1.1

Avera. (2012). *Avera medical group Pierre - Pierre, SD - Avera*. Retrieved from http://www.avera.org/clinics/pierre/index.aspx

Avgerou, C., & Cornford, T. (1993). *Developing information systems: Concepts, issues and practise*. Basingstroke, UK: Macmillan.

Balaji, P. G., & Srinivasan. (2010). Multi-agent system in urban traffic signal control. *IEEE Computational Intelligence Magazine, 5*(4), 43-51.

Bandura, A. (1977). Self-efficacy: Toward a unifying theory of behavioral change. *Psychological Review, 84*(2), 191–215. doi:10.1037/0033-295X.84.2.191

Bandura, A. (1986). *Social foundations of thought and action: A social cognitive theory*. Englewood Cliffs, NJ: Prentice Hall.

Barlett, J. G., Auwaerter, P. G., & Pham, P. (2012). *Johns Hopkins guides*. Baltimore, MD: Johns Hopkins Medicine.

Barnes, L. B., Christensen, C. R., & Hansen, A. J. (1994). *Teaching and the case method* (3rd ed.). Boston, MA: Harvard Business School Press.

Bates, D. W., & Gawande, A. A. (2003). Improving safety with information technology. *The New England Journal of Medicine, 348*(25), 2526–2534. doi:10.1056/NEJMsa020847

Baumgart, D. C. (2005). Personal digital assistants in health care: Experienced clinicians in the palm of your hand? *Lancet, 366*(9492), 1210–1222. Retrieved from http://www.ncbi.nlm.nih.gov/pubmed/16198770doi:10.1016/S0140-6736(05)67484-3

Beckley, E. T. (2005). Wellness goes wireless. *DOC News, 2*(6), 7.

Bellazzi, R. (2008). Telemedicine and diabetes management: Current challenges and future research directions. *Journal of Diabetes Science and Technology, 2*(1), 98–104.

Bell, L. M., Grundmeier, R., Localio, R., Zorc, J., Fiks, A. G., & Zhang, X. (2010). Electronic health record-based decision support to improve asthma care: A cluster-randomized trial. *Pediatrics, 125*(4), E770–E777. doi:10.1542/peds.2009-1385

Benveniste, G. (1987). *Professionalizing the organization*. San Francisco, CA: Jossey-Bass.

Berner, E. S. (2009). *Clinical decision support systems: State of the art*. Rockville, MD: Agency for Healthcare Research and Quality.

Bhuptani, M., & Moradpour, S. (2005). *RFID field guide - Deploying radio frequency identification systems*. Upper Saddle River, NJ: Prentice Hall.

Bigus, J. P., & Bigus, J. (1998). *Constructing intelligent software agents with java – A programmers guide to smarter applications*. New York, NY: Wiley.

Bloomrosen, M., & Detmer, D. E. (2010). Informatics, evidence-based care, and research: Implications for national policy: A report of an American medical informatics association health policy conference. *Journal of the American Medical Informatics Association, 2*(17), 115–123. doi:10.1136/jamia.2009.001370

Blumenthal, D. (2009). Stimulating the adoption of health information technology. *The New England Journal of Medicine, 360*(15), 1477–1479. doi:10.1056/NEJMp0901592

Compilation of References

Bodenheimer, T., & Pham, H. H. (2010). Primary care: Current problems and proposed solutions. *Health Affairs*, *29*(5), 799–805. doi:10.1377/hlthaff.2010.0026

Boehrer, J. (1995). *How to teach a case.* Boston, MA: Harvard.

Bosinski, T. J., Campbell, L., & Schwartz, S. (2004). Using a personal digital assistant to document pharmacotherapeutic interventions. *American Journal of Health-System Pharmacy*, *61*(9), 931–934.

Bourret, C., & Salzano, G. (2006). Data for decision making in networked health. *Data Science Journal*, *5*, 64–78. doi:10.2481/dsj.5.64

Broadlawns. (2010). *Broadlawns, UI hospitals and clinics share records electronically.* Retrieved July 20, 2011, from http://www.broadlawns.org/news.cfm?article=139

Broadlawns. (2011a). *Broadlawns medical center: Strategic business priorities.* Retrieved November 3, 2011, from http://www.broadlawns.org/pdfs/priorities2011.pdf

Broadlawns. (2011b). *Business service update to the finance committee.* Retrieved from http://www.broadlawns.org

Brodnik, M., McCain, M., Rinehart-Thompson, L., & Reynolds, R. (Eds.). (2009). *Fundamentals of law for health informatics and information management.* Chicago, IL: American Health Information Management Association.

Bureau of Primary Health Care. (2008, June). *Health centers: America's primary care safety net, reflections on success, 2002-2007.* Retrieved November 8, 2011 from http://www.hrsa.gov/ourstories/healthcenter/reflectionsonsuccess.pdf

Burke, L. E., Warziski, M., Starrett, T., Choo, J., Music, E., & Sereika, S. (2005). Self-monitoring dietary intake: Current and future practices. *Journal of Renal Nutrition*, *15*(3), 281–290. doi:10.1016/j.jrn.2005.04.002

Burley, L., & Scheepers, H. (2003). Emerging trends in mobile technology development: From healthcare professional to system developer. *International Journal of Healthcare Technology and Management*, *5*(3-5), 179–193. doi:10.1504/IJHTM.2003.004125

Campbell, S. (2011). XECAN and trimble partner to deliver thingmagic powered RFID oncology solution providing direct interface to EMR. *EMR Daily News.* Retrieved from http://emrdailynews.com/2011/09/28/xecan-and-trimble-partner-to-deliver-thingmagic-powered-rfid-oncology-solution-providing-direct-interface-to-emr/

Carroll, A. E., DiMeglio, L. A., Stein, S., & Marrero, D. G. (2011). Using a cell phone–based glucose monitoring system for adolescent diabetes management. *The Diabetes Educator*, *37*(1), 59–66. doi:10.1177/0145721710387163

Carroll, A. E., Marrero, D. G., & Downs, S. M. (2007). The HealthPia GlucoPack™ diabetes phone: A usability study. *Diabetes Technology & Therapeutics*, *9*(2), 158–164. doi:10.1089/dia.2006.0002

Carroll, C., Marsden, P., Soden, P., Naylor, E., New, J., & Dornan, T. (2002). Involving users in the design and usability evaluation of a clinical decision support system. *Computer Methods and Programs in Biomedicine*, *69*, 123–135. doi:10.1016/S0169-2607(02)00036-6

Cathy, H. (2010). *Cadiometabolic risk management: Addressing metabolic syndrome.* Health Dialog.

CDC. (2011). *National diabetes fact sheet, 2011.* Atlanta, GA: U.S. Department of Health and Human Services, Centers for Disease Control and Prevention.

CDC. (2012). *National diabetes prevention program.* Retrieved from http://www.cdc.gov/diabetes/prevention/about.htm

Centers for Medicare & Medicaid Services. (2009). *Revised appendix A: Interpretive guidelines for hospital.* Pub. 100-07 State Operations Provider Certification, Transmittal 47. Washington, DC: Centers for Medicare & Medicaid Services. Retrieved November 26, 2011, from https://www.cms.gov/transmittals/downloads/R47SOMA.pdf

Cercone, N., An, X., Li, J., Gu, Z., & An, A. (2011). Finding best evidence for evidence-based best practice recommendations in health care: The initial decision support system design. *Knowledge and Information Systems, 29*(1), 159–201. doi:10.1007/s10115-011-0439-8

Chignell, M., Yesha, Y., & Lo, J. (2010). *New methods for clinical decision support in hospitals.* Paper presented at the 2010 Conference of the Center for Advanced Studies on Collaborative Research. Toronto, Canada.

Chin, W. W. (1998a). Commentary: Issues and opinion on structural equation modeling. *Management Information Systems Quarterly, 22*(1), 7–16.

Chin, W. W. (1998b). The partial least squares approach for structural equation modelling. In Marcoulides, G. A. (Ed.), *Modern Methods for Business Research.* Hillsdale, NJ: Lawrence Erlbaum Associates.

Clark, J. S., & Klauck, J. A. (2003). Recording pharmacists' interventions with a personal digital assistant. *American Journal of Health-System Pharmacy, 60*(17), 1772–1774. Retrieved from http://www.ncbi.nlm.nih.gov/pubmed/14503114

Clark, T. D., Jones, M. C., & Armstrong, C. P. (2007). The dynamic structure of management support systems: Theory development, research focus and direction. *Management Information Systems Quarterly, 31*(3), 579–615.

Cline, J. (2007). *Growing pressure for data classification.* Retrieved from http://www.computerworld.com/action/article.do?articleId=9014071&command=viewArticleBasic

cms.gov. (2010). *CMD finalizes definition of meaningful use of certified electronic health records (EHR) technology.* Retrieved November 2, 2011, from https://www.cms.gov/apps/media/press/factsheet.asp?Counter=3794

cms.gov. (2011). *Overview EHR incentive programs.* Retrieved from https://www.cms.gov/ehrincentiveprograms/

Coiera, E. (1997). Artificial intelligence in medicine. In *Guide to Medical Informatics, the Internet and Telemedicine.* London, UK: Arnold.

Coiera, E. (2003). *Guide to health Informatics.* London, UK: Arnold.

Co, J. P. T., Johnson, S. A., Poon, E. G., Fiskio, J., Rao, S. R., & Van Cleave, J. (2010). Electronic health record decision support and quality of care for children with ADHD. *Pediatrics, 126*(2), 239–246. doi:10.1542/peds.2009-0710

Community Partners HealthNet, Inc. (2011). *Website.* Retrieved October 17, 2011, from http://www.cphealthnet.org/index.htm

Compilation of References

Compeau, D. R., & Higgins, C. A. (1995a). Application of social cognitive theory to training for computer skills. *Information Systems Research, 6*(2), 118–143. doi:10.1287/isre.6.2.118

Compeau, D. R., & Higgins, C. A. (1995b). Computer self-efficacy - Development of a measure and initial test. *Management Information Systems Quarterly, 19*(2), 189–211. doi:10.2307/249688

Crilly, P., & Muthukkumarasamy, V. (2010). Using smart phones and body sensors to deliver pervasive mobile personal healthcare. In *Proceedings of the 2010 Sixth International Conference on Intelligent Sensors Sensor Networks and Information Processing*, (pp. 291-296). IEEE Press.

Cronbach, L. (1951). Coefficient alpha and the internal structure of tests. *Psychometrika, 16*, 297–334. doi:10.1007/BF02310555

CSC. (2010). CSC mobile insurance. *Insurance Solutions*. Retrieved from http://assets1.csc.com/insurance/downloads/mobile_insurance_solutions.pdf

Dagogo-Jack, S. (2002). Preventing diabetes-related morbidity and mortality in the primary care setting. *Journal of the National Medical Association, 94*(7), 549–560.

Davenport, T. H., & Glaser, J. (2002). Just-in-time delivery comes to knowledge management. *Harvard Business Review, 80*(7), 107–111.

Davis, F. D. (1989). Perceived usefulness, perceived ease of use, and user acceptance of information technology. *Management Information Systems Quarterly, 13*(3), 319–340. doi:10.2307/249008

Dee, C. R., Teolis, M., & Todd, A. D. (2005). Physicians' use of the personal digital assistant (PDA) in clinical decision making. *Journal of the Medical Library Association, 93*(4), 480–486. Retrieved from http://www.pubmedcentral.nih.gov/articlerender.fcgi?artid=1250324&tool=pmcentrez&rendertype=abstract

DeFronzo, R., & Ferrannini, E. (1991). Insulin resistance: A multifaceted syndrome responsible for NIDDM, obesity, hypertension, dyslipidemia, and atherosclerotic cardiovascular disease. *Diabetes Care, 14*, 173–194. doi:10.2337/diacare.14.3.173

Department of Health and Human Services, Centers for Medicare and Medicaid Services. (2011). Medicare and medicaid programs: Changes affecting hospital and critical access hospital conditions of participation: Telemedicine credentialing and privileging. *Federal Register, 76*(87), 25550–25565. Retrieved from http://www.gpo.gov/fdsys/pkg/FR-2011-05-05/pdf/2011-10875.pdf

Department of Health and Human Services, Centers for Medicare and Medicaid Services. (2011). *Medicare learning network: Telehealth services, rural health fact sheet series*. Retrieved from https://www.cms.gov/MLNProducts/downloads/Telehealth-Srvcsfctsht.pdf

Department of Health and Human Services. (2011). *Website.* Retrieved November 14, 2011, from http://www.hhs.gov/ocr/privacy/hipaa/administrative/breachnotificationrule/index.html

DesRoches, C. M., Campbell, E. G., Rao, S. R., Donelan, K., Ferris, T. G., & Jha, A. (2008). Electronic health records in ambulatory care: A national survey of physicians. *The New England Journal of Medicine, 359*(1), 50–60. doi:10.1056/NEJMsa0802005

DiabeticsAnonymous. (2012). *Types of diabetes*. Retrieved May 7, 2012, from http://www.diabeticsanonymous.org/types.html

Dishaw, M. T., & Strong, D. M. (1999). Extending the technology acceptance model with task-technology fit constructs. *Information & Management*, *36*(1), 9. doi:10.1016/S0378-7206(98)00101-3

Do, H., & Rahin, E. (2002). Coma: A system for flexible combination of schema matching approaches. In *Proceedings of 28th Conference on Very Large Databases*, (pp. 610-621). San Francisco, CA: Morgan Kaufmann.

Doan, A.-H., Lu, Y., Lee, T., & Han, J. (2003). Profile-based object matching for information integration. *IEEE Intelligent Systems Magazine*, *18*(5), 54–59. doi:10.1109/MIS.2003.1234770

Doenges, M. E., Moorhouse, M. F., & Murr, A. C. (2010). Nurse's pocket guide. *F.A. Davis Company*. Retrieved from http://www.unboundmedicine.com/products/nurses_pocket_guide

Dolan, B. (2010). Number of smartphone health apps up 78 percent. *MobiHealthNews*. Retrieved from http://mobihealthnews.com/9396/number-of-smartphone-health-apps-up-78-percent/

Donaldson, M. S., Yordy, K. D., Lohr, K. N., & Vanselow, N. A. (Eds.). (1996). *Primary care: America's health in a new era*. Washington, DC: National Academy Press.

Doolan, D., Bates, D., & James, B. (2003). The use of computers for clinical care: A case series of advanced US sites. *Journal of the American Medical Informatics Association*, *10*, 94–107. doi:10.1197/jamia.M1127

Dorr, D., Bonner, L. M., Cohen, A. N., Shoai, R. S., Perrin, R., Chaney, E., & Young, A. S. (2007). Informatics systems to promote improved care for chronic illness: A literature review. *Journal of the American Medical Informatics Association*, *14*(2), 156–163. doi:10.1197/jamia.M2255

DPPRG. (2002). Diabetes prevention program research group: The diabetes prevention program: Reduction in the incidence of type 2 diabetes with lifestyle intervention or metformin. *The New England Journal of Medicine*, *346*, 393–403. doi:10.1056/NEJMoa012512

Drolet, B. C., & Johnson, K. B. (2008). Categorizing the world of registries. *Journal of Biomedical Informatics*, *41*(6), 1009–1020. doi:10.1016/j.jbi.2008.01.009

Dye, C. F. (2010). *Leadership in healthcare: Essential values and skills* (2nd ed.). Chicago, IL: Health Administration Press.

Dye, C., & Garman, A. (2006). *Exceptional leadership*. Chicago, IL: Health Administration Press.

Editor, A. (2011). App wrap. *Pharmacy Times*. Retrieved from http://www.pharmacytimes.com/publications/career/2011/PharmacyCareers_Spring2011/AppWrap

Edwards, J. (2009). PositiveID deal advances use of micrchip implants in Florida health system. *CBS News*. Retrieved from http://www.cbsnews.com/8301-505123_162-42843647/positiveid-deal-advances-use-of-microchip-implants-in-florida-health-system/

Einbinder, J. S., & Bates, D. W. (2007). Leveraging information technology to improve quality and safety. *Yearbook of Medical Informatics*, *2007*, 22–29.

Compilation of References

Eldar, R. (2002). Health technology: Challenge to public health. *Croatian Medical Journal, 43*(4), 470–474.

El-Gayar, O. F., Deokar, A. V., & Wills, M. (2009a). Evaluating task-technology fit for an electronic health record system. *International Journal of Healthcare Technology and Management, 11*(1/2), 50–65. Retrieved from http://www.inderscience.com/search/index.php?action=record&rec_id=33274doi:10.1504/IJHTM.2010.033274

El-Gayar, O. F., Deokar, A. V., & Wills, M. (2009b). Evaluating task-technology fit for an electronic health record system. In *Proceedings of the 15th Americas Conference on Information Systems*. San Francisco, CA: IEEE.

Elwyn, G., Greenhalgh, T., & Macfarlane, F. (2001). *Groups: A guide to small group work in healthcare, management, education and research*. Abingdon, UK: Radcliffe Publishing.

Ely, J., Osheroff, J., Ebell, M., Chambliss, M., Vinson, D., Stevermer, J., & Pifer, E. (2002). Obstacles to answering doctors' questions about patient care with evidence: Qualitative study. *British Medical Journal, 324*(7339), 710. doi:10.1136/bmj.324.7339.710

Epocrates. (2012). *Epocrates*. Retrieved from http://itunes.apple.com/us/app/epocrates/id281935788?mt=8

Espinoza, A., Garcia-Vazquez, J. P., Rodriguez, D. M., Andrade, A. G., & Garcia-Pena, C. (2009). Enhancing a wearable help button to support the medication adherence of older adults. *Web Congress*, 3-7.

Evangelista, L. S., & Shinnick, M. A. (2008). What do we know about adherence and self-care? *The Journal of Cardiovascular Nursing, 23*, 250–257.

Fahrni, J. (2009). *Tablet PCs in pharmacy practice*. Retrieved from http://www.jerryfahrni.com

Falk, R., & Miller, N. E. (1992). *A primer for soft modeling*. Akron, OH: University of Akron Press.

Faridi, Z., Liberti, L., Shuval, K., Northrup, V., Ali, A., & Katz, D. L. (2008). Evaluating the impact of mobile telephone technology on type 2 diabetic patients' self-management: The NICHE pilot study. *Journal of Evaluation in Clinical Practice, 14*(3), 465–469. doi:10.1111/j.1365-2753.2007.00881.x

Farmer, A., Gibson, O., Hayton, P., Bryden, K., Dudley, C., Neil, A., & Tarassenko, L. (2005). A real-time, mobile phone-based telemedicine system to support young adults with type 1 diabetes. *Informatics in Primary Care, 13*(3), 171–178.

Feature, S. (2008). Medication therapy management in pharmacy practice: core elements of an MTM service model (version 2.0). *Journal of the American Pharmacists Association, 48*(3), 341–353. Retrieved from http://www.ncbi.nlm.nih.gov/pubmed/16295642doi:10.1331/JAPhA.2008.08514

Feldstein, A. C., Vollmer, W. M., Smith, D. H., Petrik, A., Schneider, J., Glauber, H., & Herson, M. (2007). An outreach program improved osteoporosis management after a fracture. *Journal of the American Geriatrics Society, 55*(9), 1464–1469. doi:10.1111/j.1532-5415.2007.01310.x

Ferraiolo, D. F., & Kuhn, D. R. (1992). Role based access control. In *Proceedings of the 15th National Computer Security Conference*, (pp. 554-563). ACM.

Ferratt, T. W., & Vlahos, G. E. (1998). An investigation of task-technology fit for managers in Greece and the US. *European Journal of Information Systems*, *7*(2), 123. doi:10.1057/palgrave.ejis.3000288

Fichman, R., & Kemerer, C. (1997). The assimilation of software process innovations: An organizational learning perspective. *Management Science*, *43*(10), 1345–1363. doi:10.1287/mnsc.43.10.1345

Finkenzeller, K. (1999). *RFID handbook*. New York, NY: John Wiley and Sons Ltd.

Fischer, S., Stewart, T. E., Mehta, S., Wax, R., & Lapinsky, S. E. (2003). Handheld computing in medicine. *Journal of the American Medical Informatics Association*, *10*(2), 139–149. Retrieved from http://www.pubmedcentral.nih.gov/articlerender.fcgi?artid=150367&tool=pmcentrez&rendertype=abstractdoi:10.1197/jamia.M1180

Fishbein, M., & Ajzen, I. (1975). *Belief, attitude, intention and behavior: An introduction to theory and research*. Reading, MA: Addison-Wesley.

Ford, E., Giles, W., & Dietz, W. (2002). Prevalence of the metabolic syndrome among U.S. adults: Findings from the third national health and nutrition examination survey. *Journal of the American Medical Association*, *287*, 356–359. doi:10.1001/jama.287.3.356

Ford, S., Illich, S., Smith, L., & Franklin, A. (2006). Implementing personal digital assistant documentation of pharmacist interventions in a military treatment facility. *Journal of the American Pharmacists Association*, *46*(5), 589–593. doi:10.1331/1544-3191.46.5.589.Ford

Forjuoh, S. N., Reis, M. D., Couchman, G. R., & Ory, M. G. (2008). Improving diabetes self-care with a PDA in ambulatory care. *Telemedicine and e-Health*, *14*(3), 273-279.

Forjuoh, S. N., Reis, M. D., Couchman, G. R., Ory, M. G., Mason, S., & Molonket-Lanning, S. (2007). Incorporating PDA use in diabetes self-care: A central Texas primary care research network (CenTexNet) study. *Journal of the American Board of Family Medicine*, *20*(4), 375–384. doi:10.3122/jabfm.2007.04.060166

Fornell, C., & Larcker, D. F. (1981). Structural equation models with unobservable variables and measurement error - Algebra and statistics. *JMR, Journal of Marketing Research*, *18*(3), 382–388. doi:10.2307/3150980

Fox, B. I., Felkey, B. G., Berger, B. A., Krueger, K. P., & Rainer, R. K. (2007). Use of personal digital assistants for documentation of pharmacists' interventions: A literature review. *American Journal of Health-System Pharmacy*, *64*(14), 1516–1525. Retrieved from http://www.ncbi.nlm.nih.gov/pubmed/17617503doi:10.2146/ajhp060152

FreeDictionary. (2012). *Diabetes management*. Retrieved 05, 2012, from http://medical-dictionary.thefreedictionary.com/knowledge%3A+diabetes+management

Freund, A., Johnson, S. B., Silverstein, J., & Thomas, J. (1991). Assessing daily management of childhood diabetes using 24-hour recall interviews: Reliability and stability. *Health Psychology*, *10*(3), 200. doi:10.1037/0278-6133.10.3.200

Compilation of References

Fukuo, W., Yoshiuchi, K., Ohashi, K., Togashi, H., Sekine, R., & Kikuchi, H. (2009). Development of a hand-held personal digital assistant–based food diary with food photographs for japanese subjects. *Journal of the American Dietetic Association, 109*(7), 1232–1236. doi:10.1016/j.jada.2009.04.013

Gardner, D. G. (Ed.). (2011). *Greenspan's basic & clinical endocrinology* (9th ed.). New York, NY: McGraw Hill Medical.

Garg, A. X., Adhikari, N. K. J., McDonald, H., Rosas-Arellano, M. P., Devereaux, P. J., & Beyene, J. (2005). Effects of computerized clinical decision support system on practitioner performance and patients outcomes. *Journal of the American Medical Association, 293*(10), 1223–1238. doi:10.1001/jama.293.10.1223

Gefen, D., & Straub, D. (2005). A practical guide to factorial validity using PLS-GRAPH: Tutorial and annotated example. *Communication of the AIS, 16*, 91–109.

Global Medicine, A. M. D. Inc. (2012). *Telemedicine equipment and telehealth technologies*. Retrieved from http://www.amdtelemedicine.com

Glover, B., & Bhatt, H. (2006). *RFID essentials*. New York, NY: O'Reilly Media.

Goodenough, S. (2009). Semantic interoperability, e-health and Australian health statistics. *Health Information Management Journal, 2*(38), 41–45.

Goodhue, D. L. (1988). IS attitudes: Toward theoretical and definition clarity. *Database, 19*(3-4), 6–15.

Goodhue, D. L. (1995). Understanding user evaluations of information systems. *Management Science, 41*(12), 1827. doi:10.1287/mnsc.41.12.1827

Goodhue, D. L. (1998). Development and measurement validity of a task-technology fit instrument for user evaluations of information systems. *Decision Sciences, 29*(1), 105. doi:10.1111/j.1540-5915.1998.tb01346.x

Goodhue, D. L., Klein, B. D., & March, S. T. (2000). User evaluations of IS as surrogates for objective performance. *Information & Management, 38*(2), 87. doi:10.1016/S0378-7206(00)00057-4

Goodhue, D. L., & Thompson, R. L. (1995). Task-technology fit and individual performance. *Management Information Systems Quarterly, 19*(2), 213. doi:10.2307/249689

Graham, M., Chignell, M., & Takeshita, H. (2002). *Design of documentation for handheld ergonomics: Presenting clinical evidence at the point of care*. Paper presented at the 20th Annual International Conference on Computer Documentation. Toronto, Canada.

Greaves, P., Sullivan, C., Nguyen, H., McBride, J., Rawlins, L., & Kragh, J. ... David, B. (2007). *Florida health information network architectural considerations for state infrastructure draft white paper*. Prepared for Governor's Health Information Infrastructure Advisory Board. Retrieved November 14, 2011 from http://www.oregon.gov/OHA/OHPR/HIIAC/WebOnlyMaterials/FloridaWhitePaper4.19.07.pdf?ga=t

Greenhalgh, T., Potts, H. W. W., Wong, G., Bark, P., & Swinglehurst, D. (2009). Tensions and paradoxes in electronic patient record research: A systematic literature review using the meta-narrative method. *The Milbank Quarterly, 87*(4), 729–788. doi:10.1111/j.1468-0009.2009.00578.x

Grimson, J., Grimson, W., & Hasselbring, W. (2001). The SI challenge in healthcare. *Communications of the ACM, 43*(6), 49–55.

Grover, F. L. (2001). A decade's experience with quality improvement in cardiac surgery using the veterans affairs and society of thoracic surgeons national databases. *Annals of Surgery, 4*(234), 464–474. doi:10.1097/00000658-200110000-00006

Gupta, A. (2007). Information systems and healthcare XVII: A HL7v3-based mediating schema approach to data transfer between heterogeneous health care systems. *Communications of the Association for Information Systems, 19*, 622–636.

Gururajan, R., & Murugesan, S. (2005). *Wireless solutions developed for the Australian healthcare: A review.* Retrieved from http://portal.acm.org/citation.cfm?id=1084254

Gustafson, K. L., & Branch, R. M. (2002). What is instructional design? In Reiser, R. A., & Dempsey, J. V. (Eds.), *Trends and Issues in Instructional Design and Technology.* Columbus, OH: Merrill Prentice Hall.

Hair, J. F., Black, B., Babin, B., Anderson, R. E., & Tatham, R. L. (2006). *Multivariate data analysis* (6th ed.). Upper Saddle River, NJ: Prentice Hall.

Halamka, J. D. (2007). A chip in my shoulder. *Life as a Healthcare CIO.* Retrieved from http://geekdoctor.blogspot.com/2007/12/chip-in-my-shoulder.html

Hammermeister, K. E., Johnson, R., Marshall, G., & Grover, F. L. (1994). Continuous assessment and improvement in quality of care: A model from the department of veterans affairs cardiac surgery. *Annals of Surgery, 219*(3), 281–290. doi:10.1097/00000658-199403000-00008

Hammond, W. E. (2010). Connecting information to improve health. *Health Affairs, 29*(2), 285–290. doi:10.1377/hlthaff.2009.0903

Hanauer, D. A., Wentzell, K., Laffel, N., & Laffel, L. M. (2009). Computerized automated reminder diabetes system (CARDS): E-mail and SMS cell phone text messaging reminders to support diabetes management. *Diabetes Technology & Therapeutics, 11*(2), 99–106. doi:10.1089/dia.2008.0022

Harris, M. (1995). *Summary in diabetes in America* (2nd ed.). Bethesda, MD: National Institute of Diabetes and Digestive and Kidney Diseases, National Institutes of Health.

Haux, R. (2006). Health information systems - Past, present, future. *International Journal of Medical Informatics, 75*(3-4), 268–281. Retrieved from http://www.ncbi.nlm.nih.gov/pubmed/16169771doi:10.1016/j.ijmedinf.2005.08.002

Haywood, J., Haywood, B., & Jeff, C. (2004). *Patients like me.* Retrieved from http://www.patientslikeme.com

Health Resources and Services Administration. (2011a). *What are the benefits of a health center controlled network?* Retrieved October 18, 2011, from http://www.hrsa.gov/healthit/toolbox/HealthITAdoptiontoolbox/OpportunitiesCollaboration/benefitsofhccn.html

Health Resources and Services Administration. (2011b). *What is a health center controlled network?* Retrieved October 17, 2011, from http://www.hrsa.gov/healthit/toolbox/HealthITAdoptiontoolbox/OpportunitiesCollaboration/abouthccns.html

Health Resources and Services Administration. (2011c). *Program requirements.* Retrieved October 19, 2011, from http://bphc.hrsa.gov/about/requirements/hcpreqs.pdf

Healthcare Information and Management Systems Society. (2011). *Electronic health record*. Retrieved November 9, 2011, from http://www.himss.org/ASP/topics_ehr.asp

Hedgepeth, W. O. (2007). *RFID metrics: Decision making tools for today's supply chains*. Boca Raton, FL: CRC Press.

hhs.gov. (2009). *HITECH act enforcement interim final rule*. Retrieved November 7, 2011, from http://www.hhs.gov/ocr/privacy/hipaa/administrative/enforcementrule/hitech-enforcementifr.html

hhs.gov. (2010). *Secretary Sebelius announces final rules to support 'meaningful use' of electronic health records*. Retrieved November 7, 2011, from http://www.hhs.gov/news/press/2010pres/07/20100713a.html

HIMSS. (2011). *HIMSS mobile technology survey*. Retrieved from http://www.longwoods.com/blog/wp-content/uploads/2012/04/HIMSS-Mobile-Technology-Survey-FINAL-Revised-120511-Cover.pdf

HIMSS. (2011). *Improving outcomes with clinical decision support: An implementer's guide* (2nd ed.). Chicago, IL: HIMSS.

himssanalytics.org. (2011a). *U.S. EMR adoption model trends*. Retrieved October 25, 2011, from http://www.himssanalytics.org/docs/HA_EMRAM_Overview_ENG.pdf

Hinder, S., & Greenhalgh, T. (2012). This does my head in: Ethnographic study of self-management by people with diabetes. *BMC Health Services Research, 12*, 83. doi:10.1186/1472-6963-12-83

Hirsch, L., & Gandolf, S. (2011). Nothing personal, but doctors still fear social media in physician marketing. *Healthcare Success*. Retrieved from http://www.healthcaresuccess.com/blog/physician-marketing/nothing-personal-but-doctors-still-fear-social-media-in-physician-marketing.html

Holly, J. L. (2010). *The importance and content of a diabetes prevention program (DPP)*. Chicago, IL: Healthcare Information and Management Systems Society (HIMSS).

Holzman, T. G. (1999). Computer-human interface solutions for emergency medical care. *Interaction, 6*(3), 13–24. doi:10.1145/301153.301160

Hunt, D., Haynes, R., Hanna, S., & Smith, K. (1998). Effects of computer based clinical decision support systems on physician performance and patient outcomes: A systematic review. *Journal of the American Medical Association, 280*(15), 1339–1346. doi:10.1001/jama.280.15.1339

Hussain, I. (2011). Emergency room doctors number one consumers of mobile, pathologists last, per report of physician mobile use. *iMedicalApps: Moible Medical App Reviews & Commentary by Medical Professionals*. Retrieved from http://www.imedicalapps.com/2011/04/doctors-consumers-mobile-use/

IDF. (2011). *About world diabetes day*. Retrieved from http://www.idf.org/worlddiabetesday/about

iHealthBeat. (2009). More physicians use smartphones, PDAs in Clinical care. *California HealthCare Foundation*. Retrieved from http://www.ihealthbeat.org/Articles/2009/1/6/More-Physicians-Use-Smartphones-PDAs-in-Clinical-Care.aspx

Inami, M., Kawakami, N., Sekiguchi, D., & Yanagida, Y. (2000). Visuo-haptic display using head-mounted projector. In *Proceedings IEEE* (IEEE Press.). *Virtual Reality (Waltham Cross), 2000*, 233–240.

Inmon, W. H. (2005). *Building the data warehouse* (4th ed.). Indianapolis, IN: Wiley.

Inmon, W. H. (2011). Corporate information factory. *Glossary of Data Warehousing*. Retrieved November 10, 2011, from http://www.inmoncif.com/library/glossary/#D

Institute of Medicine. (2001). *Crossing the quality chasm: A new health system for the 21st century*. Washington, DC: National Academy Press.

iowa.gov. (2010). *Iowacare medical home model*. Retrieved November 1, 2011, from http://www.idph.state.ia.us/hcr_committees/common/pdf/prevention_chronic_care_mgmt/082710_model.pdf

iowa.gov. (2011). *IowaCare - Medicaid reform*. Retrieved October 25, 2011, from http://www.ime.state.ia.us/IowaCare/

Istepanian, R. S. H., Zitouni, K., Harry, D., Moutosammy, N., Sungoor, A., Tang, B., & Earle, K. A. (2009). Evaluation of a mobile phone telemonitoring system for glycaemic control in patients with diabetes. *Journal of Telemedicine and Telecare, 15*(3), 125–128. doi:10.1258/jtt.2009.003006

Ivanov, I. E., Gueorguiev, V., Bodurski, V., & Trifonov, V. (2010). Telemedicine and smart phones as medical peripheral devices (computational approaches). In *Proceedings of the 2010 Developments in Esystems Engineering,* (pp. 3-6). IEEE Press.

Jenner, J. (2011). *Report to the community*. Retrieved November 2, 2001, from http://www.broadlawns.org/pdfs/REPORT_TO_COMMUNITY_09_10.pdf

Johnson, S. B., Silverstein, J., Rosenbloom, A., Carter, R., & Cunningham, W. (1986). Assessing daily management in childhood diabetes. *Health Psychology, 5*(6), 545. doi:10.1037/0278-6133.5.6.545

Jones, D., & Curry, W. (2006). Impact of a PDA-based diabetes electronic management system in a primary care office. *American Journal of Medical Quality, 21*(6), 401–407. doi:10.1177/1062860606293594

Junglas, I., Abraham, C., & Watson, R. T. (2008). Task-technology fit for mobile locatable information systems. *Decision Support Systems, 45*(4), 1046. doi:10.1016/j.dss.2008.02.007

Kaiser Permanente. (2012). *Kaiser Permanente: On the go? Use our mobile app to stay connected*. Retrieved from http://mydoctor.kaiserpermanente.org/ncal/facilities/region/santarosa/area_master/members/mobile_app.jsp

Kanouse, D. E., Kallich, J. D., & Kahan, J. P. (1995). Dissemination of effectiveness and outcomes research. *Health Policy (Amsterdam), 34*(3), 167–192. doi:10.1016/0168-8510(95)00760-1

Kanter, R. M. (2001). *Evolve: Succeeding in the digital culture of tomorrow*. Boston, MA: Harvard Business Publisher.

Kaplan, B. (2001). Evaluating informatics applications - Some alternative approaches: Theory, social interactionism, and call for methodological pluralism. *International Journal of Medical Informatics, 64*(1), 39–55. doi:10.1016/S1386-5056(01)00184-8

Compilation of References

Kawamoto, K., Houlihan, C. A., Balas, E. A., & Lobach, D. F. (2005). Improving clinical practice using decision support systems: A systematic review of trials to identify features critical to success. *British Medical Journal, 330*(7494). doi:10.1136/bmj.38398.500764.8F

Khuri, S. F. (1998). The department of veterans affairs NSQIP – The first national, validated, outcome-based, risk-adjusted and peer-controlled program for the measurement and enhancement of the quality of surgical care. *Annals of Surgery, 228*(4), 491–507. doi:10.1097/00000658-199810000-00006

Kimball, R., & Caserta, J. (2004). *The data warehouse ETL toolkit: Practical techniques for extracting, cleaning, conforming, and delivering data*. Indianapolis, IN: Wiley.

King, H., Aubert, R., & Herman, W. (1998). Global burden of diabetes, 1995-2025. *Diabetes Care, 21*, 1414–1431. doi:10.2337/diacare.21.9.1414

Kinkade, S., & Verclas, K. (2008). Wireless technology for social change: Trends in mobile use by NGOs authors. *Communication, 2*(2), 1–59.

Kirk, J. K., Bertoni, A. G., Grzywacz, J. G., Smith, A., & Arcury, T. A. (2008). Evaluation of quality of diabetes care in a multiethnic, low-income population. *Journal of Clinical Outcomes Management, 15*(6), 281–286.

Kizer, K. W., & Dudley, R. A. (2009). Extreme makeover: Transformation of the veterans health care system. *Annual Review of Public Health, 30*, 313–339. doi:10.1146/annurev.publhealth.29.020907.090940

klasresearch.com. (1996). *Company - KLAS helps healthcare providers by measuring vendor performance.* Retrieved November 4, 2011, from http://www.klasresearch.com/About/Company.aspx

Klopping, I., & McKinney, E. (2004). Extending the technology acceptance model and the task-technology fit model to consumer e-commerce. *Information Technology, Learning and Performance Journal, 22*(1), 35.

Koch, S. (2010). Healthy ageing supported by technology-A cross-disciplinary research challenge. *Informatics for Health & Social Care, 35*(3-4), 81–91. doi:10.3109/17538157.2010.528646

Kohn, L. T., Corrigan, J. M., & Donaldson, M. S. (1999). *To err is human: Building a safer health system.* Washington, DC: National Academy Press.

Kollmann, A., Riedl, M., Kastner, P., Schreier, G., & Ludvik, B. (2007). Feasibility of a mobile phone–based data service for functional insulin treatment of type 1 diabetes mellitus patients. *Journal of Medical Internet Research, 9*(5). doi:10.2196/jmir.9.5.e36

Konstantas, D. (2007). An overview of wearable and implantable medical sensors. *Yearbook of Medical Informatics.* Retrieved from http://www.ncbi.nlm.nih.gov/pubmed/17700906

Korhonen, I., Pärkkä, J., & Van Gils, M. (2003). Health monitoring in the home of the future. *IEEE Engineering in Medicine and Biology Magazine, 22*(3), 66–73. doi:10.1109/MEMB.2003.1213628

Kowalke, M. (2006). RFID vs. WiFi for hospital inventory tracking systems. *TMCnet Wireless Mobility Blog*. Retrieved from http://blog.tmcnet.com/wireless-mobility/rfid-vs-wifi-for-hospital-inventory-tracking-systems.asp

Krishna, S., & Boren, S. A. (2008). Diabetes self-management care via cell phone: A systematic review. *Journal of Diabetes Science and Technology, 2*(3), 509.

Krogh, P. R., Rough, S., & Thomley, S. (2008). Comparison of two personal-computer-based mobile devices to support pharmacists' clinical documentation. *American Journal of Health-System Pharmacy, 65*(2), 154–157. doi:10.2146/ajhp070177

Kubben, P. L., Van Santbrink, H., Cornips, E. M. J., Vaccaro, A. R., Dvorak, M. F., Van Rhijn, L. W., et al. (2011). An evidence-based mobile decision support system for subaxial cervical spine injury treatment. *Surgical Neurology International, 2*, 32. Retrieved from http://www.pubmedcentral.nih.gov/articlerender.fcgi?artid=3086168&tool=pmcentrez&rendertype=abstract

Laerhoven, K. V., Lo, B. P. L., Ng, J. W. P., Thiemjarus, S., King, R., Kwan, S., et al. (2004). Medical healthcare monitoring with wearable and implantable sensors. *UbiHealth Workshop*. Retrieved from http://www.healthcare.pervasive.dk/ubicomp2004/papers/final_papers/laerhoven.pdf

Lakkaraju, S., & Moran, M. (2011). A framework to investigate the role of mobile technology in the healthcare organizations. In *Proceedings of MWAIS*. MWAIS.

Landro, L. (2010). How life's details help patients. *The Wall Street Journal: The Informed Patient*. Retrieved from http://online.wsj.com/article/SB10001424052748703960004575427531544486778.html

Lapinsky, S., Mehta, S., Varkul, M., & Stewart, T. (2000). Qualitative analysis of handheld computers in critical care. In *Proceedings of the AMIA Symposium*, (p. 1060). AMIA.

Lapinsky, S. E., Weshler, J., Mehta, S., Varkul, M., Hallett, D., & Stewart, T. E. (2001). Handheld computers in critical care. *Critical Care (London, England), 5*(4), 227–231. Retrieved from http://www.pubmedcentral.nih.gov/articlerender.fcgi?artid=37409&tool=pmcentrez&rendertype=abstractdoi:10.1186/cc1028

Leeuwen, A. M. V., Poelhuis-Leth, D. J., & Bladh, M. L. (2011). Davis's laboratory and diagnostic tests. *F.A. Davis Company*. Retrieved from www.unboundmedicine.com/products/davis_labs_diagnostic_tests

Lefkowitz, B. (2005). The health center story: Forty years of commitment. *The Journal of Ambulatory Care Management, 28*(4), 295–303.

Leong, T.-Y., Kaiser, K., & Miksch, S. (2007). Free and open source enabling technologies for patient-centric, guideline-based clinical decision support: A survey. *Yearbook of Medical Informatics, 207*, 74–86.

LeRouge, C., Mantzana, V., & Wilson, E. V. (2007). Healthcare information systems research, revelations and visions. *European Journal of Information Systems, 16*, 669–671. doi:10.1057/palgrave.ejis.3000712

Lewin, K., & Minton, J. (1986). Determining organization effectiveness: Another look and an agenda for research. *Management Science, 32*(5). doi:10.1287/mnsc.32.5.514

Compilation of References

Lewin, M. E., & Altman, S. (Eds.). (2000). *America's health care safety net: Intact but endangered*. Washington, DC: National Academy Press.

Lexicomp. (2012). *Lexicomp*. Retrieved from http://itunes.apple.com/us/app/lexicomp/id313401238?mt=8

Lin, T.-C., & Huang, C.-C. (2008). Understanding knowledge management system usage antecedents: An integration of social cognitive theory and task technology fit. *Information & Management, 45*(6), 410. doi:10.1016/j.im.2008.06.004

Logan, A. G., McIsaac, W. J., Tisler, A., Irvine, M. J., Saunders, A., & Dunai, A. (2007). Mobile phone-based remote patient monitoring system for management of hypertension in diabetic patients. *American Journal of Hypertension, 20*(9), 942–948. doi:10.1016/j.amjhyper.2007.03.020

Longman, P. (2005). The best care anywhere. *The Washington Monthly, 37*, 1–2.

Loo, G. S., & Lee, P. C. H. (2001). *A soft systems methodology model for clinical decision support systems (SSMM-CDSS)*. Paper presented at the 12th International Workshop on Database and Expert Systems Applications. Munich, Germany.

lssdata.com. (2010). *Broadlawns medical center emerges as a health IT leader in Iowa*. Retrieved September 18, 2011, from http://www.lssdata.com/news/viewnews.php?n=146

Lu, Y. C., Xiao, Y., Sears, A., & Jacko, J. A. (2005). A review and a framework of handheld computer adoption in healthcare. *International Journal of Medical Informatics, 74*(5), 409–422. doi:10.1016/j.ijmedinf.2005.03.001

Luz, P. L. D., Favarato, D., Junior, J. R. F.-N., Lemos, P., & Chagas, A. C. P. (2008). High ratio of triglycerides to HDL-cholesterol predicts extensive coronary disease. *Clinics (Sao Paulo, Brazil), 63*(4), 427–432. doi:10.1590/S1807-59322008000400003

Ma, Y., Olendzki, B. C., Chiriboga, D., Rosal, M., Sinagra, E., & Crawford, S. (2006). PDA-assisted low glycemic index dietary intervention for type II diabetes: A pilot study. *European Journal of Clinical Nutrition, 60*(10), 1235–1243. doi:10.1038/sj.ejcn.1602443

Manos, D. (2009, March 25). New study shows few hospitals have comprehensive EHR. *Healthcare IT News*.

Marcus, A., Davidzon, G., Law, D., Verma, N., Fletcher, R., Khan, A., & Sarmenta, L. (2009). Using NFC-enabled mobile phones for public health in developing countries. In *Proceedings of the 2009 First International Workshop on Near Field Communication*, (pp. 30-35). IEEE Press.

Markus, L., & Robey, D. (1988). Information technology and organizational change: Causal structure in theory and research. *Management Science, 34*(5), 583–598. doi:10.1287/mnsc.34.5.583

Mathieson, K., & Keil, M. (1998). Beyond the interface: Ease of use and task/technology fit. *Information & Management, 34*(4), 221. doi:10.1016/S0378-7206(98)00058-5

Matsumura, Y., Yamaguchi, T., Hasegawa, H., Yoshihara, K., Zhang, Q., Mineno, T., & Takeda, H. (2009). Alert system for inappropriate prescriptions relating to patients' clinical condition. *Methods of Information in Medicine, 48*(6), 566–573. doi:10.3414/ME9244

Matthews, D., Hosker, J., Rudenski, A., Naylor, B., Treacher, D., & Turner, R. (1985). Homeostasis model assessment: Insulin resistance and beta-cell function from fasting plasma glucose and insulin concentrations in man. *Diabetologia, 28*, 412–419. doi:10.1007/BF00280883

Mayo Clinic. (2012). *MayClinic app for patients: Patient app.* Retrieved from http://www.mayoclinic.org/mayo-apps/

Mcalearney, A. S., & Medow, M. A. (2004, March). Handheld computers in clinical practice: Implementation strategies and challenges. *Leadership*, 1–68.

McAlearney, A. S., Schweikhart, S. B., & Medow, M. A. (2004). Doctors' experience with handheld computers in clinical practice: qualitative study. *BMJ (Clinical Research Ed.), 328*(7449), 1162. doi:10.1136/bmj.328.7449.1162

McAuley, K. A., Williams, S. M., Jim, I., Mann, D., Walker, R. J., & Lewis-Barned, N. J. (2001). Diagnosing insulin resistance in the general population. *Diabetes Care, 24*(3), 460–464. doi:10.2337/diacare.24.3.460

McCreadie, S. R., & McGregory, M. E. (2005). Experiences incorporating tablet PCcs into clinical pharmacists' workflow. *Journal of Healthcare Information Management, 19*(4), 32–37. Retrieved from http://www.ncbi.nlm.nih.gov/pubmed/16266030

McDonald, C. J. (1997). The barriers to electronic medical record systems and how to overcome them. *Journal of the American Medical Informatics Association, 4*(3), 213–221. doi:10.1136/jamia.1997.0040213

Mcfadden, T., & Indulska, J. (2004). Context-aware environments for independent living. *Science*, 1–6. Retrieved from http://archive.itee.uq.edu.au/~pace/publications/public/mcfadden-era2004.pdf

McGinn, C. A., Grenier, S., Duplantie, J., Shaw, N., Sicotte, C., & Mathieu, L. (2011). Comparison of user groups' perspectives of barriers and facilitators to implementing electronic health records: A systematic review. *BMC Medicine, 9*(1), 46–55. doi:10.1186/1741-7015-9-46

McGlynn, E. A., Asch, S. M., Adams, J., Keesey, J., Hicks, J., DeCristofaro, A., & Kerr, E. A. (2003). The quality of health care delivered to adults in the United States. *The New England Journal of Medicine, 348*(26), 2635–2645. doi:10.1056/NEJMsa022615

McGrath, K., Hendy, J., Klecun, E., & Young, T. (2008). The vision and reality of 'connecting for health': Tensions, opportunities and policy implications of the UK national programme. *Communications of the Association for Information Systems, 23*, 603–618.

McGraw, G. (2006). *Software security.* Reading, MA: Addison-Wesley.

meditech.com. (2011a). *MEDITECH at a glance.* Retrieved October 30, 2011, from http://www.meditech.com/AboutMeditech/pages/ataglance.htm

meditech.com. (2011b). *MEDITECH mission statement.* Retrieved October 30, 2011, from http://www.meditech.com/AboutMeditech/pages/mission.htm

Menachemi, N., & Brooks, R. G. (2006). EHR and other IT adoption among physicians: Results of a large-scale statewide analysis. *Journal of Healthcare Information Management, 20*(3), 79–87.

Compilation of References

Mickey, K. (2004). RFID grew in 2002. *Traffic World, 5*, 20–21.

Miller, N. E., & Dollard. (1941). *Social learning and limitation.* New Haven, CT: Yale University Press.

Miller, R., & Sim, I. (2004). Physicians' use of electronic medical records: Barriers and solutions. *Health Affairs, 23*(2), 116–126. doi:10.1377/hlthaff.23.2.116

Mintzberg, H. (1983). *Structure in fives: Designing effective organizations.* Englewood Cliffs, NJ: Prentice Hall.

Mohammadian, M., & Jentzsch, R. (2007). Intelligent agent framework for RFID. In *Web Mobile-Based Applications for Healthcare Management* (pp. 316–335). New York, NY: IRM Publishing. doi:10.4018/978-1-59140-658-7.ch014

Mohammadian, M., & Jentzsch, R. (2008). Intelligent agent framework for secure patient-doctor profiling and profile matching. *International Journal of Healthcare Information Systems and Informatics, 1*, 1–10.

Mollon, B., Holbrook, A. M., Keshavjee, K., Troyan, S., Gaebel, K., Thabane, L., & Perera, G. (2008). Automated telephone reminder messages can assist electronic diabetes care. *Journal of Telemedicine and Telecare, 14*, 32–36. doi:10.1258/jtt.2007.070702

Mougiakakou, S. G., Kouris, I., Iliopoulou, D., Vazeou, A., & Koutsouris, D. (2009). Mobile technology to empower people with diabetes mellitus: Design and development of a mobile application. In *Proceedings of Information Technology and Applications in Biomedicine.* IEEE Press. doi:10.1109/ITAB.2009.5394344

Mulvaney, S. A., Rothman, R. L., Dietrich, M. S., Wallston, K. A., Grove, E., Elasy, T. A., & Johnson, K. B. (2012). Using mobile phones to measure adolescent diabetes adherence. *Health Psychology, 31*(1), 43. doi:10.1037/a0025543

Musen, M. A. (1997). Modelling of decision support. In Bemmel, J. H. V., & Musen, M. A. (Eds.), *Handbook of Medical Informatics* (pp. 1–26). Berlin, Germany: Springer-Verlag.

Myers, M., & Newman, M. (2007). The qualitative interview in IS research: Examining the craft. *Information and Organization, 17*(1), 2–26. doi:10.1016/j.infoandorg.2006.11.001

Nanji, K. C., Rothschild, J. M., Salzberg, C., Keohane, C. A., Zigmont, K., & Devita, J. (2011). Errors associated with outpatient computerized prescribing systems. *Journal of the American Medical Informatics Association, 18*(6), 767–773. doi:10.1136/amiajnl-2011-000205

National Association of Community Health Centers. (2010). *Fact sheet - Community health centers: The return on investment.* Retrieved October 13, 2011, from http://www.nachc.org/client/documents/CHCs%20ROI%20final%2011%2015%20v.pdf

Naumes, W., & Naumes, M. (2006). *The art & craft of case writing.* Armonk, NY: M.E. Sharpe.

NDIC. (2008). *Diagnosis of diabetes.* Washington, DC: U.S. Department of Health and Human Services, National Institutes of Health.

NDIC. (2011). *National diabetes statistics, 2011.* Retrieved from http://diabetes.niddk.nih.gov/DM/PUBS/statistics/

Newbolt, S. K. (2003). New uses for wireless technology. *Nursing Management, 22*, 22–32. doi:10.1097/00006247-200310002-00006

Niazkhani, Z., Pirnejad, H., Berg, M., & Aarts, J. (2009). The impact of computerized provider order entry systems on inpatient clinical workflow: A literature review. *Journal of the American Medical Informatics Association, 16*(4), 539–549. doi:10.1197/jamia.M2419

Nijland, N., Seydel, E. R., Gemert-Pijnen, J. E. W. C. V., Brandenburg, B., Kelders, S. M., & Will, M. (2009). Evaluation of an internet-based application for supporting self-care of patients with diabetes mellitus type 2. In *Proceedings of the 2009 International Conference on eHealth, Telemedicine, and Social Medicine*, (pp. 46-51). IEEE.

Nolan, L., et al. (2005). *An assessment of hospital-sponsored health care for the uninsured in Polk County/Des Moines, Iowa*. Unpublished.

North Carolina Community Health Center Association. (2011). *Fact sheet - Community health centers: Part of NC's health care solution*. Retrieved October 13, 2011, from http://ncchca.affiniscape.com/associations/11930/files/CHCs%20are%20cost-saving%20-%20UPDATED%20AUGUST%202011.pdf

Noteboom, C., & Qureshi, S. (2011). Physician interaction with electronic health records: The influences of digital natives and digital immigrants. In R. Sprague & J. Nunamaker (Eds.), *The Forty-Fourth Annual Hawaii International Conference on System Sciences*. Washington, DC: IEEE Computer Society Press.

Nunnally, J. C. (1978). *Psychometric theory* (2nd ed.). New York, NY: McGraw Hill.

O'Connor, P. (2003). Setting evidence-based priorities for diabetes care improvement. *International Journal for Quality in Health Care, 15*(4), 283–285. doi:10.1093/intqhc/mzg062

O'Connor, P. J., Sperl-Hillen, J. M., Rush, W. A., Johnson, P. E., Amundson, G. H., & Asche, S. E. (2011). Impact of electronic health record clinical decision support on diabetes care: A randomized trial. *Annals of Family Medicine, 9*(1), 12–21. doi:10.1370/afm.1196

Odell, J. (Ed.). (2000). *Agent technology*. OMG Document 00-09-01. OMG Agents Interest Group.

Office of Rural Health Policy, Health Resources and Services Administration, Department of Health and Human Services. (2006). *Comparison of rural health clinic and federally qualified health center programs*. Retrieved October 18, 2011, from http://www.ask.hrsa.gov/downloads/fqhc-rhccomparison.pdf

Ondash, E. (2004). Nurses choose PDAs over other mobile information technologies. *AMN Healthcare, Inc*. Retrieved from http://www.nursezone.com/nursing-news-events/devices-and-technology/Nurses-Choose-PDAs-Over-Other-Mobile-Information-Technologies_24474.aspx

Ondo, K. J., Wagner, J., & Gale, K. L. (2002). The electronic medical record (EMR): Hype or reality? *HIMSS Proceedings, 63*, 1–12.

Ooi, P., Culjak, G., & Lawrence, E. (2005). Wireless and wearable overview: Stages of growth theory in medical technology applications. In *Proceedings of the International Conference on Mobile Business ICMB05*, (pp. 528-536). IEEE Press.

OrthoInfo. (2002). *Patients have important role in safer health care*. Retrieved from http://orthoinfo.aaos.org/topic.cfm?topic=A00271#Additional Information

Ozdemir, Z., Barron, J., & Bandyopadhyay, S. (2011). Analysis of the adoption of digital health records under switching costs. *Information Systems Research*, *22*(3), 491–503. doi:10.1287/isre.1110.0349

Pagani, M. (2006). Determinants of adoption of high speed data services in the business market: Evidence for a combined technology acceptance model with task technology fit model. *Information & Management*, *43*(7), 847. doi:10.1016/j.im.2006.08.003

Pattath, A., Bue, B., Jang, Y., Ebert, D., Zhong, X., Ault, A., & Coyle, E. (2006). Interactive visualization and analysis of network and sensor data on mobile devices. In *Proceedings of the 2006 IEEE Symposium on Visual Analytics and Technology*, (vol. 9, pp. 83-90). IEEE Press.

PepeNavas Melara. (2012). Drug encyclopedia download review. *The Drugs Encyclopedia*. Retrieved from http://medical.appdownloadreview.com/online/drugs-encyclopedia

Perez, J. (2012). *myCVS on the go*. Retrieved from http://www.cvs.com/promo/promoLandingTemplate.jsp?promoLandingId=mobile-apps

Phillips, G., Felix, L., Galli, L., Patel, V., & Edwards, P. (2010). The effectiveness of m-health technologies for improving health and health services: A systematic review protocol. *BMC Research Notes*, *3*(1), 250. doi:10.1186/1756-0500-3-250

Physician Licensure. (2011). *Center for telehealth and e-health law*. Retrieved November 15, 2011, from http://www.ctel.org/expertise/physican-licensure/

Ping, A., Wang, Z., Shi, X., Deng, C., Bian, L., & Chen, L. (2009). Designing an emotional majormodo in smart home healthcare. In *Proceedings of the 2009 International Asia Symposium on Intelligent Interaction and Affective Computing*, (pp. 45-47). IEEE Press.

Polycom, Inc. (2011). *Polycom*. Retrieved from http://www.polycom.com/

Ponniah, P. (2010). *Data warehousing fundamentals for IT professionals* (2nd ed.). Hoboken, NJ: John Wiley & Sons. doi:10.1002/9780470604137

Poon, E. G., Blumenthal, D., Jaggi, T., Honour, M. M., Bates, D. W., & Kaushal, R. (2004). Overcoming barriers to adopting and implementing computerized physician order entry systems in US hospitals. *Health Affairs*, *23*(4), 184–190. doi:10.1377/hlthaff.23.4.184

Poon, E. G., Gandhi, T. K., Sequist, T. D., Murff, H. J., Karson, A. S., & Bates, D. W. (2004). I wish I had seen this test result earlier! Dissatisfaction with test result management systems in primary care. *Archives of Internal Medicine*, *164*(20), 2223–2228. doi:10.1001/archinte.164.20.2223

Pramatari, K. C., Doukidis, G. I., & Kourouthanassis, P. (2005). Towards 'smarter' supply and demand-chain collaboration practices enabled by RFID technology. In Vervest, P., Van Heck, E., Preiss, K., & Pau, L. F. (Eds.), *Smart Business Networks* (pp. 197–210). Berlin, Germany: Springer. doi:10.1007/3-540-26694-1_14

Prensky, M. (2001). Digital natives, digital immigrants. *Horizon*, *9*(5). doi:10.1108/10748120110424816

Prestigiacomo, J. (2011). Mobile healthcare anywhere: A proliferation of mobile devices means specific wireless challenges for healthcare organizations. *Healthcare Informatics, 28*(3), 34, 36.

Privacy Rule and Research. (2011). *How can covered entities use and disclose protected health information for research and comply with the privacy rule?* Retrieved November 5, 2011, from http://privacyruleandresearch. nih.gov/pr_08.zip

Products, R. N. K. Inc. (2011). *Telehealth technologies.* Retrieved from http://www. telehealthtechnologies.com/

Qiu, R., & Sangwan, R. (2005). Toward collaborative supply chains using RFID. In *CIO Wisdom II: More Best Practices* (pp. 127–144). Upper Saddle River, NJ: Prentice-Hall.

Quinn, C. C., Clough, S. S., Minor, J. M., Lender, D., Okafor, M. C., & Gruber-Baldini, A. (2008). WellDoc™ mobile diabetes management randomized controlled trial: Change in clinical and behavioral outcomes and patient and physician satisfaction. *Diabetes Technology & Therapeutics, 10*(3), 160–168. doi:10.1089/dia.2008.0283

Raghupathi, V., & Tan, J. (2008). Information systems and healthcare XXX: Charting a strategic path for health information technology. *Communications of the Association for Information Systems, 23*, 501–522.

Räisänen, T., Oinas-Kukkonen, H., Leiviskä, K., Seppänen, M., & Kallio, M. (2010). Managing mobile healthcare knowledge: Physicians' perceptions on knowledge creation and reuse. In *Proceedings of Health Information Systems: Concepts, Methodologies, Tools, and Applications,* (pp. 733-749). IEEE.

Randrup, N. (2007). *The case method: Road map for how best to study, analyze and present cases.* Rodovre, Denmark: International Management Press.

Rao, S. R., DesRoches, C. M., Donelan, K., Campbell, E. G., Miralles, P. D., & Jha, A. K. (2011). Electronic health records in small physician practices: Availability, use, and perceived benefits. *Journal of the American Medical Informatics Association, 18*(3), 271–275. doi:10.1136/amiajnl-2010-000010

Reuters, T. (2012). Micromedex drug information. *Thomson Reuters.* Retrieved from http://healthcare.thomsonreuters.com/ micromedexMobile/

Rigla, M., Hernando, M. E., Gómez, E. J., Brugués, E., García-Sáez, G., & Torralba, V. (2007). A telemedicine system that includes a personal assistant improves glycemic control in pump-treated patients with type 1 diabetes. *Journal of Diabetes Science and Technology, 1*(4), 505.

Robbins, S. P., & Judge, T. A. (2011). *Organizational behavior* (14th ed.). Upper Saddle River, NJ: Prentice Hall.

Rogers, E. M. (2003). *Diffusion of innovations* (5th ed.). New York, NY: Free Press.

Rosenfeld, S. Koss, Caruth, & Fuller. (2006). Evolution of state health information exchange: A study of vision, strategy, and progress. *The Agency for Healthcare Research and Quality.* Retrieved November 14, 2011 from http://www.avalerehealth.net/ research/docs/State_based_Health_Information_Exchange_Final_Report.pdf

Rosenthal, K. (2003). Touch vs. tech: Valuing nursing specific PDA software. *Nursing Management, 34*(7). doi:10.1097/00006247-200307000-00017

Ryan, J. (2007). Will patients agree to have their literacy skills assessed in clinical practice? *Advance Access, 23*(4), 603–611.

Sacket, D. L., Straus, S. E., Richardson, W. S., Rosenberg, W., & Haynes, R. B. (2000). *Evidence based medicine: How to practice & teach EBM*. New York, NY: Churchill Livingstone.

Satyanarayanan, M. (1996). *Fundamental challenges in mobile computing*. Retrieved from http://www.cs.cmu.edu/~coda/docdir/podc95.pdf

Saverno, K. R., Hines, L. E., Warholak, T. L., Grizzle, A. J., Babits, L., & Clark, C. (2011). Ability of pharmacy clinical decision-support software to alert users about clinically important drug-drug interactions. *Journal of the American Medical Informatics Association, 18*(1), 32–37. Retrieved from http://www.ncbi.nlm.nih.gov/pubmed/21131607doi:10.1136/jamia.2010.007609

Schillinger, D. (2002). Association of health literacy with diabetes outcomes. *Journal of the American Medical Association, 288*(4). doi:10.1001/jama.288.4.475

Schneider, D. K. (2006). *Case-based learning*. Retrieved October 31, 2010, from http://edutechwiki.unige.ch/en/Case-based_learning

Schuster, E. W., Allen, S. J., & Brock, D. L. (2007). *Global RFID: The value of the EPC-global network for supply chain management*. Berlin, Germany: Springer.

Shaalana, K., El-Badryb, M., & Rafeac, A. (2004). A multiagent approach for diagnostic expert systems via the Internet. *Expert Systems with Applications, 27*(1), 1–10. doi:10.1016/j.eswa.2003.12.018

Shah, N. R., Seger, A. C., Seger, D. L., Fiskio, J. M., Kuperman, G. L., & Blumenfeld, B. (2006). Improving acceptance of computerized prescribing alerts in ambulatory care. *Journal of the American Medical Informatics Association, 13*(1), 5–11. doi:10.1197/jamia.M1868

Shepard, S. (2005). *RFID: Radio frequency identification*. New York, NY: McGraw-Hill.

Shim, S. (2011). *The evolution of health information exchanges*. Paper presented at the meeting of the Florida Health Information Management Association. Orlando, FL.

Shirani, A. I., Tafti, M. H. A., & Affisco, J. F. (1999). Task and technology fit: A comparison of two technologies for synchronous and asynchronous group communication. *Information & Management, 36*(3), 139. doi:10.1016/S0378-7206(99)00015-4

Shroyer, A. L. (2008). Improving quality of care in cardiac surgery: Evaluating risk factors, processes of care, structures of care, and outcomes. *Seminars in Cardiothoracic and Vascular Anesthesia, 3*(12), 140–152. doi:10.1177/1089253208323060

Simon, H. (1997). *Models of bounded rationality*. Cambridge, MA: The MIT Press.

Simon, H. A. (1977). *The new science of management decision*. Englewood Cliffs, NJ: Prentice-Hall.

Sitterson & Barker, P. A. (2010, June 30). *Financial statements*. Snow Hill, NC: Greene County Health Care, Inc.

Skyler, J. S., Lasky, I. A., Skyler, D. L., Robertson, E. G., & Mintz, D. H. (1978). Home blood glucose monitoring as an aid in diabetes management. *Diabetes Care, 1*(3), 150–157. doi:10.2337/diacare.1.3.150

Skyscape. (2012). *Skyscape medical resource.* New York, NY: Skyscape, Inc.

Smith, D. (2009). *A practical approach: Network-based economies of scale for community health.* Paper presented at the Annual Conference and Exhibition of the Healthcare Information and Management Systems Society (HIMSS). Chicago, IL.

Smith, D., & Rachman, F. D. (2008). *Economies of scale in HCCN EHR implementations.* Paper presented at Management Track, National Association of Community Health Centers (NACHC) 2008 Community Health Institute (CHI). Retrieved March 8, 2012 from http://www.softconference.com/nachc/sessionDetail.asp?SID=118996

Smith, D. H., Perrin, N., Feldstein, A., Yang, X. H., Kuang, D., & Simon, S. R. (2006). The impact of prescribing safety alerts for elderly persons in an electronic medical record—An interrupted time series evaluation. *Archives of Internal Medicine, 166*(10), 1098–1104. doi:10.1001/archinte.166.10.1098

Smith, S. A., Murphy, M. E., Huschka, T. R., Dinneen, S. F., Gorman, C. A., & Zimmerman, B. R. (1998). Impact of a diabetes electronic management system on the care of patients seen in a subspecialty diabetes clinic. *Diabetes Care, 21*(6), 972–976. doi:10.2337/diacare.21.6.972

Smith, S. D. (2009). E-prescribing 101. *Minnesota Medicine.* Retrieved from http://www.minnesotamedicine.com/PastIssues/PastIssues2009/January2009/QualityRoundsJanuary2009.aspx

Sommers, M. S. (2010). Diseases and disorders. *F.A. Davis Company.* Retrieved from http://www.unboundmedicine.com/products/diseases_disorders

Sprague, R. H. (1980). A framework for the development of DSS. *Management Information Systems Quarterly, 4*(4), 1–26. doi:10.2307/248957

Stanford, V. (2002). Using pervasive computing to deliver elder care. *IEEE Pervasive Computing / IEEE Computer Society (and) IEEE Communications Society, 1*(1), 10–13. doi:10.1109/MPRV.2002.993139

Staurovsky, R. (2004). *Broadlawns medical center hospital information system and physician practive management system selection. Request for Proposal.* Southfield, MI: Superior Consultant Company, Inc.

Stier, M. (2008). *Polk county residents gain access to latest seizure diagnosis video technology.* Community News From Broadlawns Medical Center.

Stier, M. (2009). *Patients give Broadlawns medical center higher satisfaction scores.* Community News From Broadlawns Medical Center.

Stier, M. (2010). *Broadlawns earns HIMSS EMR certification.* Community News From Broadlawns Medical Center.

Stier, M. (2011a). *Broadlawns by the numbers.* Des Moines, IA: Broadlawns Medical Center.

Stier, M. (2011b). *Broadlawns installs first-in-Iowa patient identity security system.* Des Moines, IA: Broadlawns Medical Center.

Stier, M. (2011c). *Economic impact.* Des Moines, IA: Broadlawns Medical Center.

Stier, M. (2011d). *Mission.* Des Moines, IA: Broadlawns Medical Center.

Straub, D. W. (1989). Validating instruments in MIS research. *Management Information Systems Quarterly, 13*(2), 147–169. doi:10.2307/248922

Compilation of References

Straub, D. W., Boudreau, M.-C., & Gefen, D. (2004). Validation guidelines for IS positivist research. *Communications of the AIS*, *13*(24), 380–427.

Stross, R. (2012). Chicken scratches vs. electronic prescriptions. *The New York Times*. Retrieved from http://www.nytimes.com/2012/04/29/business/e-prescriptions-reduce-errors-but-their-adoption-is-slow.html

Stroud, S. D., Erkel, E. A., & Smith, C. A. (2005). The use of personal digital assistants by nurse practitioner students and faculty. *Journal of the American Academy of Nursing Management*, *17*(2), 67–75. doi:10.1111/j.1041-2972.2005.00013.x

Stroud, S. D., Smith, C. A., & Erkel, E. A. (2009). Personal digital assistant use by nurse practitioners: A descriptive study. *Journal of the American Academy of Nurse Practitioners*, *21*(1), 31–38. Retrieved from http://www.ncbi.nlm.nih.gov/pubmed/19125893doi:10.1111/j.1745-7599.2008.00368.x

Sullivan, C. (2008). *Florida's RHIO initiative: Recycling lessons learned into new strategies for health information exchange.* Paper presented at the HIMSS 2008 RHIO/HIE Symposium. Orlando, FL.

Swayne, L. (2009). *Case writers newcomers' workshop.* Paper presented at the North American Case Research Association Conference. Santa Cruz, CA.

Takach, M., & Neva, K. (2008). *Using HIT to transform health care: Summary of a discussion among state policy makers.* State Health Policy Briefing. Retrieved November 14, 2011 from http://nashp.org/sites/default/files/shpbriefing_usinghit.pdf?q=Files/shp-briefing_usinghit.pdf

Tatara, N., Arsand, E., Nilsen, H., & Hartvigsen, G. (2009). A review of mobile terminal-based applications for self-management of patients with diabetes. In *Proceedings of eHealth, Telemedicine, and Social Medicine.* IEEE Press. doi:10.1109/eTELEMED.2009.14

Taylor, S., & Todd, P. A. (1995). Understanding information technology usage - A test of competing models. *Information Systems Research*, *6*(2), 144–176. doi:10.1287/isre.6.2.144

Teo, T. S. H., & Men, B. (2008). Knowledge portals in Chinese consulting firms: A task-technology fit perspective. *European Journal of Information Systems*, *17*(6), 557. doi:10.1057/ejis.2008.41

Thielst, C. B. (2010). *Social media in healthcare: Connect, communicate, collaborate.* Chicago, IL: Health Administration Press.

Thompson, R. L., Higgins, C. A., & Howell, J. M. (1991). Personal computing - Toward a conceptual-model of utilization. *Management Information Systems Quarterly*, *15*(1), 125–143. doi:10.2307/249443

Thrall, J. (2004). Quality and safety revolution in health care. *Radiology*, *233*, 3–6. doi:10.1148/radiol.2331041059

Timmons, S. (2003). Nurses resisting information technology. *Nursing Inquiry*, *10*(4), 257–269. Retrieved from http://www.ncbi.nlm.nih.gov/pubmed/14622372doi:10.1046/j.1440-1800.2003.00177.x

Tindal, S. (2008). One in ten RFID projects tag humans. *ZDNet Australia*. Retrieved from http://www.zdnet.com.au/news/hardware/soa/RFID-people-tagging-benefits-health-sector-/0,130061702,339285273,00.htm

Triandis, H. C. (1977). *Interpersonal behavior*. Monterey, CA: Brooke Cole.

Trossen, D., & Pavel, D. (2007). Sensor networks, wearable computing, and healthcare applications. *IEEE Pervasive Computing / IEEE Computer Society (and) IEEE Communications Society, 6,* 58–61. doi:10.1109/MPRV.2007.43

Tuomilehto, J., Lindstrom, J., Eriksson, J. G., Valle, T. T., Hamalainen, H., & Ilanne-Parikka, P. (2001). Finnish diabetes prevention study group: Prevention of type 2 diabetes mellitus by changes in lifestyle among subjects with impaired glucose tolerance. *The New England Journal of Medicine, 344,* 1343–1350. doi:10.1056/NEJM200105033441801

Turner, C. (2011). *Florida HIE subscription agreements and policies*. State Consumer Health Information and Policy Advisory Council Interoffice Memorandum. Retrieved November 14, 2011 from http://b.ahca.myflorida.com/schs/AdvisoryCouncil/AC062211/TABDLegalWorkgroupReport.pdf

U.S. Department of Health & Human Services. (2011). *Summary of the HIPAA privacy rule*. Retrieved October 22, 2011, from http://www.hhs.gov/ocr/privacy/hipaa/understanding/summary/index.html

U.S. Department of Health & Human Services. (2011). *The office of the national coordinator for health information technology*. Retrieved November 14, 2011 from http://healthit.hhs.gov/portal/server.pt?open=512&objID=1488&mode=2

U.S. Wireless Quick Facts. (2011). *CTIA consumer info*. Retrieved from http://www.ctia.org/consumer_info/index.cfm/AID/10323

Ulrich, R. S., Zimring, C., Quan, X., Joseph, A., & Choudhary, R. (2004). The role of the physical environment in the hospital of the 21st century: A once-in-a-lifetime opportunity. *Environment*. Retrieved from http://scholar.google.com/scholar?hl=en&btnG=Search&q=intitle:The+role+of+the+physical+environment+in+the+hospital+of+the+21st+century:+a+once-in-a-lifetime+opportunity#0

Unbound Evidence. (2011). Evidence central. *Wiley Blackwell*. Retrieved from www.unboundmedicine.com/products/evidence_central

University of Maryland. (2009). Medical encyclopedia. *Maryland Medical Systems*. Retrieved from itunes.apple.com/us/app/medical-encyclopedia/id313696784?mt=8

Venkatesh, V., & Bala, H. (2008). Technology acceptance model 3 and a research agenda on interventions. *Decision Sciences, 39*(2), 273–315. doi:10.1111/j.1540-5915.2008.00192.x

Venkatesh, V., Bala, H., Venkatraman, S., & Bates, J. (2007). Enterprise architecture maturity: The story of the veterans health administration. *MIS Quarterly Executive, 2*(6), 79–90.

Venkatesh, V., & Davis, F. D. (2000). A theoretical extension of the technology acceptance model: Four longitudinal field studies. *Management Science, 46*(2), 186–204. doi:10.1287/mnsc.46.2.186.11926

Venkatesh, V., Morris, M. G., Davis, G. B., & Davis, F. D. (2003). User acceptance of information technology: Toward a unified view. *Management Information Systems Quarterly, 27*(3), 425–478.

Compilation of References

Venkatraman, S., Bala, H., Venkatesh, V., & Bates, J. (2008). Six strategies for electronic medical record systems. *Communications of the ACM*, *51*(11), 140–144. doi:10.1145/1400214.1400243

Versel, N. (2011). Emergency room patients tracked with RFID tags. *Information Week Healthcare*. Retrieved from http://www.informationweek.com/news/healthcare/EMR/231901224

Vijayaraghavan, K., Parpyani, K., Thakwani, S. A., & Iyengar, N. C. S. N. (2009). Methods of increasing spatial resolution of digital images with minimum detail loss and its applications. In *Proceedings of the 2009 Fifth International Conference on Image and Graphics*, (pp. 685–689). IEEE Press.

Vishwanath, A., & Scarmurra, T. (2007). Barriers to the adoption of electronic health records: Using concept mapping to develop a comprehensive empirical model. *Health Informatics Journal*, *13*(2), 119–134. doi:10.1177/1460458207076468

Vlahos, G. E., Ferratt, T. W., & Knoepfle, G. (2004). The use of computer-based information systems by German managers to support decision making. *Information & Management*, *41*(6), 763. doi:10.1016/j.im.2003.06.003

Waegemann, C. P., & Tessier, C. (2002). Documentation goes wireless: A look at mobile healthcare computing devices. *Journal of American Health Information Management Association*, *73*(8), 36–39.

WalgreensCo. (2012). *Walgreens mobile*. Retrieved from http://www.walgreens.com/topic/apps/learn_about_mobile_apps.jsp

Wallace, T., Levy, J., & Matthews, D. (2004). Use and abuse of HOMA modeling. *Diabetes Care*, *27*, 1487–1495. doi:10.2337/diacare.27.6.1487

Wang, M.-Y., Tsai, P. H., Liu, J. W. S., & Zao, J. K. (2009). Wedjat: A mobile phone based medicine in-take reminder and monitor. In *Proceedings of the 2009 Ninth IEEE International Conference on Bioinformatics and BioEngineering*, (pp. 423-430). IEEE Press.

Warner, M. (2004). Under the knife. *Business 2.0*, *5*(1), 84-89.

Wears, R., & Berg, M. (2005). Computer technology and clinical work: Still waiting for Godot. *Journal of the American Medical Association*, *293*(1261), 1–3.

Web, M. D. (2012). WebMD for android, iphone, and ipad. *WebMD.com*. Retrieved from http://www.webmd.com/webmdapp

Webahn, I. (2012). *Capzule-PHR*. Retrieved from http://capzule.com/

Weber, J. R. (2009). Nurses' handbook of health assesment. *Lippincott Williams & Wilkins*. Retrieved from http://www.unboundmedicine.com/products/nurses_handbook_health_assessment

Weick, K., & McDaniel, R. R. (1989). How professional organizations work: Implications for school organization and management. In Sergiovanni, T., & Moore, J. H. (Eds.), *Schooling for Tomorrow Directing Future Reforms to Issues that Count* (pp. 330–355). Boston, MA: Allyn and Bacon.

Weinstein, R. (2005). RFID: A technical overview and its application to the enterprise. *IT Professional Magazine*, *7*(3), 27–33. doi:10.1109/MITP.2005.69

Weinstock, M., & Hoppszallern, S. (2011, July). Most wired 2011. *Hospitals and Health Networks*.

Weitzel, M., Smith, A., Lee, D., Deugd, S., & Helal, S. (2009). Participatory medicine: Leveraging social networks in telehealth solutions. *Lecture Notes in Computer Science, 40*. Retrieved from http://portal.acm.org/citation.cfm?id=1575560

Weitzel, M., Smith, A., Deugd, S. D., & Yates, R. (2010). A web 2.0 model for patient-centered health informatics applications. *Computer, 43*(7), 43–50. doi:10.1109/MC.2010.190

Wenger, E. C., & Snyder, W. M. (2000, January-February). Communities of practice: The organizational frontier. *Harvard Business Review*.

Whiting, R. (2004). MIT = RFID + Rx. *Information Week, 988*, 16.

WHO. (2011). *Diabetes*. Retrieved April 2, 2012, from http://www.who.int/mediacentre/factsheets/fs312/en/

WHO/IDF. (2006). *Definition and diagnosis of diabetes mellitus and intermediate hyperglycemia*. Geneva, Switzerland: World Health Organization.

Wikipedia. (2012). *Mobile phone*. Retrieved from http://www.wikipedia.org

wikipedia.org. (2009). *Healthcare information and management systems society*. Retrieved November 3, 2011, from http://en.wikipedia.org/wiki/HIMSS

wikipedia.org. (2011a). *LSS data systems*. Retrieved October 28, 2011, from http://en.wikipedia.org/wiki/LSS_Data_Systems

wikipedia.org. (2011b). *MEDITECH*. Retrieved from http://en.wikipedia.org/wiki/MEDITECH

Wild, J. J. (2008). *Scanning and archiving assessment/implementation strategy for regional health*. Unpublished manuscript.

Wills, M., El-Gayar, O. F., & Deokar, A. V. (2009). Evaluating the technology acceptance model, task-technology fit and user performance for an electronic health record system. In *Proceedings of the Decision Sciences Institute 40th Annual Conference*. New Orleans, LA: Decision Sciences Institute.

Winters, J. M., Wang, Y., & Winters, J. M. (2003). Wearable sensors and telerehabilitation. *IEEE Engineering in Medicine and Biology Magazine, 22*(3), 56–65. doi:10.1109/MEMB.2003.1213627

Wooldridge, M., & Jennings, N. (1995). Intelligent software agents: Theory and practice. *The Knowledge Engineering Review, 10*(2), 115–152. doi:10.1017/S0269888900008122

Wright, A., Pang, J., Feblowitz, J. C., Maloney, F. L., Wilcox, A. R., & Ramelson, H. Z. (2011). A method and knowledge base for automated inference of patient problems from structured data in an electronic medical record. *Journal of the American Medical Informatics Association, 18*(6), 859–867. doi:10.1136/amiajnl-2011-000121

Wu, I.-L., Li, J.-Y., & Fu, C.-Y. (2011). The adoption of mobile healthcare by hospital's professionals: An integrative perspective. *Decision Support Systems, 51*(3), 587–596. doi:10.1016/j.dss.2011.03.003

Compilation of References

Wu, S., Chaudhry, B., Wang, J., Maglione, M., Mojica, W., & Roth, E. (2006). Systematic review: Impact of health information technology on quality, efficiency, and costs of medical care. *Annals of Internal Medicine, 144*(10), 742–752.

Wyne, K. (2008). Information technology for the treatment of diabetes: Improving outcomes and controlling costs. *Journal of Managed Care Pharmacy, 14*(2), 12.

Zadeh, L. A. (1965). Fuzzy sets. *Information and Control, 8*, 338–352. doi:10.1016/S0019-9958(65)90241-X

Zhou, Y. Y., Unitan, R., Wang, J. J., Garrido, T., Chin, H. L., Turley, M. C., & Radler, L. (2011). Improving population care with an integrated electronic panel support tool. *Population Health Management, 14*(1), 3–9. doi:10.1089/pop.2010.0001

Zigurs, I., & Buckland, B. K. (1998). A theory of task/technology fit and group support systems effectiveness. *Management Information Systems Quarterly, 22*(3), 313. doi:10.2307/249668

Zigurs, I., & Khazanchi, D. (2008). From profiles to patterns: A new view of task-technology fit. *Information Systems Management, 25*(1), 8. doi:10.1080/10580530701777107

About the Contributors

Surendra Sarnikar is an Associate Professor in Information Systems at the College of Business and Information Systems, Dakota State University. He holds a Bachelor's degree in Engineering from Osmania University, India, and a PhD in Management Information Systems from the University of Arizona. He teaches Healthcare Informatics, Design Research, and Knowledge Management at the Dakota State University and has published several conference and journal publications in the area of knowledge management systems, information retrieval, and healthcare information systems.

Dorine Bennett received a EdD in 2010 in Educational Administration from University of South Dakota, holds an MBA in Management of Information Systems since 1995, is Program Director of Health Information Management and an Associate Professor at Dakota State University since 1998. She has several publications.

Mark Gaynor holds a PhD in Computer Science from Harvard University and is an Associate Professor of Health Management and Policy at Saint Louis University. His research interests include sensor/RFid networks and applications, architecture promoting innovation, applying emerging technology to medical applications, IT for medical applications, standardization in the IT area, designing network-based services, and wireless Internet services. He is Co-PI and PI on several NSF grant projects studying virtual markets on a wireless grid and wireless sensor networks. He is a CTO, member of the board of directors, technical director, and network architect at 10Blade. His first book, *Network Services Investment Guide: Maximizing ROI in Uncertain Markets*, was published by Wiley.

* * *

Charles H Andrus, MHA, is a Software Developer at St. Louis Children's Hospital. After receiving Bachelors' in Science in Computer Science and Biology from Saint Louis University, Charles went on to complete a Master in Health Administration, where he became interested in clinical decision support and its use to reduce medical errors. His research interests include interoperable clinical decision support, the use of mobile phone apps in healthcare, and mitochondrial diseases. He guest lectures for Saint Louis University regarding how technology can improve patient care quality and medical outcomes. He currently programs custom modules and clinical decision support for St. Louis Children's Hospital's electronic health record system.

Aristides P. Assimacopoulos, MD, is the founding partner of the Infectious Disease Specialty Clinic in Sioux Falls, SD, and is the Medical Director of Infection Control for Avera McKennan and Select Specialty Hospital. Dr. Assimacopoulos received his Medical degree and completed his Infectious Disease Fellowship at the University of Minnesota in 1996. He is board certified in Infectious Disease. He has been involved in research and clinical trials through the Avera Research Institute. Dr. Assimacopoulos is a member of the Clinical Faculty at the University of South Dakota School of Medicine. He has authored several articles on infectious diseases. Dr. Assimacopoulos is a member of the Infectious Disease Society of America, South Dakota State Medical Society, and the Society for Healthcare Epidemiology of America.

Leigh W. Cellucci (celluccie@ecu.edu) is Associate Professor, Department of Health Services and Information Management, East Carolina University, Greenville, NC. Her research interests focus on the management of health care organizations, including the introduction and use of Electronic Health Records in health care settings. She is currently examining the role of organizational culture as a critical variable for effective strategy implementation regarding Health-IT initiatives. She serves as editor for the *Journal of Case Studies* and is a member on the board of directors for Society for Case Research. She received a PhD in Sociology from the University of Virginia, a Master's in Sociology from the College of William and Mary, and an MBA from Idaho State University.

Mary DeVany is the Outreach Director for the Great Plains Telehealth Resource and Assistance Center (GPTRAC), within the Institute of Health Informatics at the University of Minnesota. She has been involved with telemedicine activities since 1993 when she served as the statewide telemedicine activities coordinator for the state of South Dakota. Since then, she has served as the Director of Avera Telehealth and before that as the Telemedicine Coordinator for Sanford Health. Mary is a member of the American Telemedicine Association and also serves on the Board of Directors for the Center for Telehealth and E-Health Law. She earned her B.S. in Mass Communications from the University of South Dakota.

Elizabeth J. Forrestal (forrestale@ecu.edu) is Professor, Department of Health Services and Information Management, East Carolina University, Greenville, NC. Her research interests include health care reimbursement, health informatics research, ethics, leadership, and work redesign. She is co-author of *Health Informatics Research Methods: Principles and Practice and Principles of Healthcare Reimbursement*. She is a Fellow of the American Health Information Management Association and, in 2007, received its Legacy Award. She received a PhD in Higher Education from Georgia State University, a Master's in Organizational Leadership from the College of St. Catherine, and a Post-Baccalaureate certificate in Health Information Management from the College of St. Scholastica.

Sherrilynne Fuller, Ph.D., is Professor, Department of Biomedical Informatics and Medical Education, School of Medicine, Professor (Adjunct) Health Services, School of Public Health, and Professor (Joint), Information School, all at the University of Washington (UW), Seattle, Washington. She received her BA (Biology) and MLS (Information Science) degrees from Indiana University, Bloomington, Indiana, USA, and her PhD (Library and Information Science) from the University of Southern California, Los Angeles, California, USA. Fuller served as the founding head of the Division of Biomedical and Health Informatics, School of Medicine, UW, and has led several large-scale campus and regional research and development projects in the areas of biomedical informatics and telemedicine. As Co-Director, Center for Public Health Informatics, Fuller has contributed to the development of innovative information systems and tools to improve public health practice. Fuller has authored teaching cases and frequently uses cases in her teaching of health informatics topics at UW and beyond. She has lectured, taught courses, and worked on health information systems development in resource-constrained countries around the world.

Jennifer Gholson, RHIT, is an Applications Supervisor in the Information Technology Department at Regional Health in Rapid City, SD, where she oversees the clinical applications team who support the clinical modules within the main HCIS. Some of the modules include Computerized Physician Order Entry (CPOE), electronic physician documentation, bedside medication verification. Prior to this, she was an Assistant Director in the Health Information Management Department at Rapid City Regional Hospital, where she served as Project Manager for the Regional Health Scanning Project. She has been with Regional Health for 18 years. She holds an Associate's degree in Health Information Technology and a Bachelor of Science degree in Health Informatics.

Biswadip Ghosh is Assistant Professor of Computer Information Systems at MSCD. Dr. Ghosh received his Ph.D. in Information Systems from the University of Colorado. His research interests include healthcare IS, knowledge management, enterprise systems, business processes management, and analytics. His teaching areas are enterprise systems (SAP-ERP), Netweaver tools, MIS, Java, VB, systems analysis and networking. Prior to joining MSCD, he had worked with AT&T/Lucent/Avaya for over 19 years on multimedia messaging, systems, and processes for global service delivery in multiple roles including analyst, project manager, and architect/developer. He has consulted for over 4 years on Healthcare Information Technology (HIT), analytics, and decision support systems. His research is published in AIS, IEEE, ACM, and IFIP sponsored conference proceedings and journals such as *MIS Quarterly, Communications of the AIS, Journal of Information Systems Education, International Journal of Technology Management, IEEE Transactions on IT in BioMedicine, IEEE Networks*, and *Information Systems Management*.

Michael H. Kennedy (kennedym@ecu.edu) is Associate Professor and Director of the Health Services Management Program in the Department of Health Services and Information Management at East Carolina University. His research interests focus on health services decision support, simulation, and modeling. He has 35 years experience in teaching and health services administration that have been divided between academic positions and operational assignments in the military health system culminating as the Chief Operating Officer of a small hospital. He earned a PhD in Decision Sciences and Engineering Systems from Rensselaer Polytechnic Institute and a Master of Health Administration from Baylor University, and he is a Fellow in the American College of Healthcare Executives.

Sandeep Lakkaraju holds a Baccalaureate of Engineering degree in Information Technology from Laki Reddy Bali Reddy College of Engineering/JNTU, India, and a Master of Science degree in Information Systems from Dakota State University, USA. His research interests include healthcare informatics and health information technology. He is a Doctoral student and also a graduate assistant at the Dakota State University, USA. He is a continuous member of AIS and MWAIS and has publications in HICSS and MWAIS.

Santhosh Lakkaraju is a Doctoral student at Dakota State University. He holds a BE in Computer Science and Information Technology from SSIET/JNTU, India, and a Masters degree in Information Systems from Dakota State University. His current research interests include healthcare informatics, decision support systems, and predictive analytics. He is working with the Department of Business and Information Systems at Dakota State University. He is a member of AIS and MWAIS.

Cynthia LeRouge, Ph.D., M.S., C.P.A., is an Associate Professor at Saint Louis University in the Department of Health Policy and Management at the School of Public Health. She holds a joint appointment in the Decision Sciences and Information Technology Management Department, John Cook School of Business. She recently served as a Visiting Scholar at the Center of Disease Control with the Public Health Informatics Fellowship Program. She has over 60 publications including academic journal articles, edited chapters in research-based books, and peer-reviewed conference proceedings. Dr. LeRouge has been recognized with teaching, research, and service awards. Her primary research interests relate to telemedicine, consumer health informatics, and public health informatics. Dr. LeRouge has chaired health care mini-tracks for various information systems conferences and served as guest editor for multiple journal special issues on healthcare related topics. She is currently Co-Editor in Chief of *Health Systems Journal*. She served as executive officer of the Association of Information Systems Special Interest Group for Healthcare Research for four years. Dr. LeRouge has held various senior management roles in industry, including roles in software and healthcare industry prior to joining academia. She completed her Ph.D. at the University of South Florida.

Karla Ludwig, RN, has served as the Clinical Nurse/Office Manager for Infectious Disease Specialists, PC, since 2010. She began her career in infectious disease and telemedicine within the Infectious Disease Specialist Clinical Office as a Clinical RN in 2005 and later served as a Telemedicine Clinical Coordinator with the Avera Health System, working extensively to enhance and improve the telemedicine services and available resources at the remote and specialist sites. Karla received her Nursing degree from Augustana College in Sioux Falls, SD.

Kelly McLendon, RHIA, CHPS, is a Founder of CompliancePro Solutions, which has developed a state-of-the-art privacy product called PrivacyPro™. Kelly McLendon is also President of Health Information Xperts, a consultancy specializing in healthcare privacy, security, and HIM automation. Kelly's scope of practice also includes Legal Health Records and EHRs. He currently serves as an analyst for AHIMA on issues ranging from HITECH privacy to meaningful use. Kelly is considered an innovator and is well known for his contributions to the migration of HIM into the electronic environment. He is a well-known speaker and author, recently publishing a new book for AHIMA entitled *The Legal Health Record: Regulations, Policies, and Guidelines*. He has been recognized with numerous awards, including the 2003 AHIMA Visionary Award and the 2008 FHIMA Distinguished Member, as well as numerous literary awards.

Sergey Motorny is a Ph.D. candidate at Dakota State University, Madison, SD, with specialization in Healthcare Information Systems. Sergey has worked in the field of information technology for almost ten years. His professional experience includes design and implementation of information systems solutions for prominent universities and Fortune 300 companies. Sergey holds a Bachelor's degree in Business Administration and Master's in Computer Information Systems from Nova Southeastern University. His current research interests include electronic health records, clinical collaboration and communication support tools, consumer health informatics, and mobile technology in health care. Sergey lives in Des Moines, Iowa, with his wife Sarah and one-year-old son Phillip.

Nina Multak is an Assistant Clinical Professor in the College of Nursing and Health Professions. She has held faculty appointments at the University of Florida College of Medicine, NOVA Southeastern University, and the Philadelphia College of Osteopathic Medicine. Nina Multak is a 1988 graduate of the Hahnemann University Physician Assistant Program. Her Masters in Physician Assistant Studies was awarded from the University of Nebraska with an emphasis on educational innovation for physician assistant students. Nina Multak maintains professional affiliations with the American Academy of Physician Assistants, Pennsylvania Academy of Physician Assistants, Physician Assistant Education Association, Society for Simulation in Healthcare, ACM, and HIMMS. A Doctoral student in the Drexel University College of Information Science, Nina Multak is advancing her studies in Health Information Technologies.

Alice Noblin is the Undergraduate Health Informatics and Information Management Program Director at the University of Central Florida. She is an instructor in the program as well as in the Masters in Health Care Informatics Program. She received her MBA from Georgia State University and her PhD in Public Affairs from UCF. Dr. Noblin has work experience in both hospitals and physician offices. Dr. Noblin is credentialed by the American Health Information Management Association (AHIMA) as a Registered Health Information Administrator (RHIA) and a Certified Coding Specialist (CCS). She is certified as an ICD-10 Trainer by AHIMA as well. Dr. Noblin is active in the regional, state, and national HIM organizations. She is also a panel reviewer for the Commission on Accreditation for Health Informatics and Information Management Education. Dr. Noblin is a co-author on the textbook *Learning to Code with CPT/HCPCS*. She has several peer-reviewed publications and has presented her research at academic and practitioner conferences. Her research interests include electronic health records, personal health records, and health information exchanges.

Cherie Noteboom is an Assistant Professor at the College of Business and Information Systems at Dakota State University. She holds a Ph.D. in Information Technology from University of Nebraska-Omaha. In addition, she has earned an Education Doctorate in Adult and Higher Education and Administration and an MBA from the University of South Dakota. She has a BS degree in Computer Science from South Dakota State University. Her industry experience runs the continuum from technical computer science endeavors to project management and formal management assignments. She has significant experience working with management information systems, staff development, project management, application development, education, healthcare, mentoring and leadership. She has served on several nursing college advisory boards, YMCA board of directors, and K12 school boards. Cherie is a member of the Project Management Institute and participates in the Special Interest Groups of Healthcare, Information Technology, and Education. She has held the Project Management Professional (PMP) designation since 2000. Noteboom enjoys running, fishing, reading, and travelling.

Marilyn Dahler Penticoff, RN, BSN, has a background in rural nursing, education, and performance improvement. She became involved with telehealth in 1995 as a rural facility site coordinator, where she implemented education and clinical telehealth services. In 2000, Ms. Dahler Penticoff assumed the role of Telehealth Clinical Coordinator at a tertiary medical center and was responsible for policy development, and assisting providers and rural sites in the development of their telehealth practice. Ms. Dahler Penticoff is a Consulting Member of the Great Plain Telehealth Resource and Assistance Center and a Member of the American Telemedicine Association. She earned her BSN from Mount Marty College, Yankton, SD.

Ann Pommer is a Registered Health Information Technician (RHIT), a Certified Coding Specialist (CCS) and a Certified Professional Coder (CPC). She has been working in the health information technology field since 2009. She spent more than two years working with health insurance, claim denials, and reimbursement. She currently works as a medical coder. She has a Bachelor's degree in Health Information Administration with a minor in Sociology from Dakota State University. She is a member of the American Health Information Management Association and the American Academy of Professional Coders. She was the recipient of a 2010 Scholarship Award from the South Dakota Health Information Management Association.

Steven Shim is the Chief Healthcare Solutions Architect for Commercial Managed Services, Harris IT Services. Harris is an industry leader in providing mission-critical IT support services to healthcare, defense, intelligence, and civil clients. Prior to joining Harris, Mr. Shim was Vice President of IT for Health First, a nationally recognized Integrated Health Network comprised of four hospitals supporting a trauma level II center, a commercial insurance plan, and a host of ancillary outpatient and ambulatory services. Mr. Shim holds a Bachelor of Science degree in Industrial Engineering from the University of Central Florida. He is an active member of the American College of Healthcare Executives, Health Information Management System Society, and American Health Information Management Association (AHIMA). He serves on the UCF Community Advisory Board for Department of Health Management and Informatics and is a member of the AHIMA Privacy and Security Practice Council.

Sarin Shrestha is a Doctoral student in College of Business and Information Systems at Dakota State University, Madison, SD. He holds a Bachelor degree in Computer Engineering from Tribhuvan University, Nepal, and Master of Science in Software Engineering from Fairfield University, CT. He is currently working as a Research Assistant in National Center for the Protection of the Financial Infrastructure at Dakota State University. His fields of particular interest are privacy and security issues in healthcare domain.

Doug Smith (dsmith@greenecountyhealthcare.com) is CEO/CIO of Community Partners HealthNet, Inc., a health-center-controlled network of sixteen community/ migrant and rural health centers. He was responsible for securing the network's EMR system that has gotten national recognition. Smith is also CEO of Greene County Health Care (GCHC), an $8 million dollar a year diversified healthcare corporation. GCHC, Inc. has primary care, dental, student health, family medical therapy, and farmworker divisions, and employs over 165 individuals. An Adjunct Professor in the Department of Family Medicine of the Brody School of Medicine at East Carolina University, he has made over 100 presentations at meetings at the national and state levels, including such organizations as the National Association of Community Health Centers, the Health Resources and Services Administration, the Towards an Electronic Patient Record (now known as the mHealth Alliance), and the Healthcare Information Management and Systems Society. He earned his MBA from Wharton School of Business.

Stuart M. Speedie, Ph.D., is a Professor of Health Informatics, a Co-Director for Minnesota's Institute for Health Informatics, and Director of Graduate Studies in Health Informatics at the University of Minnesota Medical School. Dr. Speedie holds a B.S. in Computer Science and a Ph.D. in Educational Research from Purdue University, and is a Fellow in the American College of Medical Informatics. He was the principal investigator on a long-running grant from the Office for Advancement of Telehealth to establish and evaluate the Fairview-University Telemedicine Network and the current Great Plains Telehealth Resource and Assistance Center grant. He is a member of the ATA policy committee and co-authored several policy papers for the group. Dr. Speedie is particularly interested in the intersection of telehealth and health information technology. He has worked on several projects to extend the reach of telemedicine into the home that involve home videoconferencing, the Internet, and home monitoring.

Heidi Tennyson, MAOM, is an Applications Analyst in the Information Technology Department at Regional Health in Rapid City, South Dakota. She supported the medical records and scanning module in Regional Health's main HCIS system and has recently switched to supporting reference lab applications. She was part of the team that converted Regional Health from the old character-based HCIS to the newer Windows-based HCIS. After graduating with her Bachelor's degree, she worked for American Express as a Project Manager, then later became a consultant for System Engineering Services and worked with Perot Systems. She has been with Regional Health for eight years. She holds a Bachelor of Arts in Business with an emphasis in Information Systems and Masters Degree in Organizational Management.

Herman Tolentino, M.D., serves as the Chief of the Public Health Informatics Fellowship Program (PHIFP) at the Centers for Disease Control and Prevention (CDC). After being trained as a physician and anesthesiologist at the University of the Philippines, he attended medical informatics training at the Division of Biomedical and Health Informatics at the University of Washington in 1997 and his Public Health Informatics (PHI) training at CDC in 2006. He has led innovations in public health informatics practice through development and implementation of an award-winning community-based electronic health record (http://www.chits.ph/web/) and an innovative Semantic Web application that tracks disease outbreaks and disasters called EpiSPIDER (http://www.epispider.net/). He has advanced competency-based PHI workforce development through game-based learning, development of case studies, and use of systems-based problem solving in collaborative PHI projects. He teaches PHI as Adjunct Associate Professor at the School of Public Health, University of Illinois in Chicago.

Seth Trudeau has been employed at Sanford Health for over 10 years. As a Database Administrator for 6 of those years, he was involved in many large system implementations including: Epic Electronic Medical Record system with an Intersystems Cache database and an Oracle reporting database, Lawson Enterprise Resource Planning software with an Oracle database, and a Business Objects Enterprise implementation. As an Interface Analyst, Seth was involved in merging clinical trial data from another application into Sanford Health's Velos Clinical Trial Management System. He also worked with the CoRDS team to setup the CoRDS participant portal. Seth currently holds certifications as an Oracle Certified Professional, Epic Cache Administrator, and Epic Clarity ETL Administrator.

Allison Tuma, M.H.A., is a recent graduate of Saint Louis University's School of Public Health. She earned a Master of Healthcare Administration and was the recipient of a two-year Graduate Research Assistantship award. Before moving to St. Louis, she received her undergraduate degree in Psychology from Miami University in Oxford, Ohio. She has worked in healthcare settings including major academic medical centers, a children's hospital, mental health organizations, and a community care clinic. She will soon begin an Administrative Fellowship in the Division of Surgical Services at Cincinnati Children's Hospital Medical Center in Cincinnati, Ohio.

Matthew Wills is an Assistant Professor of informatics at Indiana University East in Richmond, IN. His primary interest in the field of informatics is health care. He has published papers and book chapters on a number of topics, including clinical decision support systems, clinical knowledge management systems, cyberinfrastructure for comparativeness effectiveness research systems, and electronic health records. Matthew is an active member of his professional community, having presented at numerous national and international information systems and decision sciences conferences. His research goals include developing effective systems for the support of clinical decision-making and evaluation of health information technologies.

Xiaoming Zeng (zengx@ecu.edu) is Associate Professor and Chair of the Department of Health Services and Information Management in the College of Allied Health Sciences at East Carolina University (ECU). He earned his MD degree from Peking Union Medical College in Beijing, China, in 1997 and PhD in Health Information Management from the University of Pittsburgh in 2004. He also earned a certificate in Biomedical Informatics from the University of Pittsburgh. He has been teaching health information technologies and informatics related courses since he joined the faculty at ECU in 2004. Dr. Zeng has research interests in Health Information Technology workforce training, social media for online education and patient empowerment, consumer informatics, and e-Health care information systems.

Index

CPSIA information can be obtained
at www.ICGtesting.com
Printed in the USA
BVOW04*1527010917

493572BV00009B/6/P